NEW ADVANCES IN THE GENETICS AND TREATMENT OF TYPE 1 DIABETES MELLITUS AND LATE DIABETIC COMPLICATIONS

NEW ADVANCES IN THE GENETICS AND TREATMENT OF TYPE 1 DIABETES MELLITUS AND LATE DIABETIC COMPLICATIONS

DIMITRY A. CHISTIAKOV

Nova Biomedical Books
New York

LIBRARY OF CONGRESS CATALOGING-IN-PUBLICATION DATA

Chistiakov, Dimitry A.
New advances in the genetics and treatment of type 1 diabetes mellitus and late diabetic complications / Dimitry A. Chistiakov.
p. ; cm.
Includes bibliographical references and index.
ISBN 13: 978-1-30021-410-3
ISBN 10: 1-60021-410-X
1. Diabetes—Genetic aspects. 2. Diabetes—Complications. I. Title.
[DNLM: 1. Diabetes Mellitus, Type 1—genetics. 2. Diabetes Mellitus, Type 1—therapy. WK 810 C542n 2006]
RC660.C442 2006
616.4'62042—dc22 2006025701

Published by Nova Science Publishers, Inc. ✢ New York

CONTENTS

Chapter 1

INTRODUCTION

In lovely memory of my family:
father Alexander,
mother Emma and
brother Pavel

Type 1 diabetes (T1D) is caused by the autoimmune destruction of pancreatic β cells and is characterized by absolute insulin insufficiency. The disease was thought to be the prevalent type of diabetes in children and adolescents, affecting up to 0.1% of the world population. T1D is a typical complex and heterogeneous pathology, occurred in genetically predisposing subjects as a result of harmful influence of non-genetic (environmental) factors.

Recent years have witnessed an explosive growth in available biological data. This includes a tremendous quantity and quality of analytic tools and sequence data (i.e., biological structures, genetic maps and polymorphisms, metabolic and signaling pathways) generated by genome and transcriptome projects focused on humans, mice, and a multitude of other species. Diabetes research and treatment stands to greatly benefit from those advances. Creating a non-obese diabetic (NOD) mouse resulted in producing large-scale data sets that significantly improved our understanding of the precise pathophysiology and genetics of diabetes and disease treatment. To date, more than 22 loci, predisposing to T1D, have been mapped in the human genome, but only a half of them was later confirmed. Four of them are already defined as follows: the HLA region on chromosome 6p21, a variable number of tandem repeats within the insulin gene (INS-VNTR; chromosome 11p15), the CTLA-4 (2q33) and PTPN22 (1p13) genes. For those four loci, multiple and consistent genetic and functional evidences suggesting for their strong involvement in T1D have been obtained. In addition, there are three more loci, containing likely positional and functional candidate genes that are close now to be fully defined as susceptibility genes for T1D. Those three include the CD25 (10p15.1), IF1H1 (2q24) and IL7RA (5p14-p12) genes. Genetic studies strongly suggest for the contribution of these genes to T1D susceptibility, but more data from functional analyses are needed to complete the evaluation of their role in the etiology of T1D.

The monocellular nature of T1D and endocrine action of insulin make this disease an excellent candidate for cellular therapy. Furthermore, precedent for cellular therapies has been set by successful cadaveric whole pancreas and islet transplantation. In order to expand the supply of cells to meet current and future needs, several novel cell sources have been proposed, including human β cells or islets expanded in culture, islet xenografts and pancreatic ductal progenitor cells. Surrogate β cells derived from hepatocytes, intestinal K cells or non-endodermal cell types have also been suggested.

Finding the etiological variants of susceptibility genes should strongly benefit the prediction of T1D, which is a prerequisite for disease prevention. The prediction is currently performed on three levels, which include the genetic susceptibility for disease, the identification of preclinical T1D by way of circulating islet autoantibodies and the use of metabolic tests to stage preclinical disease into late or early prediabetes. Combinations of genetic markers, such as HLA genotype, INS-VNTR genotype and if and how much family history of T1D is present, can stratify disease risk more than 1000-fold and can be used for selection of first-degree relatives of patients with T1D for primary intervention trials. Measurement of autoantibodies in genetically at-risk subjects identifies future cases of T1D. Further stratification of diabetes risk in autoantibody-positive subjects can be made on the basis of autoantibody characteristics that correspond to the magnitude of the autoantibody response.

Chapter 2

TYPE 1 DIABETES MELLITUS: CLASSIFICATION, DIAGNOSIS, CLINICAL SYMPTOMS AND MANAGEMENT

CLASSIFICATION

The current classification of type 1 diabetes (T1D) is based on pathogenesis rather than on the requirement for insulin therapy. Type 1 diabetes previously defined as insulin-dependent (IDDM) or juvenile diabetes is caused by β cell destruction, often immune-mediated, that leads to loss of insulin secretion and absolute insulin deficiency. However, T1D also includes cases that resulted in non-immune-mediated insulin deficiency [1].

An expert committee of the American Diabetes Association (ADA) has published etiological diagnostic criteria [2], which recognize that most patients with type 1 diabetes are not children at onset [3], and that not all individuals at onset are insulin-dependent [4] or have an immune-mediated form of diabetes [2]. Thus, the terms juvenile onset, or IDDM are no longer used. The ADA committee recommended using the term type 1A diabetes for immune-mediated diabetes and type 1B for non-immune diabetes with severe insulin deficiency [1]. Type 2 diabetes is a term to be used for idiopathic forms of diabetes with insulin resistance and without severe insulin deficiency or dramatic loss of β cells. Gestational diabetes was classified in a separate category. Specific genetic syndromes (i.e., mutations of the hepatocyte nuclear factor and glucokinase genes) contribute to the final category for classification of other specific forms of diabetes.

Type 1A (autoimmune) diabetes is a well-defined form of T1D [5], whereas type 1B (not immune-mediated) is a form that remains poorly designated [6]. Type 1A is the most common form of diabetes among children and adolescents of European origin usually characterized by acute onset and dependence on exogenous insulin for survival. In adults, the disease is nearly as frequent as in children, but often less dramatic onset may lead to misclassification as type 2 and a delayed insulin treatment. About 60% of persons with type 1 diabetes are diagnosed as adults.

Diagnosis

The diagnosis of diabetes is performed on the basis of hyperglycaemia. Anti-islet autoantibody determination with specific assays based on detection of four major islet autoantigens (insulin, glutamic acid decarboxylase (in particular GADA65), ICA512/IA2A and IA2B) can be used to diagnose Type 1A diabetes [7,8]. About 90% of white children will have at least one of these autoantibodies at disease diagnosis. Around 50% of children from other ethnic groups with diabetes do not have type 1A diabetes, indeed most have type 2 diabetes.

T1D is not a disorder limited to young people, and the rate of disease may be equally prevalent in adults. Type 1 diabetes has historically been considered a disorder predominately of children and young adults (the disease is commonly referred to as juvenile diabetes because it has peak expression between ages 10-14 years). However, recent studies support a different model, in which the disease can occur at any age. Specifically, 5-30% of patients initially diagnosed with type 2 diabetes actually have type 1 diabetes [4,9]. Such patients are best identified by the expression of anti-islet autoantibodies, in particular, GADA. Clinically, these individuals are commonly treated with oral agents, do not respond to oral hypoglycaemic therapy, and are unable to maintain adequate glucose control. The slow onset and protracted disease course has led to the disease designation of such individuals as latent autoimmune diabetes of adults (LADA) [9]. Given the large numbers of patients diagnosed with type 2 diabetes (estimated to be ten times greater than type 1 diabetes), patients with LADA are likely to comprise about half all patients with type 1 diabetes. Furthermore, in some countries, such as Japan, most cases of type 1 diabetes develop during adulthood [10].

Except for immunological tests, measuring glucose, fructosamine, glycated haemoglobin (HbA1C), C peptide and some other metabolites are important for diagnosis and monitoring diabetes [5].

Clinical Symptoms

The process that destroys the insulin-producing βcells can be a long and insidious one. At the point, when insulin production bottoms out, however, T1D usually appears suddenly and progresses quickly. Warning signs of T1D include:

- Frequent urination (in children, a recurrence of bed-wetting after toilet training has been completed).
- Unusual thirst, especially for sweet, cold drinks.
- Extreme hunger.
- Sudden, sometimes dramatic, weight loss.
- Weakness.
- Extreme fatigue.
- Blurred vision or other changes in eyesight.
- Irritability.
- Children with T1D may also be restless, apathetic, and have trouble functioning at school.

- Nausea and vomiting are acute symptoms.
- In severe cases, diabetic coma may be the first sign of type 1 diabetes [11].

Diabetic Ketoacidosis

The goals for the management of T1D in adolescents are to (i) prevent diabetic ketoacidosis (DKA); (ii) prevent severe hypoglycemia; (iii) maintain normal growth and development; and (iv) prevent long-term diabetic complications. DKA is the most commmon hyperglycemic emergency in type 1 diabetic patients. In USA, DKA is responsible for for more than 100,000 hospital admissions per year, and accounts for 4-9% of all hospital discharge summaries among patients affected with diabetes [12]. DKA develops when insulin stores are depleted. It is almost always caused by noncompliance with insulin treatments. The use of implanted insulin pumps have also been associated with DKA, possibly because short-acting insulin is used in the pumps, and if its delivery is interrupted there is no reserve to control blood sugar levels [13]. Other contributing factor is intentionally reducing insulin levels in order to lose weight. DKA is usually triggered in insulin-deficient patients by a stressful event, most often pneumonia or urinary tract infections. Other triggers include alcohol abuse, physical injury, pulmonary embolism, heart attacks, or other illnesses [14]. In addition, severely low insulin levels cause excessive amounts of glucose in the bloodstream (hyperglycemia). Fat metabolism breakdown could accelerate and increase the production of fatty acids, which further are converted into so-called ketone bodies that are toxic at high levels [15].

DKA symptoms and complications include the following:

- Nausea and vomiting.
- Breathing may be abnormally deep and rapid with frequent sighing.
- The heartbeat may be rapid.
- Cerebral edema, or brain swelling, is a rare but very dangerous complication that occurs in 1% of ketoacidosis cases and results in coma, brain damage, or death in many cases [16].
- Aspiration pneumonia and adult respiratory distress syndrome.

Management of patients with DKA includes monitoring and measurement of intrabody electrolytes (sodium, potassium, magnesium, bicarbonate, phosphate), insulin treatment, blood glucose, rehydration and other procedures [17]. For preventing DKA, the following strategies should be applied: diabetic education among patients, blood glucose monitoring, home monitoring of ketones and hydroxybutyrate, easily digestible liquid diets when sick, supplemental short-term insulin regiments and others [17,18].

Diabetic Hypoglycaemia (Insulin Shock)

Intensive insulin control increases the risk of hypoglycemia (also called insulin shock), which occurs if blood glucose levels fall below normal. Hypoglycemia may also be caused by insufficient intake of food or excess exercise or alcohol. Usually the condition is manageable, but occasionally, it can be severe or even life threatening, particularly if the patient fails to recognize the symptoms [19].

People at highest risk for severe hypoglycemia are those who intensively control blood glucose and also have long-term diabetes or previous history of severe hypoglycemia [20]. Hypoglycemia unawareness is a condition, in which people become insensitive to hypoglycemic symptoms. It affects about 25% of those, who use insulin. In such cases, hypoglycemia appears suddenly, without warning, and can escalate to a severe level. Even a single recent episode of hypoglycemia may make it more difficult to detect the next episode. With vigilant monitoring and by rigorously avoiding low blood glucose levels, such patients can often regain the ability to sense the symptoms. It is important to note, however, that even very careful testing may fail to detect a problem, particularly one that occurs during sleep.

Mild symptoms of hypoglycemia usually occur at moderately low and easily correctable levels of blood glucose and include sweating, trembling, hunger and rapid heartbeat. Severe hypoglycemia is usually associated with confusion, weakness, disorientation and combativeness [21,22].

To prevent hypoglycemia, some special tasks should be taken into account. Hypoglycemia is a common problem during sleep, particularly for children, even those, who are on non-intensive insulin therapy. Bedtime snacks may be helpful. In addition, the use of the insulin pump may help prevent hypoglycemic episodes [22]. For patients taking insulin, various insulin regimens are available that can reduce the risk. For example, taking fast acting insulin before the evening meal may be particularly helpful in preventing hypoglycemia [23]. Patients, who intensively control their blood sugar, should monitor blood levels as often as possible, four times or more per day. This is particularly important for patients with hypoglycemia unawareness. Diabetic patients on therapies that put them at risk for hypoglycemia should always carry hard candy, juice, sugar packets or commercially available glucose substitutes designed for diabetic individuals. Family and friends of the patient should be aware of the symptoms and be prepared to provide an essential sugar-containing food, be able to inject intravenously glucose and glucagon, a hormone, which raises blood glucose [24].

Chapter 3

TYPE 1 DIABETES: EPIDEMIOLOGY

PREVALENCE OF TYPE 1 DIABETES

Evaluation of a disease initially starts with cross-sectional data on its prevalence. The prevalence of a disease is the number of people in the population, who have the disease at a given point in time). According to the data of International Diabetes Federation (IDF) in 2003 among 1.8 billion children aged under 15 years, 430,000 have T1D. More than a quarter come from South East Asian region, and more than a fifth from Europe (Table 1). A world-wide prevalence of T1D is 0.02%. The highest prevalence of disease is observed in North America and Europe, while Africa and particularly the Western Pacific region show the lowest rates (Table 1).

Countries of Northern Europe have the highest prevalence of T1D, which is 7-14-fold higher than the average prevalence in the globe. High prevalence of disease is also occurred in UK, Ireland and a number of former British colonies, such as Canada, Australia, New Zealand and some others (Table 2). In contrast, oriental countries, such as Vietnam, Malaysia, Indonesia, Cambodia, Thailand and China show the lowest rates, ranging from 0.0013 to 0.0031. However, comparisons of prevalence data may be subject to considerable bias, since prevalence is determined not only by disease incidence, but also by case survival, which may vary markedly across populations. However, prevalence data are useful in determining the public health impact of type 1 diabetes. For example, the number of T1D patients in France was increased from 120,000 in 1995 to 140,000 in 1999 [25]. In the early 1990's, the number of T1D patients 0-19 years of age in USA was estimated at approximately 123,000 individuals. However, in 2000, with the growth of this segment of the U.S. population to over 80 million, there were approximately 160,000 children with type 1 diabetes [26].

Table 1. Number of prevalent cases of type 1 diabetes in children by region estimated by IDF in 2003

Region	Number of children aged under 14 years (x 10^3)	Number of children affected with T1D (x 10^3)	T1D prevalence by region (%)
South East Asia	412,237	104.8	0.025
Europe	161,462	90.2	0.056
North America	105,192	64.6	0.061
Eastern Mediterranean and Middle East	205,821	46.4	0.023
South and Central America	126,039	40.4	0.032
Africa	295,038	35.1	0.012
Western Pacific	516,198	21.5	0.004

Table 2. Countries with the highest prevalence of type 1 diabetes in children as estimated by IDF in 2003*

Country	Number of children aged under 14 years (x 10^3)	Number of children affected with T1D (x 10^3)	T1D prevalence (%)
Finland	899	2.5	0.278
Sweden	1,498	3.1	0.207
Iceland	64	0.1	0.156
Canada	5,759	9.1	0.158
Norway	876	1.3	0.148
Kuwait	540	0.8	0.148
UK	10,923	13.7	0.125
Denmark	982	1.2	0.122
Luxembourg	84	0.1	0.119
Puerto Rico	934	1.1	0.117
Australia	3,931	4.4	0.112
Ireland	817	0.9	0.110
Haiti	3,305	3.6	0.109
Dominican Republic	2,806	3.0	0,107
New Zealand	864	0.9	0.104

* Only countries with prevalence of T1D of higher than 0.1 are shown.

INCIDENCE OF TYPE 1 DIABETES: GEOGRAPHIC, RACIAL AND ETHNIC VARIABILITY

The incidence indicates how often a disease occurs. More precisely, it corresponds to the number of new cases of a disease among a certain group of people for a certain period of a time. T1D is characterized by large geographic variability in the incidence. Scandinavian countries and the Mediterranean island of Sardinia have the highest incidence rates in the world (Table 3). Most countries and territories of the Western Pacific region show the lowest incidence of T1D ranging between 0.1-0.7 cases per 100,000 children aged under 14 years per year. While there is a strong south-north gradient in the incidence, 'hot-spots' in warm climates have been reported (Sardinia, Puerto Rico, Dominican Republic, Haiti, Malta and Kuwait) are reported [27-29]. The geographic and ethnic variations in type 1 diabetes reflect the prevalence of susceptibility genes or that of causal environmental factors, or both.

Table 3. Countries with the highest incidence of type 1 diabetes in children as estimated by IDF in 2003

Country	Incidence rates (cases per 100,000 population Per year) 0-14 years
Finland	37.4
Sardinia (Italy)	35.0
Sweden	28.0
Canada	24.1
Norway	22.5
Kuwait	20.9
Denmark	19.4
UK	18.9
Australia	17.8
Dominican Republic	17.4
Puerto Rico	17.4
Haiti	17.4
Ireland	16.3
Malta	15.6
New Zealand	15.2

* Only countries with incidence of T1D of higher than 15.2 are shown.

It is estimated that around 65,000 children under 15 years of age annually develop T1D worldwide. The incidence of type I diabetes is increasing worldwide both in low and high incidence populations. An estimated increase in global incidence of T1D is 3.0% per year, and that the incidence of disease will be 40% higher in 2010 than in 1998 [30]. In Finland, where the incidence of T1D is the highest in the world, the annual incidence rate has increased from 18 per 100,000 in 1965 to 45 per 100,000 in 2000 [31]. By the year 2010, if this trend continues, the incidence in Finland will be of 50 per 100,000 a year, and also in many other populations it will exceed 30 per 100,000 a year [30].

A significant racial difference in T1D risk is observed in multiracial populations, although not of the same magnitude as the geographic differences. In the US, non-Hispanic whites are reported to be able to develop type 1 diabetes about 1.5 times more likely than African Americans or Hispanics [32,33]. Among 86,000 relatives of type 1 diabetic patients screened for the Diabetes Prevention Trial-Type 1 diabetes (DPT-1), lower prevalence of islet autoantibodies was observed in Asian Americans (2.6%) and in Hispanics (2.7%) compared to African Americans (3.3%) or non-Hispanic whites (3.9%) [34]. Frequency of GAD antibodies was shown to be lower in Asian populations compared to Caucasians [35,36].

However, a rising trend in T1D was observed not only for non-Hispanic white population, but also among Hispanic and African American children [33,37]. An annual increase in incidence of disease is reported in sub-Saharan African countries, although the incidence rate remains low compared to European and North American regions [38]. Epidemiological analysis of different ethnic groups, living in Israel, revealed a marked increase in T1D incidence since 1985 among Jewish subgroups, but not in Arab population [39].

Incidence of Type 1 Diabetes: Age-Related Differences

The highest rate of incidence of T1D is observed in the 10-14 age group, while the highest annual increase is in the 0-4 years age children [26,40,41]. Multiple anti-islet antibodies are also detected by age 14 years [42]. The incidence decreases in the third decade of life [43,44] to increase again in the fifth to seventh decades of life [45,46]. However, there is no hard evidence of increase of incidence at the 50-70 years age group, since it is difficult to separate between adult-onset T1D and type 2 diabetes in older individuals [47].

The increase in T1D incidence affects all age groups and, particularly, the youngest children aged under 5 years [48, 49]. The incidence is increasing in individuals of 15-29 years old, despite this age group is characterized by the lowest incidence of disease compared to other age cohorts [50-52]. The rising T1D incidence is reported in all age groups of children and young adult in both low and high incidence populations. Over the past 30 years, the incidence is doubled in countries with high incidence (Finland, Sweden, Denmark) [50,51,53] and even is tripled in countries known as a moderate risk area (Poland, Israel) [40,54].

Incidence of Type 1 Diabetes: Gender-Related Differences

Generally, both sexes have equal risk to develop T1D [55]. However, populations with high incidence of T1D show male preponderance: male/female ratio among diabetic patients from Scandinavian countries ranges from 1.32:1 (Norway, age 15-29 years) [43] to 1.69 (Sweden, age 15-34 years) [56]. In contrast, in low-risk (mostly oriental) populations, there is female excess [57-59]. Whether male excess among T1D diabetic young adults in high-risk populations resulted from the preferable interaction between harmful environment and male sex is unclear. For example, in Norway, population data show a clear male excess in diabetes in childhood and early adult life for the period 1925-1954 [60] and 1978-1982 [43], suggesting that the male excess is an inherent characteristic of Norwegian and probably other Scandinavian populations.

Interestingly, except Scandinavian young adults, male excess is also a consistent finding in other European populations aged 15-40 years, with an approximate 1.5:1 male:female ratio [55]. This ratio remained constant in young adults over two or three generations in some populations. Male excess in type 1 diabetic young adults seems to be a paradox phenomenon, because the 15-40 years age range corresponds to female childbearing life. In pregnancy, the cellular immune responses of the mother are down-regulated to prevent immunity directed against the fetus and, therefore, pregnant women are more sensitive to a variety of autoimmune disorders [61]. Additionally, sex hormones could significantly affect the behavior of the immune system, particularly in pregnancy, and modify balance between immune responses mediated by T helper type 1 (Th1) and T helper type 2 (Th2) cells as strongly scheduled from experiments with mouse models of autoimmunity [62]. However, extrapolation from mouse to man should be cautious, because the Th1/Th2 paradigm might have limited relevance in humans, in whom immune reactions are much less polarized than in mice [63].

Male sex was shown to be associated with prediabetic state (i.e., appearance of β-cell autoimmunity and presence anti-islet antibodies ICA and ICA512), but not with the development T1D [64]. This finding therefore suggests that the male sex represents an independent risk factor for the development of anti-islet autoimmunity, but not for overt disease. In addition, male relatives with autoimmunity are less likely compared to female relatives to progress to clinical diabetes [64]. A possible explanation of this phenomenon is that men could develop disease slower than women or that women develop diabetes, expressing different antibody responses. The latter suggestion is supported by the observation, demonstrating lower titers and less frequency of GAD antibodies in newly diagnosed male vs. female subjects [65].

Early studies among diabetic families based on the analysis limited data sets (240-2,000 offspring) showed that offspring of men with T1D are more likely to have diabetes-related autoantibodies [66] and high risk for disease [67,68]. However, recent DPT-1 screening of 21,579 offspring found no significant effect of the sex of the parent with ICA [64]. These data were consistent with the report from Austria, showing no sex differences in risk for T1D among families with only one affected child [69].

Chapter 4

NON-GENETIC RISK FACTORS IN SUSCEPTIBILITY TO TYPE 1 DIABETES

Environmental triggers play the important role in the etiology of T1D, facilitating the appearance of β-cell autoimmunity and subsequent development of disease in genetically predisposing subjects (Figure 1). Some non-genetic factors provide significant risk for T1D development. There are viral infections (particularly during pregnancy), fetal diet (cow's milk proteins), older maternal age, increased growth rate, stressful life, N-nitroso compounds (in animal models of diabetes). Other non-genetic triggers, such as low birth weight, short birth length, breast feeding, early vitamin D supplementation and atopic diseases, are associated with reduced risk of T1D [70,71].

VIRAL INFECTIONS

To date, 13 different viruses have been reported to be associated with the development of T1D in humans and in various animal models [72]. Enteroviruses, particularly coxsackie virus B4, have been implicated as possible agents in the pathogenesis of type 1 diabetes. Early studies showed the detection of antibodies against these viruses in newly diagnosed T1D patients and especially in the 10-18 year-old age group [73,74]. A case report described the isolation of coxsackie virus B4 from the pancreas of a child died from DKA, and this virus caused diabetes when transferred into a susceptible murine strain [75]. Enterovirus RNA was detected in the blood of 27-64% of newly diagnosed T1D patients compared to 0-4% in healthy controls [76-78]. Detection of enterovirus RNA was associated with increased levels of interferon-α production in Langerhans' cells, suggesting for acute and persistent viral infection [79,80].

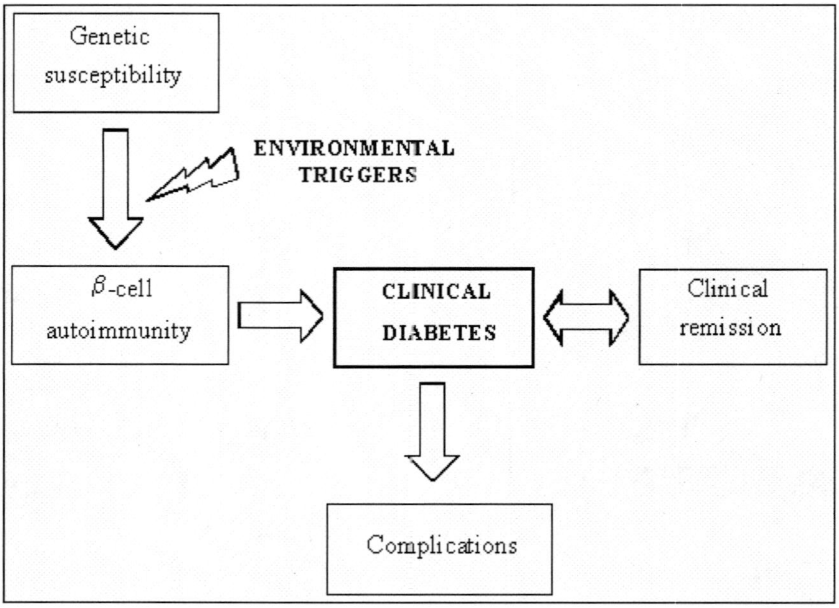

Figure 1. Natural history of type 1 diabetes. Disease may be caused by harmful influence of one or several environmental risk factors in genetically predisposing individuals. Initially, the induction of autoantibodies against insulin-producing islet β-cells occurs that leads to the loss of β-cells and the development of clinical diabetes. Diabetic patients have increased risk to develop various diabetic complications, such as macroangiopathies (coronary heart disease, heart attack, atherosclerosis, cerebrovascular stroke, diabetic foot) and microangipathies (diabetic nephropathy, diabetic retinopathy and diabetic neuropathy).

Coxsackie virus can induce diabetes directly through the cytotoxic activity of immune cells against infected β-cells, leading to depletion of the insulin-producing cells, or indirectly through the destruction of surrounding non-infected β-cells by the release of immune mediators, such as cytokines [81], cross-reactivity with β-cell antigen (molecular mimicry) and activation of autoreactive T cells by viral superantigen or by cytokines (Figure 2) [80]. A popular model of virus-induced diabetes is very popular involves a mechanism of molecular mimicry. This model was proposed for coxsackie virus-induced T1D based on the significant sequence similarity between the viral capsid protein P2C and GAD that could provoke immune response to destroy self-tissue after clearance of the virus [82]. Anti-P2C antibodies were detected in serum of T1D patients, and 80% of these patients reacted with the islet isoform of glutamate decarboxylase (GAD65; residues 256-268) [83]. However, later studies showed that this sequence is a T cell recognition epitope but T cell clones, recognizing this epitope, did not cross-react with the relevant GAD65 peptide [84,85]. Furthermore, autoreactive T cells, recognizing the immunogenic GAD65 epitope, showed cross-reactivity with the relevant homologous epitope of cytomegalovirus, but not with the coxsackie viral peptide [86]. A putative ability to induce T1D via the mechanism of molecular mimicry was suggested for another enterovirus strain, coxsackievirus A9, a capsid protein VP1 of which showed cross-reactivity with diabetes-related autoantibodies against certain epitopes of tyrosine phosphatase IA-2/IAR and heat shock protein 60 [87]. A potential involvement of echovirus 3, a human enterovirus B species, in the initiation of β-cell autoimmunity was recently proposed, when this virus was isolated from an individual, who soon after virus isolation developed IA-2 and islet autoantibodies [88]. A likely role of enteroviruses in inducing T1D was supported by experiments in animal models, in which β-cell autoimmunity was induced after enterovirus infection of β cells through molecular mimicry or bystander activation of autoreactive T cell clones [89-91].

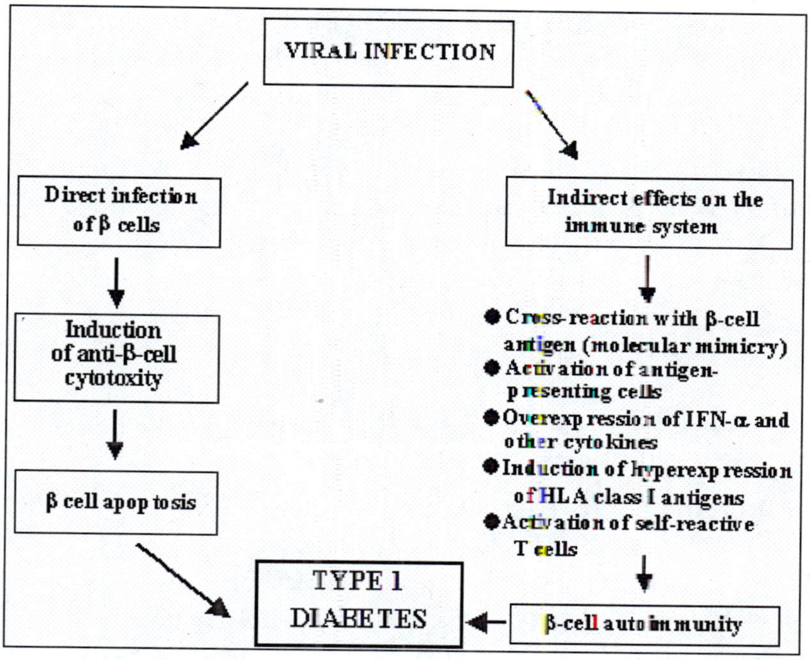

Figure 2. Mechanisms of virus-induced type 1 diabetes. Viruses may cause disease by two ways - through the direct infection of β cells and through indirect effects altering immune responses. Viral infection is followed by the initiation of antiviral immune response that kills infected β cells and therefore could lead to inducing type 1 diabetes as a consequence of dramatic loss in the population of β cells. Indirect effects of viruses on the immune system include several pathogenic mechanisms that can cause the induction of β-cell autoimmunity, insulitis and diabetes.

Other viruses (mumps, rubella, measles, cytomegalovirus and retroviruses) have been also studied, but the evidence is less convincing than that for enterovirus [92]. One of the best characterized model is the encephalomyocarditis (EMC) virus induction of diabetes mellitus in mice [93]. The EMC-D variant of virus causes diabetes in infected SJL mice by direct β-cell destruction. Infection with EMC-B does not cause diabetes and interferes with the production of diabetes by EMC-D due to the greater ability of EMC-B than of EMC-D to induce interferon in mice [94]. The EMC-induced diabetes happened in genetically susceptible murine strains. Another vary interesting model is Kilham rat virus induced diabtes in rats [95]. The virus initiates diabetes, altering immune response in rats that leads to an autoimmune attack against β cells.

Viral infection is associated with the induction of expression of interferons and other cytokines mediated antiviral immunity. IFN-α plays an important role in initiating antiviral response, involving a variety of mechanisms, such as activation of T cell response, upregulation of expression of chemokines and major compatibility complex (MHC) class I molecules, stimulation of natural killer cells, dendritic cells and CD8+ T cell proliferation [96]. The expression of IFN-α could be induced by viruses, bacteria, hypoxia, polyanions (DNA or RNA), interleukin-2 and other agents. Since association between entrovirus infection and elevated levels of IFN-α in type 1 diabetic patients was documented [78], coxsackie virus could stimulate production and even overproduction of IFN-α by β cells [79,97]. Overexpression of IFN-α can induce β-cell autoimmunity through inducing hyperexpression of MHC class I antigens in human islets, apoptosis of β cells and activation of Th1-mediated autoimmune response [98,99]. In addition, IFN-α therapy of tumors and viral infections caused by hepatitis B and C viruses could induce autoimmune responses [100]. Several studies reported the development of T1D in genetically predisposing patients with chronic hepatitis C treated with IFN-α [101-103]. Treatment with IFN-α is reported to induce diabetes-related pancreatic autoantobodies in subjects affected with hepatitis C [104,105]. These findings suggest that the overproduction of IFN-α in Langerhans' islets could represent a mechanism, by which viral infection may cause autoimmune diabetes, and IFN-α therapy could be considered as an independent risk factor in the development of T1D.

Dietary Factors

Cow's Milk Proteins and Breast Feeding

Experiments in animal models genetically susceptible to T1D clearly showed a significant positive correlation between the consumption of unfermented milk protein and induction of disease in non-obese diabetic (NOD) mice and BioBreeding (BB) rats [106-108]. In humans, an increased risk of the development of type 1 diabetes was associated with short breast-feeding duration (less than 4 months) and early child exposure to supplemental cow milk before the age of 2-3 months [109,110]. An association between inducing β-cell autoimmunity and a short breast-feeding, shorter than two months, was found in Finnish children susceptible to diabetes [111]. Exposure to cow's milk (CM) proteins is related to increased risk of the development of diabetes not only in young children but also during a whole period of infancy, when a high dietary intake of CM proteins occurs [112].

The mechanism of diabetogenicity of CM proteins is likely to be related to the structural sequence homology between those and β-cell antigens that could provoke T cells to recognize self-antigens and induce autoimmune response against islet cells. The diabetogenic effect of bovine serum albumin (BSA) is suggested from the similarity between the sequence of BSA and β-cell membrane protein ICA69 [113]. It was shown that antibodies to BSA cross-react with a ICA [107]. At the molecular level, a region of BSA has distinct homology to the beta-subunits of the MHC class II proteins Ia, DQ and DR, and antibodies raised against this BSA region identified the same β-cell membrane protein ICA69, in the same manner as antibodies to the third hypervariable region of DR-β did [107].

An enhanced cellular immune response and elevated levels of antibodies to another milk protein, β-lactoglobin, was detected in patients, who recently developed T1D [114-116]. The antibodies were found not only in individuals with newly diagnosed diabetes, but also in their subling [117]. This suggests for an important role of CM β-lactoglobin as an environmental (dietary) trigger of β-cell autoimmunity.

Increased T cell-mediated immunity to bovine β-casein was reported in subjects with newly diagnosed diabetes [118-120]. Interestingly, high titers of anti-β-casein antibodies were also shown in patients with other autoimmune disorder, celiac disease, that could reflect common mechanisms of the induction of T1D- and celiac disease-related autoimmunity linked to impaired mucosal immune function in the mucosa-associated lymphoid system (Figure 3) [120,121]. Bovine β-casein shows structural relationship to an islet cell protein, glucose transporter 2 (GLUT-2). One of nine β-casein-specific T cell lines isolated from the serum of patients with newly diagnosed T1D was recently reported to react also to the homologous peptide from GLUT-2, whereas three of four tested T cell lines reacted also to extracts of the human insulinoma cell line [122]. This could suggest for potential mechanisms of bovine β-casein-induced autoimmunity directed against the islet insulin-producing cells.

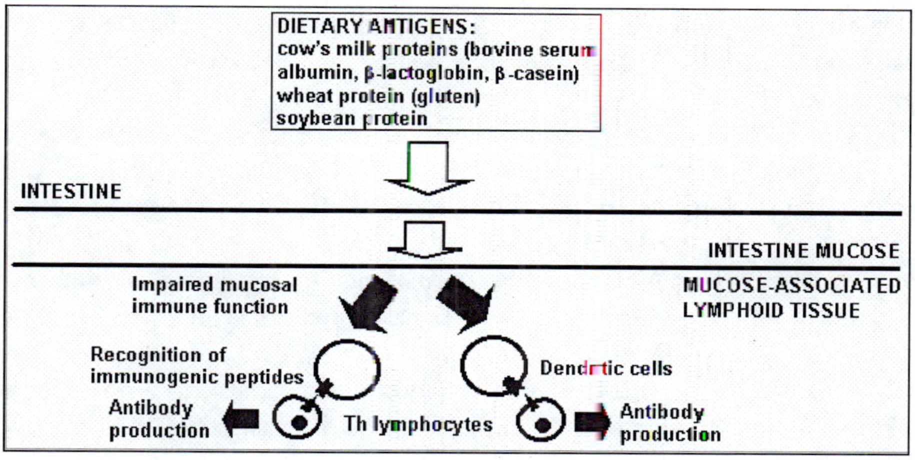

Figure 3. Potential mechanisms of the association between infant diet and β-cell autoimmunity. Early exposition to cow's milk proteins, wheat protein and some other dietary antigens is associated with increased production of antibodies, recognizing these antigens, in individuals with impaired function of immune-associated lymphoid tissue. Due to the sequence homology with certain islet antigens, dietary antigens may provoke T helper (Th) cells to induce immune response against host β cells. This may lead to T cell-mediated β-cell autoimmunity and type 1 diabetes.

Gluten

The diabetogenic effect of dietary gluten, a wheat protein, was demonstrated in animal models. Gluten addition to the food resulted in increased incidence of diabetes in BB rats [123,124] and NOD mice [125,126]. In humans, anti-gluten antibodies and enhanced T cell reactivity to gluten were detected at the time of diagnosis of T1D [127,128]. However, other researchers reported low or normal levels of these antibodies at diabetes onset [129,130].

Coincidence of T1D and celiac disease is well known. Endomysial antibodies are found in 5% of diabetic patiens and identify a subgroup of T1D individuals with clinically silent from of celiac disease. Similarly, around 5% of subjects with celiac disease have anti-islet antibodies, but they rarely develop clinical T1D [124]. In a 10-year follow-up study, 4 of 21 children with celiac disease and on gluten-free diet showed an impaired insulin secretion rate, but only one of those developed T1D [131]. Gluten-free diet was shown to result in disappearing anti-islet antibodies in patients with celiac disease, suggesting that intestinal inflammation could lead to the induction of β-cell autoimmunity [132].

Vitamin D Supplementation

Multiple studies, involving NOD mice or BB rats, reported that supplementation with the active form of vitamin D, 1,25-dihydroxyvitamin D3 and its analogs, prevents autoimmune insulitis and diabetes [133,134]. The EURODIAB Substudy 2 Study Group showed protective effects of dietary vitamin D supplementation for the first year of life against T1D in all age groups of children [135]. Daily intake of 2,500 IU of vitamin D or via use of cod liver oil in early life significantly reduced risk of childhood-onset of T1D [136,137]. Vitamin D intake during pregnancy also protected against the rapid development of β-cell autoimmunity [138].

Vitamin D is likely to provide its antigiabetogenic effects, influencing the immune system. Vitamin D suppresses the antigen-presenting capacity of dendritic cells and macrophages and inhibits expression of interleukin-12 (IL-12) by antigen-presenting cells that prevents the development of Th1-mediated immune response [139]. Since Th1 way of autoimmunity is predominant in T1D, suppression of this way by vitamin D could explain its protective role in T1D. In addition, vitamin D may also protect insulin-producing βcells from damage and dysfunction through the downregulation of synthesis of proinflammatory cytokines IFN-γ and IL-1β, which inhibit β-cell function (synthesis and secretion of insulin) [140-142] and stimulate expression of surface antigens by islet cells [143]. Thus, dietary vitamin D intake represents an important protective factor, which is significant for improving β-cell function and preventing autoimmune insulitis and diabetes.

Nitrates and Nitrites

A Finnish case-control study demonstrated positive association between dietary intake of nitrates and nitrites and risk of the development of T1D, and this association was independent from other environmental risk factors [144]. Another population study performed in Sweden showed that child's consumption of meals with high content of nitrate and nitrite is related to increased risk of diabetes [145]. A moderate positive correlation between the incidence of childhood T1D and the nitrate content of drinking water was observed in the ecological study in Colorado, USA [146]. Another ecological study (Yorkshire, England) reported the incidence of T1D in children was positively associated with raised mean nitrate levels in drinking water [147].

Nitrate and nitrite themselves are not risk factors for T1D. In the gut, nitrate is reduced to nitrite, which can be further transform, by reaction with amines and amides, into N-nitroso compounds, i.e. nitrosamines and nitrosamides, respectively [148]. N-nitroso compounds are substances, showing toxic effects on tissues and cells. These chemicals could be diabetogenic, causing damage and death of β cells via the involvement of free radical-mediated mechanisms.

TOXIC COMPOUNDS

Alloxan

Alloxan (2,4,5,6,-tetraoxypyrimidine) is a chemical agent that is commonly using to induce experimental diabetes in animal models. Alloxan is able to cause specific necrosis of pancreatic islets. Human islets are considerably more resistant to harmful action of alloxan than those of the rat and mouse [149]. In rodents, alloxan exerts its diabetogenic action when it is administrated parenterally.

The mechanism of alloxan action was intensively studied. This substance is shown to cause a sudden rise in insulin secretion independently from whether glucose presents or not [150]. However, the insulin release is of short duration and is followed by full inhibition of the islet response to glucose, even at high concentrations (16.6 mM) of this disaccharide [151]. A first key point in the pathogenic mechanism of alloxan action against pancreatic islets is the phenomenon of fast uptake of alloxan by β cells [152]. Another aspect of alloxan-induced diabetogenicity concerns the formation of reactive oxygen species. In β cells, alloxan is reduced through the interaction with various reducing agents, such as SH-containing cellular compounds (reduced glutathione, cysteine and thiol groups of proteins and enzymes), vitamin C and other natural antioxidants [153,154].

When reduced, alloxan forms dialuric acid, which could be reoxidized back to alloxan (Figure 4) [155]. These reactions are followed by generation of highly reactive superoxide radicals, which can release Fe^{3+} ions from ferritin and reduce them to Fe^{2+} [156]. In parallel, superoxide radicals undergo to hydrogen peroxide in the reaction of dismutation that may occur spontaneously or may be catalyzed by superoxide dismutase.

In presense of Fe^{2+} and hydrogen peroxide, highly reactive and cytotoxic hydroxyl radicals are then formed:

$$Fe^{2+} + H_2O_2 \rightarrow Fe^{3+} + OH^- + OH^{\cdot}$$

One of the preferable targets of alloxan-induced oxidizing effects in the islet cells is glucokinase, an enzyme, containing two SH-groups in the glucose-binding site. Alloxan reacts with these groups that leads to the formation of the disulfide bond and subsequent inactivation of the enzyme [157]. Alloxan-induced reactive oxygen species are shown to cause DNA damage and fragmentation in β cells [156].

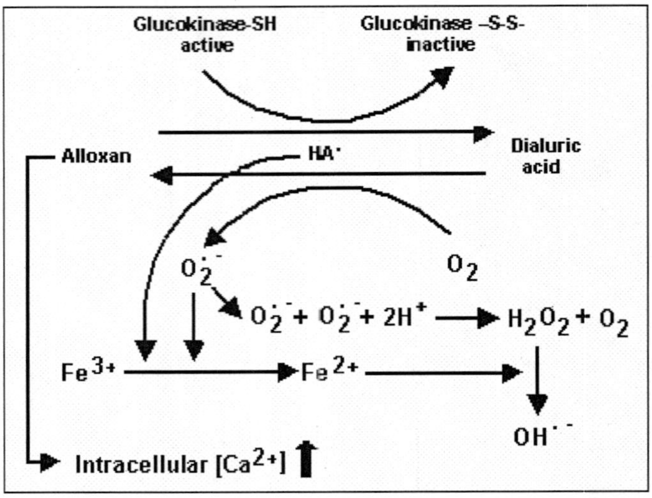

Figure 4. Mechanism of alloxan-induced formation of reactive oxygen species in rat islet β cells. Alloxan is reduced into dialuric acid after reaction with SH-containing compounds, including enzyme glucokinase. Oxidation of two SH-groups in sugar-binding site of the enzyme causes inactivation of glucokinase. Dialuric acid can be oxidized back to alloxan followed by generation of intermediate alloxan radicals (HA·) and superoxide radicals ($O_2^{·-}$), which are able to resolve Fe^{3+} ions from ferritin and reduce them to Fe^{2+}ions. Two superoxide radicals undergo dismutation to hydrogen peroxide (H_2O_2) that can react with Fe^{2+} to generate highly reactive hydroxyl radicals ($OH^{·-}$). These radicals are very toxic, causing the oxidation of proteins and lipids and fragmentation of DNA in pancreatic islets. In addition, alloxan-induced β-cell cytotoxicity can be induced through accelerated increase in intracellular calcium (Ca^{2+}) concentration, which is associated with the subsequent sudden rise in release of insulin from β cells.

Glucose is able to protect islet cells from harmful effects of alloxan. For example, this carbohydrate can protect glucokinase from the inactivation, hampering the access of alloxan to the SH-groups of the enzyme [157]. The protective effect of glucose against alloxan is not only limited by the protection of glucokinase. Glucose provides a total protection of β cells from alloxan-induced death through different mechanisms. This sugar may interact with glucose transporter GLUT-2 that results in limited alloxan uptake [158]. Glucose metabolism is linked to increased formation of NADH and NADPH, accelerating recirculation of glutathione. Glutathione, an important intracellular antioxidant, can react with hydrogen peroxide and therefore prevent formation of hydroxyl radicals [159]. Moreover, Sakurai and Ogiso [160] observed that generation of hydroxyl radicals in the presense of alloxan strongly depends on concentration of reduced glutathione (GSH). The reaction between GSH and hydroxyl radical results in the formation of thyil radical (GS·). Two thyil radicals then convert to glutathione (GSSG):

$$GSH + OH^{·-} \rightarrow GS^{·} + H_20$$

$$GS^{·} + GS^{·} \rightarrow GSSG$$

In addition to glutathione, other non-enzymatic scavengers of hydroxyl radicals and antioxidant enzymes, such as superoxide dismutase and catalase, could protect against alloxan-induced cytotoxicity [161,162].

Alloxan uptake by pancreatic islets is followed by increase of cytosolic Ca^{2+} concentration in β cells [163]. This effect results from the mobilization of Ca^{2+} from intracellular stores and accelerating Ca^{2+} influx from extracellular fluid due to the ability of alloxan to depolarize pancreatic β cells [164]. Depolarization of the cell plasma membrane activates voltage-dependent calcium channels and stimulates Ca^{2+} entry into the cell. The phenomenon of sudden rise in insulin release from β cells treated with alloxan could result from increase in intracellular Ca^{2+} concentration [151].

Thus, the toxic effect of alloxan to β cells is the sum of several processes, such as oxidation of enzymatic SH-groups, inactivation of glucokinase, generation of free radicals and alteration of inracellular calcium homeostasis.

Streptozotocin

Streptomycetes achromogenes produces streptozotocin (2-deoxy-2-(3-(methyl-3-nitrosoureido)-D-glucopyranoside), a compound that is used to induce both type 1 and type 2 diabetes in animal models. For inducing diabetes, rats should be injected with streptozotocin intravenously or intraperitoneally [165].

Two hours post-injection, streptozotocin causes hyperglycemia in treated rats. Six hours later, severe hypoglycemia occurs due to the sudden rise in serum insulin concentration. Finally, hyperglycemia develops, with reducing insulin levels [166]. These changes in glucose concentrations and insulin levels reflect the harmful influence of streptozotocin on β cells. Streptozotocin alters glucose oxidation and suppress insulin production [167,168]. The diabetogenic agent enters into the β cells through glucose transporter GLUT-2. When administered in multiple doses, streptozotocin restricts expression of GLUT-2 in vitro and in vivo [169].

DNA is a major target of streptozotocin-mediated β-cell toxicity. Treatment with streptozotocin causes DNA alkylation, especially at O^6 position of guanine [170], and subsequent fragmentation (Figure 5) [171,172]. Streptozocin-induced DNA damage induces poly ADP-ribosylation, a process, participating in DNA repair. This process leads to reduction of cellular NAD^+ and ATP content and subsequent inhibition of insulin synthesis and secretion [167]. The involvement of poly ADP-ribosylation into diabetogenic action of streptozotocin was suggested by using 3-aminobenzamide and nicotinamide, which are strong inhibitors of poly(ADP-ribose)synthase. Treatment with these inhibitors of rats injected with streptozotocin prevented the development of diabetes in the animals [173]. Experiments in the poly(ADP-ribose)synthase-deficient mouse showed the inhibition of poly(ADP-ribose)synthase itself prevents streptozotocin-induced β cell damage and hyperglyacemia, suggesting the activation of poly ADP-ribosylation of greater importance for the diabetogenicity of streptozotocin than generation of free radicals and DNA damage per se [174].

Streptozotocin is a nitric oxide (NO) donor, and NO mediates cytotoxic effects of this agent. Pancreatic β cells exposed to streptozotocin manifested changes characteristic for NO action, i.e. stimulation of guanylyl synthase and enhanced production of cyclic GMP [175]. NO synthase is not envolved in NO formation from streptozotocin. Nitric oxide releases, when streptozotocin is metabolised within the cells. NO scavengers can effectively protect β cells against streptozotocin-induced diabetes [176].

However, NO is not only molecule responsible for cytotoxicity of streptozotocin. Streptozotocin can generate reactive oxygen species, which contibute to DNA damage and other deleterious effects of streptozotocin on pancreatic β. cells [168]. The formation of superoxide anions results from both streptozotocin action on mitochondria and activation of xanthine oxidase. Streptozotocin inhibits Krebs' cycle and significantly decreases oxygen intake by mitochondria [167,175]. These effects strongly limit ATP production and lead to the depletion of this nucleotide in β cells [167]. NO plays a significant role in suppression of ATP generation by mitochondria. Nitric oxide is shown to bind to the Fe^{2+}-containing aconitase that causes inactivation of the enzyme [177].

Islet β cells display a high activity of xanthine oxidase. Dephosporylation of ATP leads to the formation of ADP, which is a supply of substrate for xanthine oxidase. This enzyme catalyzes a reaction followed by generation of superoxide anion that then transforms into hydrogen peroxide and hydroxide radicals [167,178]. The inhibition of xanthine oxidase by allopurinol restricts cytotoxic effect of streptozotocin in vitro.

DNA damage caused by streptozotocin results not only from its alkylation but also from deleterious effects of NO, reactive oxygen species and highly toxic peroxynitrate (ONOO), which is formed in the reaction between NO and superoxide anion (Figure 5).

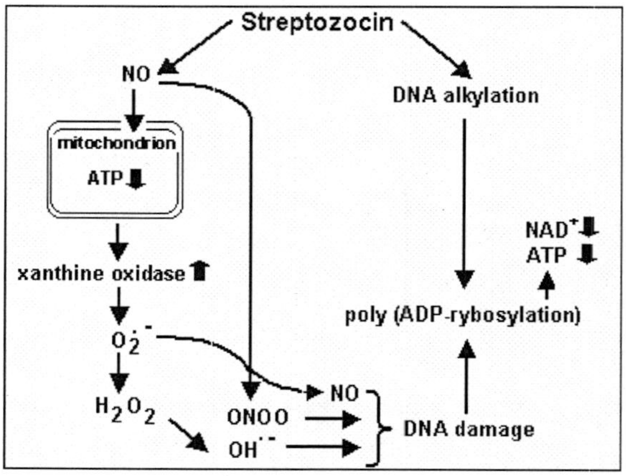

Figure 5. Toxic effects of streptozotocin in rat pancreatic β cells. Streptozotocin is a donor of nitric oxide (NO), a molecule that is cytotoxic itself, but also induces generation of other toxic substances, such as peroxynitrate (ONOO), hydroxyl radical ($OH^{\cdot}$), superoxide radical ($O_2^{\cdot}$) and hydrogen peroxide (H_2O_2). In mitochondria, NO causes the dephosphorylation and depletion of ATP that activates xanthyne oxidase, an enzyme, participaiting in the metabolic pathway of oxidative degradation of ATP to uric acid. The enzyme generates superoxide radical, which takes part in the formation of other highly toxic compounds, such as peroxynitrate and hydroxyl radical. These substances attack and cause fragmentation of cellular DNA. Streptozotocin is also able to induce direct DNA damage through DNA alkylation. DNA damage induces DNA repair system, including poly ADP-rybosylation that further reduces ATP content and leads to the depletion of cellular NAD^+.

Ca^{2+} does not seem to play an important role in cell death evoked by streptozotocin, because Ca^{2+}-channel antagonists do not protect β cells against streptozotocin [165

N-Nitroso Compounds

N-nitroso compounds are structurally related to streptozotocin and provide their deleterious effects on β cells through DNA alkylation and generation of highly toxic free oxygen radicals and peroxides. As mentioned above, they are formed in the gut by the reaction of nitrate with amines and amides.

First report on the effect of N-nitroso compounds, possibly affecting the incidence of T1D, was presented by Helgason and Jonasson [179] who tried to explain increased incidence of disease in Iceland among boys born in October by the intake of smoked mutton by the parents after Christmas. This food was shown to contain considerable concentrations of N-nitroso compounds [179]. Later, an association between intake of selected foods contained high levels of N-nitroso compounds and T1D was found in Canada [180] and Sweden [145].

A study of a role of dietary N-nitroso compounds as a factor, increasing risk of the incidence of T1D, needs more research to find a dose, timing and age-dependent differences. Excess of dietary N-nitroso compounds is likely to represent a risk factor for children, starting from the second year of life, when infants receive any foods, containing nitrate or nitrite. Comsuption of food, containing natural antioxidants (i.e. vitamin C, vitamin E) definetely protects infants from harmful action of dietary N-nitroso compounds.

GROWTH

An increased weight gain in infancy is associated with higher risk of diabetes. Such relationship was reported by Johansson et al. [181], who observed a positive correlation between inhanced increase in weight and incidence of T1D in girls at the age of up to 30 months. An association between increased infant body mass index rate before onset of T1D and presense of islet autoantibodies IA-2 [182] and daily insulin dose [183] was also found. Bruining [182] suggested that increased growth in infancy occurs with more rapid decay of pancreatic islet function, since IA-2 antibodies are present, and this combination should additionally increase risk of early onset of T1D.

Comparative case-control analyses in Finland showed a strong correlation between enhanced infant growth, obesity in childhood and risk of T1D [184,185]. A 10% gain in relative weight was associated with 50-60% increase in the risk of T1D before 3 years of age, and 20-40% increase from 3-10 years of age [184]. Obesity (relative weight exceeding 120%) after 3 years of age was related to a more than two-fold risk of the development of T1D [185].

According to the hypothesis of Wilkin [186], body constitution could influence accelerated loss of β cells through apoptosis. Increased growth in infancy needs more insulin that can lead to early exhaustion of insulin-producing cells and their depletion. Thus, accelerated weight gain in early childhood and overweight could be independent risk factor, explaining rising incidence of type 1 and type 2 diabetes in industrialized countries [186].

STRESSFUL LIFE

Stressful life events could also contribute to early onset of diabetes. Severe psychological stress, such as loss of a family member, was found to be more common during the year preceeding the diagnosis among children, who developed disease, than among controls during the corresponding time period [187]. In Italy, an association between social deprivation and increased incidence of diabetic ketoacidosis was observed [188]. Psychological stress early in life may increase the risk for T1D, because intense stress would promote overt diabetes by increasing the requirements of endogeneous insulin due to the stress-induced release of counteracting hormones (cortisol and catecholamines) [189]. Prospective observations of individuals at high risk of T1D up to disease manifestation would be helpful in the estimation of a role of psychosocial factors and stress events in the development of diabetes.

PREGNANCY AND PRENATAL FACTORS

Pathogenic process, leading to T1D, can start in the prenatal period of fetal life. Studies in Sweden among children, who became diabetic in 1978-88, showed increased relative risk (OR) in several groups of children, particularly in the age group of 0-4 years and among those, whose mothers were older than 35 years [190]. The highest OR of 4.13 was observed for maternal-child blood group incompatibility. The incompatibility was associated with neonatal β cell dysfunction and could act as immunological trigger for T1D [190]. Studies in the UK confirmed the association of increased risk of β-cell autoimmunity with old maternal age and reported new risk factors, including excessive weight gain in pregnancy [191].

Maternal enterovirus infections during pregnancy can be associated with late onset of diabetes in the offspring. In Sweden, analysis of maternal sera revealed presense of IgM against coxsackie B virus type 3 closely related to the incidence of T1D in children [192]. In Finland, tested sera showed strong association between coxsackie B virus type 5 and disease in offspring under the age of 3 years but not in those older than 3 years [193].

INTERACTION BETWEEN GENETIC PREDISPOSITION TO TYPE 1 DIABETES AND ENVIRONMENTAL TRIGGERS

Due to the complexity of T1D etiology, disease can be induced not only by a certain environmental factor, but be resulted from the harmful action of a combination of several environmental triggers. For example, a combination of the usually non-diabetogenic EMC-B variant and single low doses of streptozotocin can cause diabetes in male mice, while these agents are not able to induce disease when administrated alone [194].

High variability in the incidence of T1D in Europe reflects differences in environmental risk factors (nutrition, lifestyle) specific for a certain country/region that are important in determining a country's incidence rate [195]. Different genetic and non-genetic factors could interact to initiate disease in different individuals. For each individual, there is a unique diabetogenic combination of genetic and environmental triggers causing disease. Some of those like CM proteins and viral infections induce diabetes through the damage of β cells. Other factors, such as accelerated growth rate and stressful life promote the development of T1D.

In humans, susceptibility to diabetogenic enteroviruses appears to be genetically restricted by HLA-DR and DQ alleles [196]. Early observations found increased T-cell mediated response against Coxsackie B4 virus or elevated levels of virus-specific antibodies in T1D patients with predisposing HLA-DR4 and DR4 alleles [197,198]. These results have been confirmed in recent case-control studies. In Finnish diabetic patients, who carried DR3 and/or DR4 alleles, levels of antibodies against Coxsackie B4 virus were significantly higher than those in subjects with the protective DR2 allele [199]. Studies in Linkoping region (where the highest incidence for T1D was detected) showed increased titers of antibodies against CBV in individuals, who have DR3/DR4 genotypes and additionally carry alleles 5 and 5.1 of the Major Histocompatibility Complex (MHC) class I chain-related gene-A (MICA) associated with higher risk of T1D in Caucasians [200]. The results suggest that HLA-DR3/DR4 alleles can modulate antiviral immune response. This phenomenon could have pathogenetic significance, i.e. by exaggerating immune pathology and cell damage in pancreatic islets in enterovirus-infected subjects, who are positive for these HLA-DR alleles associated with diabetes.

Several studies evaluated a possibility of an interaction between the HLA genes and dietary factors but produced controversial results. An early exposure to cow's milk of children, carrying HLA-DR3/4 and HLA-DQ8 genotypes, is shown to be associated with the development of β-cell autoimmunity [201, 202]. However other studies showed no relation between HLA genotypes and consumption of CM proteins [116,203,204].

Genetic background determines predisposing or protective genetic markers associated with higher or lower risk of diabetes. Genetic susceptibility/protection may play a role in the initiation of pathogenetic process, or later, either accelerating or delaying the autoimmune response, when a new insult (of the same or another agent causing the initial lesion) occurs [205].

Chapter 5

Prediabetes and Islet Autoimmunity: Islet Self-Antibodies and Mechanisms of the Breakage of Peripheral Self-Tolerance

Tolerance to Pancreatic Islet Autoantigens

Self-reactive T cells specific to β cell autoantigens are present in most normal individuals but are kept under control by a number of immune tolerance mechanisms. Among them, thymic or central deletion of β-cell reactive T cell clones is one major potential mechanism. Numerous autoantigens, including islet autoantigens (insulin, GAD, I-A2, pancreatic polypeptide, C-reactive protein and others), are expressed in the thymus [206]. T cells, displaying high affinity to these antigens, are likely to be deleted through negative selection, while autoreactive low-affinity T cells could survive and circulate in peripheral blood of normal individuals. Self-reactive cells, escaping central deletion, are kept under control of peripheral tolerance that includes indifference, peripheral deletion, anergy and immunoregulation.

Deletion of autoreactive cells is a major mechanism of maintaining peripheral self-tolerance. Studies on transgenic mice, expressing high doses of antigen (ovalbumin) in β cells, showed that tolerance to ovalbumin-specific CD8+ T cells is developed through the peripheral deletion of these cells [207]. Tolerance to self-reactive CD8+ T cells is induced with the cross-presentation of self-antigens within the complex with MHC class I molecules by professional antigen-presenting cells (APCs), taking place in the draining lymph nodes. This leads to CD95-mediated deletion of the T cells responding to high dose of self-antigen [208]. Low dose self-antigens are not cross-presented and are consequently ignored by T cells.

A subset of T lymphocytes namely regulatory T cells (Tregs) are responsible for the immune regulation of self-reactivity. In thymectomized animals, autoimmunity may be prevented by the administration of selected T cell subsets from non-thymectomized animals, such as CD25+ T cells in mice [209] and RT6+ or CD62L+ cells in rats [210]. Tregs may be demonstrated in the prediabetic stage in animal models of diabetes. When transferred into the spleen or thymus of the immunoincompetent hosts, such as NOD mouse, regulatory cells are able to suppress the development of T1D [211]. Further studies revealed that the regulatory cells are CD4+ CD62L+ and/or CD25+ [212, 213]. The regulatory function of these cells does not rely to the production of Th2 cytokines (IL-4) [214]. The mechanism of immunosuppressive action of Tregs will be considered in details below, in the section, discussing on the role of immunoregulation in loss of the tolerance to β cell antigens.

PATHOGENIC ACTIVATION OF SELF-REACTIVE T CELLS

β-cell autoantigen(s)-driven T cell activation is a mandatory step for the emergence of the aggressive diabetogenic lymphocyte response. The activation involves certain MHC molecules, presenting pathogenic β-cell epitopes to T cells. Experiments in NOD mice showed a substantial role of Th1 cells, since T cell activation is accelerated by administration of IL-12 [215] and impaired by treatment with monoclonal antibody against IFN-γ [216]. The privileged role of CD8+ T cells in β-cell autoimmunity was revealed from the treatment of very young NOD mice (2-5 weeks old) with a depleting CD8 antibody prevented insulitis [217]. An unbalanced activation of CD4+ and CD8+ lymphocytes with predominant activation of the CD8+ lymphocyte subset was found in patients with recently diagnosed diabetes [218]. Intra-islet inflammation may also play a role independently on the nature of primary insult. The inflammation could be primary in the induction of anti-islet autoimmune response, when caused by viral infection [219], or secondary as a result of cytotoxic action of pathogenic CD4+ Th1 or CD8+ cells [220].

Several mechanisms of the activation of self-reactive T cells are suggested. The mechanism of molecular mimicry was proposed to explain how viral antigens, sharing homology with islet antigens, could provoke T cells to initiate the immune response against host β cells. Information, supporting the hypothesis of molecular mimicry, is coming from observations of sharing T cell epitopes and sequence homology between GAD and Coxsackie B3 virus protein but needs additional confirmation [221,222]. As mentioned above, a sequence homology between certain CM and plant proteins and β-cell antigens exists that can induce islet antibodies in subjects with impaired mucosal immune function [107,122].

An aberrant expression of MHC molecules by islet β cells described in patients with newly diagnosed T1D could also lead to the induction of β-cell autoimmunity [223,224]. However, this observation should be consistently confirmed, since the aberrant expression of HLA class II molecules may be a secondary to the cytokine release induced by the initial immune response. The role of inflammation-induced abnormal expression of molecules involved in the antigen presentation and recognition is likely to result in inducing the initial autoimmune response or in accelerating it through the antigen spreading [225].

T cell autoreactivity may be induced by a viral superantigen [226]. Human endogeneous retrovirus type K (HERV-K) was isolated from the culture supernatants of leukocyte-infiltrated islets of two diabetic patients [227]. The retrovirus was shown to be implicated in expression as a superantigen. Detection of a novel viral sequence $IDDMK_{1,2}22$, which was similar to HERV-K10/K18 subfamilies and contained a Vβ7-specific superantigen sequence, could explain the predominance of T cell repertoire, bearing a Vβ7 receptor in two pancreases from diabetic patients [228].

This observation led to the hypothesis that a human endogeneous virus, belonging to the HERV- K family might express as a superantigen, initiating or triggering islet autoimmunity, and the identification of the $IDDMK_{1,2}22$ sequence in serum of patients should predict an increased risk for T1D. However, data of Conrad et al. [227] have not been replicated. Muir at al. [229] failed to detect the $IDDMK_{1,2}22$ viral sequence in genomic DNA, lymphocyte, or plasma RNA in any (diabetic and non-diabetic) subject. In other investigation, viral mRNA of this virus was detected in patients with recent diagnosis of diabetes and with long-term diabetes and in healthy controls, while there was no significant difference in levels of virus-specific antibodies between diabetic patients and control subjects [230].

A ROLE OF IMMUNOREGULATION

Naturally Occurring Regulatory CD4+CD25+ T Cells

Autoimmune process that follows T cell activation by islet self-antigens is under control of immunoregulatory CD4+ T cells. This population of Tregs includes approximately 10% of CD4+ T cells that coexpressed the CD25 antigen, or IL-2 receptor α-chain [231]. Depletion of this CD4+CD25+ T-cell subset from normal murine tissues resulted in the induction of a variety of organ-specific autoimmune diseases, such as thyroiditis, gastritis, insulitis, adrenalitis, glomerulonephritis and others. Autoimmune disease in these mice could be prevented by cotransfer of the CD4+CD25+ Tregs. Similarly, the induction of disease post-day 3 thymectomy may be prevented by reconstitution of the animals with CD4+CD25+ but not CD4+CD25- T cells by days 10 through 14 of life [232].

Naturally occurring CD4+CD25+ Tregs are likely to represent a major subset of cells that play a unique role in the regulation of the immune response. Studies in humans showed that T1D patients have lower Tregs counts in their peripheral blood compared to normal controls and type 2 diabetics [233,234]. Immunosuppressive function of CD4+CD25+ Tregs in patients affected with T1D was significantly reduced in comparison with normal subjects [235]. Additionally, in patients with T1D, cocultures of Tregs displayed in vitro a more proinflammatory phenotype, with increased secretion of IFN-γ and decreased IL-10 production. These data demonstrate that deficiency in the number or function of the CD4+CD25+ Treg population may influence the pathogenesis of type 1 diabetes.

In NOD mice, a reduced frequency of CD4−CD25+ Tregs is shown [213]. However, another study reported that prediabetic NOD mice have intact CD4+CD25+ Treg compartment [236]. CD4+CD25+ Tregs from the prediabetic NOD mouse are regulatory, because transfer of autoreactive T cells from prediabetic NOD mice to NOD.Scid mice that do not have any T cells, including Tregs, induces a rapid progression of severe diabetes. In contrast, cotransferring CD4+CD25+ Tregs from the prediabetic NOD mice with self-reactive T cells prevents the induction of disease in the recipient NOD.Scid mouse [237].

Despite the presense of CD4+CD25+ Tregs with normal regulatory properties in prediabetes, NOD mice develop T1D. It is not clear what happens with naturally occurring

Tregs in diabetic NOD mice, while they are not able to prevent the development of disease. No studies so far have demonstrated that transfer of CD4+CD25+ Tregs can protect normal immune-competent NOD mice in vivo.

The mechanism of suppression mediated by CD4+CD25+ Tregs still remains unclear. These cells suppress the proliferation and cytokine production of conventional CD4+ and CD8+ lymphocytes, antigen-presenting B cells and innate immune cells (dendritic cells and monocytes) [238]. Once stimulated, regulation by naturally occurring T regs is independent of the antigen specificity of the target cells. Stimulation with IL-2 and T cell receptor (TCR) is required for suppression mediated by these regulatory cells [239].

IL-2 and other regulatory molecules (CD28, CD40 and forkhead transcription factor FoxP3) are crucial for CD4+CD25+ Tregs development and survival [239]. Among them, FoxP3 is probably the most crucial molecule in the generation and function of Tregs. FoxP3-deficient mice lack subpopulation of CD4+CD25+ Tregs, and CD4+ T cells from these mice are hyperresponsive to stimulation, produce a variety of cytokines and cause a devastating lymphoproliferative disease [240]. In humans, FOXP3 is also specifically expressed in CD4+CD25+ Tregs and thymocytes [241]. The human FOXP3 gene is likely to have the same function as its murine orthologue, since mutations within FOXP3 result in severe autoimmune polyendocrinopathy referred to as IPEX [242].

Inducible Regulatory CD4+ T Cells

Naturally occurring Tregs provide their suppressive action through the direct cell-cell interaction with the target cells. Supernatants from activated CD4+CD25+ Tregs did not exhibit detectable suppressive properties [243]. Interaction between the regulatory T cell and the target cell involves cytotoxic effector functions associated with the synthesis of perforin, granzyme A and CD18 [244].

It has been recently demonstrated that CD4+CD25+ Tregs could suppress conventional CD4+CD25- T cells (Th1 and Th2) via LAG-3-mediated mechanism [245]. Lymphocyte activation gene-3 (LAG-3) is a CD4-related molecule that binds to MHC class II and is selectively expressed on Tregs. Th1 and Th2 cells do not express significant levels of LAG-3 when activated. Transduction of LAG-3 onto CD4+CD25- T cells switched them to anergic phenotype. Addition of a LAG-3-specific monoclonal antibody prevented LAG-3/MHC class II interactions that led to the proliferation of T cells, T cell expansion and Th1, but not Th2 cytokine production [246]. These results indicate that LAG-3 signaling inhibits early events in primary activation of human CD4 and CD8 T cells and further support a role for LAG-3 signaling in regulating the expansion of activated effector or memory T cells, either directly or indirectly through Treg suppressor activity.

The suppression of Th1 and Th2 cells by Tregs may involve the ligation of B7 molecule on target T cells, which delivers a negative signal [247]. Target cells deficient in the B7 molecules (CD80 and to less degree CD86) were resistant to Treg suppression. Interaction between naturally occurring Tregs and APCs is shown to be followed by the downregulation of costimulatory molecules on APCs,thus rendering them ineffective [243]. Probably, Tregs suppress immune responces in multiple ways, which may involve negative signals produced by inhibitory Treg surface molecules, cytotoxicity, APC function downregulation and induction of other regulatory cells.

While CD4+CD25+ Tregs appear to be present at a relatively low level in normal subjects, studies in animal models showed that another type of CD4+ Tregs called Th2-like Tregs act at lower baseline. These cells are antigen-induced, and their protective function is substantial only after external immunization [248,249]. Once CD4+ Tregs have been induced, they can move to the appropriate tissue (organ) and inhibit autoreactive T cells through the mechanism of bystander suppression. Bystander suppression is mediated by the production of anti-inflammatory cytokines, such as IL-4, IL-10 and transforming growth factor (TGF-β) (Figure 6). Whereas CD4+CD25+ Tregs inhibit many immune responses via cell-cell contact and are of unknown antigen specificity, Th2-like Tregs suppress only certain autoimmune responses through the production of effector cytokines [250,251].

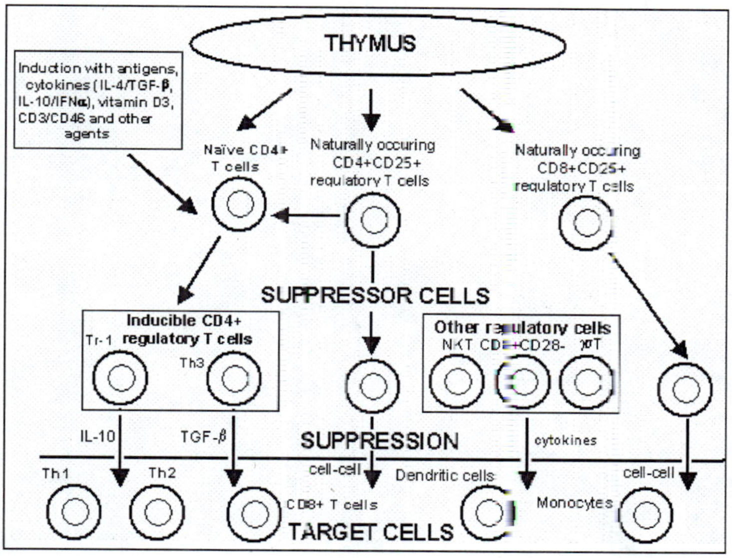

Figure 6. Targets for immune suppression and mechanisms of suppressive effects of different populations of immunoregulatory cells. Naturally occuring CD4+CD25+ regulatory T cells, CD8+CD25+ regulatory T cells and naïve T cells are generated from the thymus. Naïve CD4+ could be induced with a variety of stimulating agents to differentiate into inducible regulatory T cells that include two cells subsets – Tr-1 and Th3 cells. These populations of regulatory T cells as well other types of regulatory cells (NKT – natural killer cells, CD8+CD28-, γσ T cells, etc.) mediate suppression in a cytokine-dependent manner, while CD4+CD25+ and CD8+CD25+ regulatory T lymphocytes use cell-cell interactions for suppression.

IL-4 is shown to mediate protection against diabetes induced by DNA vaccination with GAD [252] or oral insulin administration [253]. Presense of IL-4 in the target organ, i.e. pancreas, can be very effective in preventing T1D [254]. Transgenic NOD mice, which express IL-4 in β cells, are protected from lymphocytic choriomeningitis virus-induced diabetes [255] or spontaneous diabetes [256].

IL-10 is effective against diabetes when injected with DNA vaccine [250] or viral gene transfer [257]. Defective responses to IL-10 are implicated in the pathogenesis of diseases with striking polarized Th1 versus Th2 pathological features. In humans, tolerant, non-diabetic state is characterized by autoreactive T cells that express IL-10, while in diabetes autoreactive T cells show clear proinflammatory phenotype [258]. The immune-suppressive properties of IL-10 are likely to be explained by the ability of this cytokine to inhibit APC function [259] and mediate direct antiproliferative effects on T cells [260].

Table 4. Characteristics of naturally occurring CD4+CD25+ regulatory T lymphocytes and two types of antigen-induced regulatory T cells (Tr-1 and Th3)

Phenotype	Naturally occuring CD4+CD25+ Tregs	Antigen-induced Tr-1	Antigen-induced Th3
IL-4	+/-	-	+/-
IFN-γ	+/-	+	+/-
IL-2Rα (CD25) expression	++++	+/-	+++
FoxP3 expression	++++	-	+++
LAG-3 expression	++++	?	?
IL-10 production	+/-	++++	+/-
TGF-β production	+/-	++	++++
B helper	-	-	IgA
IL-10 required for suppression	No	Yes	?
TGF-β required for suppression	No	Yes	Yes
CTLA-4 required for suppression	No	?	Yes
Growth and differentiation factors	Thymic interactions, CD28, IL-2, FoxP3	IL-10/ IFN-γ	TGF-β/IL-4

TGF-β may be induced after oral administration with islet antigens. This cytokine suppress T-cell responses, but displays pleiotropic effects to its targets. TGF-β contributes to maintaining normal immune homeostasis. TGF-β expressed transgenically in the pancreas or given as a DNA vaccine can protect NOD mice from diabetes [261,262]. On the other hand, TGF-β did not protect mice from LCMV-induced autoimmune diabetes [263]. The overexpression of this cytokine in the murine pancreas led to autoimmune pancreatitis and actually induced diabetes, while coexpressed with tumor necrosis factor-α (TNF-α) in the pancreas [264]. Similarly, some studies showed that IL-10 expressed transgenically in pancreatic islets or T cells failed to protect NOD mice from diabetes [265,266]. Thus, while anti-inflammatory Th2 cytokines can be effective in reducing self-reactive immune responses in type 1 diabetes, they may not always be beneficial.

The current classification of regulatory T cells divides antigen-induced Th2-like Tregs to regulatory type 1 (Tr-1) and T helper type 3 (Th3) cells [267]. Tr-1 cells produce IL-10, while Th3 cells secrete TGF-β. Compared to CD4+CD25+ T regs and Th3 cells, Tr-1 cells did not express FoxP3. Th3 cell, like CD4+CD25+ T regs, express cytotoxic T lymphocyte antigen-4 (CTLA-4) on their surface, the triggering of which results in the secretion of TGF-β. Unlike naturally occurring T regs, the main suppressive mechanism of Th3 cells is dependent on the production of CTLA-4 and TGF-β, which suppresses the proliferation of Th1 and Th2 cells (Table 4) [268]. Th3 cells also stimulate plasma cells to secret immunoglobulin A (IgA), while CD4+CD25+ T regs and Tr-1 do not [269].

Natural Killer T Cells

There are many other types of regulatory cells with suppressive properties, including CD8+CD25+ T lymphocytes derived from thymus, B helper cells, γσ T cells, CD8+CD28- T cells and natural killer T cells (NKTs) [270]. Among those, NKTs could play an important role in suppressing β-cell autoimmunity in prediabetes. While the NKTs cell population was first recognized to be deficient in NOD mice, augmenting NKT cell activity has been shown to suppress the development of autoimmune disease in this strain [271, 272].

CD1d-restricted NKTs have CD4+CD62L-CD25-CD122+ phenotype, representing a T cell subset characterized by the use of an invariant TCR α chain (Vα14Jα281) and MHC class I –like molecule CD1d [273]. NOD mice lacking CD1d displayed an accelerated onset and increased incidence of diabetes [274,275]. NKTs could be activated by CD1d-restricted myeloid dendritic cells, which present on their surface isoglobotrihexosylceramide (lysosomal glycosphingolipid) and other lipid ligands bound to the CD1d molecule [276]. When activated NKTs produce different cytokines, including large amount of IL-4 and IFN-γ [277]. NOD NKT cells display disturbances in the expression profile of secreted cytokines, producing low levels of IL-4, but maintaining a reduced ability to secret IFN-γ [278]. This NKT cell defect was suggested to contribute to diabetes susceptibility, which would be compatible with the protective effect of IFN-γ on diabetes development in the NOD mouse [279].

There are several mechanisms, by which NKTs can inhibit an autoimmune process in pancreatic islets. CD1d-restricted NKTs may suppress autoimmunity via the interaction with dendritic cells. Injection of myeloid DC isolated from pancreatic lymph nodes protected female NOD mice from diabetes, suggesting for the ability of NKTs to recruit tolerogenic dendritic cells to the pancreatic lymph nodes [280]. Production by NKTs of Th2 type cytokines (IL-4 and IL-10) could shift Th1-mediated immune response to Th2 type way and then prevent the development of diabetes From murine experimental models of diabetes, the suppression of autoimmunity exerted by NKT cells clearly depends on IL-4 in some settings, while the role of IL-10 requires further investigation [281, 282]. In some cases, NKTs may prevent the development of self-reactive CD8+ T cells without shifting the response to a Th2 type. Beaudoin et al. [283] demonstrated that TCR transgenic MHC class II-restricted diabetogenic T cells from BDC2.5 NOD mice were unable to induce diabetes in TCR transgenic mice with elevated NKTs numbers. BDC2.5 T cells underwent initial activation and proliferation in pancreatic lymph nodes, but did not differentiate into IFN-γ-producing cells when contacted with NKT cells [284].

Thus, NKTs play a substantial role in the regulation of diabetes pathogenesis in NOD mice. Studies, addressing a correlation between NKT cell levels in peripheral blood and T1D in humans, yielded variable results [285-287]. However, the studies of human peripheral blood lymphocytes should be interpreted with caution, since the deficiency in the inducible NKT cell population found in lymphoid organs of NOD mice is not reflected among peripheral blood lymphocytes in the same mice [288]. Therefore, further investigation should be awaited before conclusions can be drawn a similar deficiency in diabetic patients.

PREDICTIVE AUTOANTIBODIES IN TYPE 1 DIABETES

Table 5. The occurrence and predictive significance of four major diabetes-related antibodies

Islet self-antigen	Antibody frequency in diabetic patients	Predictive value for diabetes diagnosis*
GAD65	70-80%	60%
Insulin	40-80%	30%
IA-2	50-60%	30%
IA-2β	50%	30%

*The predictive values are estimated from studies of ICA-positive first-degree relatives

Several self-reactive islet antibodies have been found in patients with newly diagnosed T1D. Among those, there are four major antibodies against glutamic acid decarboxylase 65 kD isoform, insulin and islet antigens IA-2 and IA-2β, which occur in sera of diabetic patients with high frequency and can predict diabetes (Table 5). Other autoantibodies, recognizing the islet antigen of 69 kD (ICA69), glima 38, DNA topoisomerase type II, heat shock proteins, carboxypeptidase H and other islet antigens, occur significantly less frequently and are characterized with low diagnostic sensitivity. These antibodies are considered as putative diabetogenic self-antibodies. For them, detection assays need to be standardized or the detection of these antibodies should be continuously confirmed.

Antibodies to Islet Glutamic Acid Decarboxylase (GADA)

There are four self-antibodies specificities that are useful in defining islet autoimmunity. The antibodies against the 65 kD islet isoform of GAD detected as a 64 kD islet autoantigen were found in patients with recent diagnosis of diabetes in early 80's [289, 290]. There are two GAD isoforms with molecular weight of 65 and 67 kD, respectively. Both isoforms are expressed in neurons, catalizing the formation of the inhibitory neurotransmitter γ-aminobutiric acid (GABA) from glutamine. Although high activity of GAD, GAD65 mRNA and high concentrations of GABA in pancreatic islets have been detected, the role of GAD65 and GABA in Langherhans' β cells is still unclear [291]. Presumably, GABA can be used for both regulatory and throphic functions, and both paracrine and metabolic effects to islet GABA have been reported [292]. A putative significance of GABA for β cell energy metabolism by generating NADH and ATP in the GABA shunt has been speculated [293].

A total 70-80% of T1D sera recognized GAD65, whereas only 10-20% recognize GAD67 [294,295].

To detect GAD self-antibodies, a variety of assays have been developed, including ELISA, radioimmunoassay and measuring enzymatic activity in immunoprecipitates [296,297]. Cloning and producing of the recombinant GAD65 made it possible to generate a precise and reproducible radioligand-binding assays [298,299] and non-radioactive GAD65 antibody detection technique, using biotin-GAD65 fusion protein [300,301]. The availability of simple and high-resolution detecting assays allowed the analysis of GAD65 and GAD67 antibodies in a variety of disorders to better understand their diagnostic sensitivity and significance. For example, both GAD65 and GAD67 antibodies have been found in patients with autoimmune thyroid disease [302-305], celiac disease [306,307] and autoimmune polyendocrine syndrome type 1 [308], suggesting for common mechanisms of the induction of autoimmunity in early stages of these autoimmune disorders.

The highest diagnostic sensitivity of GADA has been found at onset of diabetes. Typically, 80% of patients with newly diagnosed T1D have GAD65 antibodies (Table 5). [295,309]. The frequency of GAD65 antibodies is increased among first-degree relatives and predicts T1D [310,311]. The predictive value of T1D of GAD65 antibody alone or in combination with other islet antibodies ranges between 50-60% and requires additional testing for presenting ICA antibodies and loss of β cells to diagnose diabetes. The presense of GAD65 antibodies at diagnosis is suggested to be associated with more rapid loss of β-cell mass [312]. In long-term diabetes, levels of GAD65 antibodies decrease but their prevalence remains surprisingly high [313].

GAD65 antibodies are restricted to IgG type. These monoclonal antibodies (MICA 1-10) recognize several epitopes within GAD65 molecule located at the N-terminal region (starting at position 39 for MICA 8/9), middle region (amino acids 245-449 for MICA 4/6 and 10) and C-terminal region (amino acids 450-570 for MICA 1/3 and 7) [314-317]. A study, using GAD65/67 chimeric molecules, showed that the middle and C-terminal epitopes are immunodominant [318]. The GAD epitopes are conformational, since diabetes-related GAD65 antibodies are unable to recognize linear GAD65 epitopes [319].

Because of the presenting somatic mutations in GAD65 antibody molecules, which are likely to be antigen-driven by CD4+ T cell-mediated mechanisms, the identification of GAD65 T-cell receptor epitopes was also crucial [318]. In NOD mice, proliferative T cell response in the spleen was initially confined to the C-terminal region of GAD65 (peptides 509-528 and 524-543). Using synthetic peptides, which spanned the 509-543 region of human GAD, four T cell hybridomas were produced from spleen cells of GAD (524-543)-immunized NOD mice. Four amino acid residues (alanine-530, proline-531, arginine-536 and methionine-537) were found to be critical for the activation of three of these four hybridomas, suggesting that these positions in the GAD-524-543 determinant were MHC-binding residues or conserved TCR contact sites [320]. Further study revealed at least two I-A(g7)-restricted overlapping determinants present in the GAD65(524--543) sequence, each capable of recruiting unique T cell repertoires characterized by distinct TCR Vβ gene use. All CD4+ T cells responsive to the immunization with the GAD65 peptide 530-543 used the Vβ4 gene, whereas the Vβ12 gene is preferentially used to encode the TCR of GAD65 peptide 524-543-responsive T cell populations [321].

Human studies demonstrated a complexity of T cell-mediated autoimmune responses against GAD65 in diabetic patients, carrying the HLA-DR4 haplotypes characteristic of susceptibility to T1D. Multiple immunostimulatory epitopes were identified, with diverse class II DR molecules, functioning as the restriction element. The majority of T cell responses were restricted by DRB1 molecules; however, DRB4 restricted responses were also observed [322]. After immunization with the naturally processed self-peptide of human GAD65 (552-572), T cell hybridoma was generated from mice transgenic for the susceptible HLA-DR4 allele. These autoreactive CD4+ T cells were specific for the self-peptide, but recognized it with low avidity, suggesting the predominance of low avidity recognition of self-peptide epitopes may be a characteristic feature of CD4+ T cells, responding to autoantigens [323]. However, in peripheral blood of diabetic patients, high-avidity CD4+ T-cells, coexisting with low-avidity cells directed to the same GAD65 epitope specificity have been also found. T-cell clones with high MHC-peptide avidity utilize a biased set of TCR genes that favor two combinations, Vα12-β5.1 and Vα17-Vβ4 [324]. Thus, presence of these high-avidity TCRs indicated a failure to delete autoreactive T cells that likely arised from oligoclonal expansion in response to autoantigen exposure during the progression of T1D.

Analysis of two GAD65 self-reactive T-cell clones isolated from T1D patients, using a DNA-based randomized epitope library, showed the recognition by both TCRs was significantly affected by combinations of amino acids in the antigenic peptide, although the degree of combinatorial effect differed between the two TCRs. Protein database search proved successful in identifying several microbial and self-protein-derived mimicry epitopes [325]. The homology between human GAD65 and protein P2C of Coxsackie virus B4 has been found, and immune reactivity of sera from T1D patients to both GAD65 autoantigen and viral P2C antigen has been reported [83, 326-328]. The homologous motif (PEVKEK) was highly conserved among coxsackie B-like enteroviruses, therefore suggesting for the role of enteroviral infection in inducing islet cell autoimmunity through the mechanism of molecular mimicry. This motif was shown to bind specifically to HLA-DR3, and both P2C and GAD65 peptides bind in the same position within the peptide-binding groove of the DR3 molecule, which is an essential requirement for T-cell cross-reactivity [328]. However, several later attempts failed to isolate T cell clones that specifically crossreact against the homologous peptide of both GAD65 and P2C [84, 85, 329]. The antigen-specific T-cell clones from patients with newly diagnosed T1D were reacting either with the GAD65 peptide [(amino acids 247-280) with sequence homology to Coxsackie P2C (amino acids 30-50)] or the Coxsackie P2C peptide (30-50), using different restriction elements without crossreacting to the homologous peptide [85]. So, the possible role of molecular mimicry in Coxsackie virus-induced diabetes remains unclear and needs further confirmation. It is possible that molecular mimicry may be limited to the HLA-DR3 positive subpopulation of diabetic patients, but this phenomenon requires additional investigation.

Several studies investigated the immune processing of the GAD65 antigen, reporting the identification of GAD65 epitopes, binding to certain MHC class II molecules. Two DRB1*0401-restricted T cell epitopes from human GAD65 (amino acids 274-286 and 115-127) were found. Both peptides were immunogenic in mice transgenic for the DRB1*0401 MHC class II molecule. These peptides could be naturally generated by APCs and formed complexes with the DRB1*0401 molecules [330]. The presentation of these two T-cell epitopes in the islets of DRB1*0401 individuals, who are at risk for type 1 diabetes, was suggested to allow the antigen-specific recruitment of regulatory cells to the islets following peptide immunization. When pulsed with the GAD protein, human B-lymphoblastoid cells were able to present the GAD65 274-268 epitope, but not the GAD65 115-127 epitope [331]. Blood mononuclear adherent cells, B cells or dendritic cells derived from the same individual displayed the same presentation pattern as observed in B cell lines, suggesting that the defect most likely is genetically determined. Therefore, individual differences in antigen processing may result in the presentation of distinct set of peptides derived from an autoantigen, such as GAD65. This may be an important mechanism for the deviation of the immune response either into a regulatory pathway or into an inflammatory autoimmune reactivity.

Experiments in islet endothelial cell (EC) cultures which expressed HLA class II molecules, showed the ability of the ECs, expressing the DRB1*0401 allele, to process and present whole GAD65 to the HLA-DR4-restricted murine T-cell hybridoma T33.1 that recognized the 274-286 epitope of GAD65 [332]. Additionally, T33.1 hybridoma cells and autoreactive T lymphocytes of the human T-cell clone PM1#11, which recognizes the GAD65 epitope 339-352 presented by HLA-DR3, more rapidly migrated through monolayers of islet ECs, expressing the DRB1*0401 molecule, in the presense of GAD65 [332]. These results support the hypothesis that presentation of autoantigens by islet endothelium in vivo could promote transmigration of circulating islet autoantigen-specific T-cells primed in regional lymph nodes against islet autoantigens. Stimulation of T33.1 hybridoma cells with APCs exposed to recombinant human GAD65 was greatly enhanced with sera from patients with high GAD65 antibody levels. The uptake of antibody-complexed GAD65 was Fc receptor (FcR)-medaited, because the enhancement of presentation was inhibited by monoclonal antibody against FcR [333]. These results suggest that GAD65 antibodies can modulate presentation of GAD65 to T-cells. Increased antigen uptake and heterogeneity in the autoantibody specificity may provide a mechanism for antibody-facilitated T-cell response, influencing the progression of T1D.

Insulin Autoantibodies (IAA)

In 1983, insulin autoantibodies (IAA) were detected by Palmer et al. [334] in patients with recent onset of T1D before the start of the treatment with exogenous insulin. The frequency of IAA at clinical diagnosis typically varies from 40% to 80% (Table 5) [335,336]. The prevalence of IAA correlates with age, because insulin antibodies are more frequent among young children than among adolescents or adults [335,337,338].

The first standardized radioimmunoassay for insulin, using ^{35}S-insulin as a radioligand, reached the highest diagnostic sensitivity and specificity with the elongation of incubation and the use of larger volumes of sera [339,340]. Further progress resulted in the development of a detection microassay, substantially decreasing the serum volume needed for the analysis, with no loss in sensitivity of the insulin measurement [341]. Several non-radioactive IAA detection assays are also currently available [342-344].

Recent studies indicated a primary role of insulin as an autoantigen in the initiation of T1D in mice and humans. Nakayama et al. [345] replaced the native insulin gene in the NOD mouse with an engineered gene, encoding insulin, which is hormonally active but is unable to stimulate T cell-mediated responces. The mice did not develop either β-cell autoimmunity, or diabetes. The important finding was associated with the replacement of tyrosine-to-alanine at residue 16 of the insulin molecule that negates immune response to a single fragment of the insulin B-chain (residues 9-23). CD4+ T lymphocytes in NOD mice recognize the insulin B-chain 9-23 fragment bound to the I-A^{g7} MHC class II molecule [346], whereas CD8+ T cells recognize a related fragment of the β-chain at residues 15-23 complexed to the H-K^d class I molecule [347]. The replacement of tyrosine-to-alanine at residue 16 in the mutated insulin molecule results in failure of these peptides to bind to the corresponding MHC molecule, making these insulin fragments unrecognizable to the TCR repertoire. Nakayama and coauthors [345] suggested that the epitope 9-23 might be sufficient in the induction of anti-islet autoimmunity and the absence of its recognition by autoreactive T cells prevents the development of spontaneous diabetes in NOD mice.

Studies with overlapping synthetic 20mer peptides, spanning human preproinsulin, did not reveal significant difference in binding characteristics of T1D-protective HLA-DR2 and -DQ6.2 alleles and susceptible HLA- DR4 and DQ8 alleles. Furthermore, insulin peptide implicated as a major CD4+ T-cell target in disease pathogenesis (B9-23) had high affinity binding to both protective and permissive HLA molecules but did not represent the highest affinity region of (prepro)insulin identified in either case [348]. These data suggest that peptide-binding affinity alone is unlikely to be the major determinant of disease susceptibility in relation to interactions between (prepro)insulin epitopes and HLA molecules.

Several studies reported the association between IAA and HLA-DR4 [349-352]. In Finnish diabetic patients, IAA emerged as the first detectable antibody more commonly than any other antibody specificity, implying that insulin may be the primary antigen in most cases of human type 1 diabetes associated with the DR4-DQB1*0302 haplotype [350]. In Germany, a frequency of HLA genotypes DRB1*03/04 and DRB1*04/04 was significantly increased in offspring of parents with T1D, who rapidly developed IAA (i.e., within the first two years of life) [351]. These data suggest that HLA-DR4 could represent the major HLA allele responsible for insulin bearing and antigen presentation.

Kent et al. [353] showed that about 50% of CD4+ T cell clones isolated from the pancreatic drain nodes of diabetic patients with HLA-DR4, a susceptibility allele for type 1 diabetes, recognized the N-terminal fragment (amino acids 1-15) of the insulin A-chain restricted by DR4, therefore confirming a major role of HLA-DR4 in the antigen presentation of insulin as well as a primary role of insulin in initiating the diabetogenic immune responce. To induce proliferative responces of these T cell clones, surprisingly large amount of the insulin peptide (1 mM, or about 1.6 mg/ml) were required. Insulin in such high concentrations needed to activate T cells is present in islet-cell granules (240 mg/ml) [354]. If an insulin granule was phagocytozed by a dendritic cell, the concentration in the early endosomal compartment will be extremely high, although bound peptide would dissociate rapidly. Sufficiently high concentrations are therefore obtainable for dendritic cells, carrying antigen to the draining lymph nodes, although the avidity of the T cell clones for insulin is not known.

Although the diagnostic specificity of IAA for T1D is high (99%), there are large differences in sensitivity (40-80%) dependent of the type of assay used (Table 5)

[337,355,356]. The predictive value of IAA for T1D in children and young adults in a general population is low and varied from 3 % in Germany, showing an average incidence of T1D [357], to 8% in Scandinavian countries, where T1D incidence is high [65, 337, 358]. In first-degree relatives of childrens with newly diagnosed disease, a predictive value of IAA for T1D varied from 12 to 35% [359-361]. In combination with GAD65 or ICA512 antibodies, IAA may have predictive values for T1D among first-degree relatives as high as 50-70% [362-364]. Actually, the number of autoantibodies is important in the prediction, rather than the particular autoantibody specificities present. For example, measurements of three antibodies (IAA, GADA and ICA) among first-degree relatives, the five year risk of diabetes was 0% if no autoantibody was positive, 15% if only one was positive, 44% if two were positive and 100% if all three were positive [365].

IA-2/ICA512 Antibodies

Antibodies to islet proteins were initially identified in human diabetic sera by trypsin digestion of the 64 kD immunoprecipitation product [366]. The limited proteolysis of the immunoprecipitate revealed three different antibody specificities, binding fragments of 37, 40 and 50 kD. The 50 kD fragment was able to bind to GAD65 antibodies, whereas the remaining 37 and 40 kD products bound neither GAD65 nor GAD67 antibodies [367]. Two groups independently isolated cDNA, encoding a new diabetes-related islet autoantigen designated IA-2 and ICA512 [368, 369]. The 3613-bp cDNA encodes a 979-amino acid protein with molecular weight of 106 kD structurally similar to the members of protein tyrosine phosphatase family. It contains large extracellular domain (576 amino acids) with a cystein-rich segment (residues 40-62), transmembrane domain and cytoplasmic portion with a phospatase domain (Figure 7) [370]. Comparison of the amino acid sequences of IA-2 from human, mouse and rat revealed a high conservation in the intracellular domain (over 97%) across the species, while the extracellular domain was less conserved (80-90%) [371].

IA-2 is mostly expressed in cells of the neuroendocrine system, including endocrine pancreas and brain [369,372,373]. IA-2 is located in secretory granules [372]. As secretory granules mature, the extracellular domain of IA-2 undergoes posttranslational modifications, including proteolysis of the signal peptide (amino acids 1-34), glycosylation and digestion by a furin-like protease. Processing eliminates the N-terminal fragment of the extracellular domain (amino acids 35-448) and leaves the remaining portion (amino acids 449-576) attached to the membrane [374].

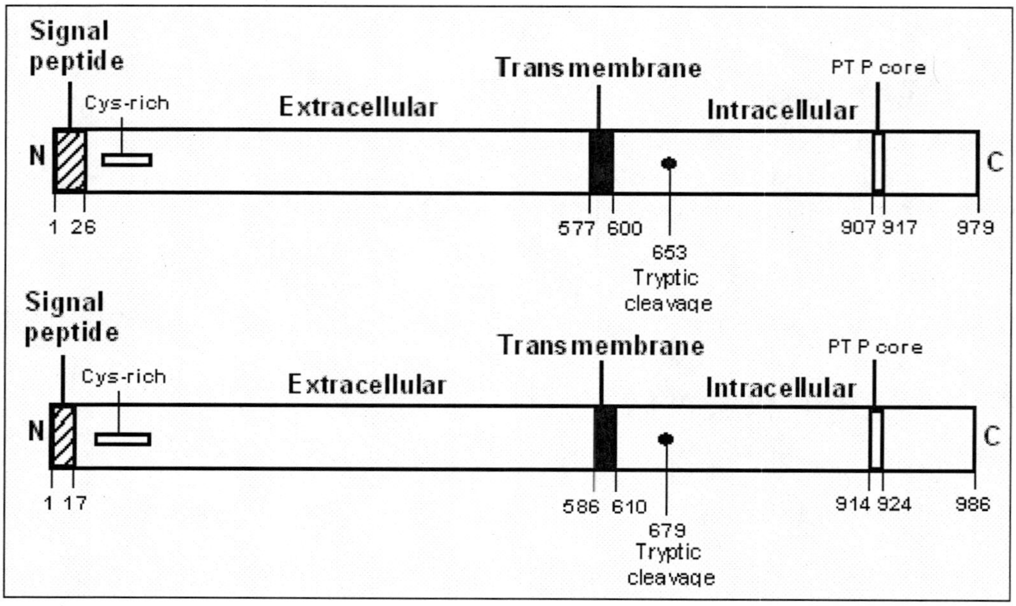

Figure 7. Structural organization of IA-2 and IA-2β antigens. IA-2/ICA512 and IA-2β islet antigens are members of the protein tyrosine kinase (PTP) family. IA-2 molecule comprises 979 amino acid residues, whereas IA-2b consists of 986 amino acids. Both antigens have a very similar structure, consisting of the extracellular, transmembrane and intracellular domains. Both molecules show high sequence homology (74%) within the intracellular domain, but only 27% identity within the extracellular domain. In the extracellular domain, a cysteine-rich segment follows a signal peptide. The intracellular domain includes juxtamembrane and PTP-like regions. Tryptic cleavage of IA-2 generates a 40 kD fragment, which represents a N-terminal portion of the intracellular domain (residues 653-979) and is responsible for antigenic properties of IA-2 and binding IA-2 –specific autoantibodies from diabetic sera. For IA-2β, digestion with trypsin releases an antigenic 37 kD product, binding diabetes-related antibodies.

IA-2 has been proposed to play a role in trafficking of secretory granules through the formation of complex with β2-syntrophin and utrophin that anchors the granules to the skeleton [375]. In INS-1 culture cells, incorporation of IA-2 into the cell membrane leads to a Ca^{2+}-dependent proteolysis of the intracellular domain of human IA-2 by by μ-calpain, releasing a fragment that translocates into the nucleus and promotes expression of the insulin gene [376]. Recent experiments of Harashima et al. [377] also confirmed an important role of IA-2 in the regulation of insulin secretion. The overexpression of IA-2 in insulin-producing MIN-6 cells resulted in a 6-fold increase in glucose- or K+-induced insulin secretion and an approximately 3-fold increase in the number of secretory vesicles and the insulin content of cells. In addition, Hu et al. showed [378] the interaction between the IA-2 molecule and numerous proteins, which form so-called IA-2 interactome that currently includes 12 proteins and is responsible for regulation of insulin secretion.

Antibodies to IA-2 are detected in the majority of the newly diagnosed T1D patients with frequency, ranging from 60 to 80% [362, 379, 380]. These antibodies are also detectable in healthy non-diabetic individuals, with frequency of less than 2% [369]. The occurrence of IA-2 antibodies varies with age, being more common in the younger population and in patients with the HLA-DQA1*0301-DQB1*0302 genotype than in diabetic patients without that genotype [380, 381]. Studies in Finnish diabetic patients also showed increased levels of AA-2 antibodies in children with newly diagnosed diabetes, carrying the DR4-DQB1*0302 high T1D risk haplotype [183,352]. In Germany, subjects with IA-2 antibodies revealed an increased frequency of the diabetes-associated HLA-DQB1 alleles *0302 and/or *02 [382].

Trypsin cleavage of the recombinant IA-2 molecule and competition studies showed that IA-2 is a precursor of the 40 kD trypic fragment, which itself represents an autoantigen, binding to IA-2 antibodies [383]. Further investigations found that antibodies from diabetic sera react exclusively with the intracellular, not extracellular domain of IA-2 [384]. The autoantibody reactivity in new-onset T1D sera is directed against at least four cytoplasmic epitopes of IA-2 [384]. Two were mapped to the juxtamembrane domain and additional two in the protein phosphatase-like domain (amino acids 777-937 and 687-979). In the juxtamembrane domain, fine mapping revealed contiguous to each other IA-2-specific epitopes JM1 (residues 611-620) and JM2 (residues 621-630) [385]. JM1 and JM2 were recognized by sera from 67% of patients with IA-2 antibodies. Antibodies to JM2, but not to JM1, were associated with HLA-DR4 in German and British Caucasian patients with T1D and found in first-degree relatives with the DR4/3, DR4/13 and DR4/1 genotypes [385]. In Japanese, only 8% sera of patients positive for IA-2 antibodies recognized the juxtamembrane region, 64% bound the protein tyrosine phosphatase-like domain of IA-2 only, and 29% bound both [386]. Autoantibodies specific to the phospatase-like domain were significantly associated with HLA-DR4, while the additional reactivity to the juxtamembrane domain of IA-2 was associated with HLA-DR9 allele in Japanese T1D subjects.

In German BABY-DIAB study, a unique role of autoantibodies, binding to the juxtamembrane domain of IA-2, was demonstrated [387]. This study revealed the juxtamembrane region of IA-2 is an early IA-2 autoantibody target, and suggested that antibodies specific to this domain are a risk factor for development of type 1 diabetes in infancy. The finding was confirmed by observations in diabetic children derived from the "Childhood Diabetes in Finland" (DiMe) Study. In this study, Hoppu and coauthors [388] also showed that the juxtamembrane domain-reactive IA-2 antibodies are associated with an increased risk of progression to overt T1D.

Park et al. [389] studied a possible role of alternative splicing of IA-2 mRNA in humoral autoreactivity to the molecule. Park and coauthors [389] observed an increased humoral immune reactivity against the full-length IA-2 isoform than against the IA-2 isoform, lacking exon 13, in all categories of patients tested (prediabetic, new-onset and long-term diabetes). Exon 13 encodes the transmembrane and juxtamembrane domains that comprise several type 1 diabetes target epitopes. Pancreatic islets were shown to express a full-length mRNA and two alternatively spliced transcripts, whereas thymus and spleen exclusively express an alternatively spliced IA-2 transcript, lacking exon 13 [390]. This supports a concept that tolerance to IA-2 epitopes not expressed in lymphoid organs may not be achieved. An interesting hypothesis, suggesting for the permissive role of differential splicing as a regulatory mechanism of gene expression in the development of autoimmune responses to IA-2, was proposed, but it has to be experimentally evaluated.

Actually, the majority of T1D sera (83%) reacted with the IA-2 phosphatase-like domain, while 39% only react with both (phosphatase-like and juxtamembrane) regions [391]. Analysis of seven other members of the protein tyrosine phosphatase family found no reactivity of these proteins with diabetic sera [392]. In contrast to the IA-2 intracellular domain resistant to trypsin treatment, the intracellular domains of these phosphatases were completely susceptible to the digestion with trypsin [391]. Sequence analysis revealed five cysteine residues within the intracellular domain of IA-2 that are not present in the other tyrosine phosphatases. Chemical modification of the cystein residues of the IA-2 molecule resulted in loss of both resistanse to tryptic digestion and reactivity with diabetic antibodies [391]. These observations argue that disulfide bond fonmation is crucial for the maitenance of antigenic structure and that the IA-2 antibodies recognize primarily conformational epitopes.

Using chimeric constructs between IA-2 and IA-2β antigens, IA-2 residues 795-889 were shown to be important for IA-2-specific antibody binding in the tyrosine phosphatase-like domain [393]. Analysis of monoclonal IA-2 specific IgG antibodies isolated from sera of patients, most of whom had been recently diagnosed for T1D, showed that these antibodies required the entire phosphatase-like domain of IA-2 for binding, but critical amino acids clustered in the N-terminal region 687-777 [394]. Nucleotide sequence analysis of one of these antibodies revealed that it used a V_H germline gene (DP-71) preferably expressed in autoantibodies associated with T1D. The presence of somatic mutations in both heavy and light chain genes and the high affinity or this antibody suggested that the immune response to IA-2 is antigen-driven [394].

The dominant T cell epitope was found at positions 805-820 of the IA-2 molecule [395]. Interestingly, this epitope showed 56% identity and 100% similarity over 9 amino acids with a sequence in VP7, a major immunogenic protein of human rotavirus. Both peptides (human IA-2 and viral) bound to HLA-DR4*0401 and are deduced to present identical amino acid residues to the TCR. The contiguous sequence of VP7 exhibited 75% identity and 92% similarity over 12 residues with a known T-cell epitope in GAD65, another autoantigen in T1D [395]. These findings suggest for a putative mechanism of T-cell activation and induction of β-cell autoimmunity by rotavirus and possibly other viruses, through molecular mimicry with IA-2 and (for rotavirus) GAD.

Harkonen et al. [87,396] identified sequence similarities between immunogenic epitopes in the enterovirus capsid protein VP1 and procapsid protein VP0 and diabetes-associated epitopes in tyrosine phosphatase IA-2. For example, the N-terminal conservative motif of 12 amino acids (residues 21-32) in the VP1 protein of coxsackievirus 9 showed a 5-amino acid sequence identity, followed by 5-amino acid sequence similarity with the C-terminal peptide 961-972 of IA-2 [396]. Several diabetes-linked epitopes in IA-2 were also recognized by CBV-4-induced antisera. Immunization of female NOD mice with formalin-inactivated purified strain of coxsackievirus B4 (CBV-4-E2) induced an increased humoral immune response to β-cell antigens, including the IA-2 diabetogenic peptide, but delayed the onset of spontaneos diabetes presumably through changing the autoantigen-specific Th1/Th2 balance [397]. Additional studies are definitely required to clarify whether the similarity between human IA-2 and viral epitopes could promote the induction of diabetes in patients affected with enteroviral infection.

IA-2β Antibodies

Using degenerated primers, Lu et al. [398] isolated cDNA for a new transmembrane protein tyrosine phosphatase from mouse insulinoma and glucagonoma cell lines. A novel protein phosphatase, designated IA-2β and also referred to as phogrin, showed a high similarity with IA-2 [399]. Human homolog of mouse IA-2β was then isolated [400]. Human IA-2β cDNA has a length of 3853 bp and encodes two isoforms of the molecule: a long version of 986 amino acids (Figure 7) and a short version of 969 amino acids. The short isoform lacks 17 amino acid residues between the positions 38 and 54 of the long isoform. IA-2β showed the expression of two transcripts differed in their size (4.0 and 5.0 kb) probably due to the alternatively splicing mechanism [401]. Similarly to IA-2, IA-2β is primarily expressed in pancreatic islets, pituitary gland and brain [400].

IA-2β is located in secretory granules in islets and other neuroendocrine tissues. Despite having tyrosine phosphatase-like structure, both IA-2 and phogrin fail to dephosphorylate artificial substrates as a result of substitution of key amino acid residues in the catalytic center [401]. IA-2 and phogrin are synthesized as precursors of over 100 kD that are cleaved within the granule lumenal domain to generate mature proteins of approximately 66 kD [402]. Like IA-2, phogrin is a subject to further post-translational modifications, including glycosylation and phosphorylation. Phogrin is phosphorylated in intact β cells on stimulation of insulin secretion, suggesting that the protein is a target for secretagogue-activated protein kinases [403]. Whereas IA-2 is regulated by locally secreted insulin, which stimulates its biosynthesis, as well as by glucose and elevated cAMP at the mRNA level, phogrin expression is insensitive to factors that modify β-cell function [404]. In contrast to IA-2, administration of ghrelin, a recently discovered peptide ligand for endogenous ligand for growth hormone secretagogue receptor, stimulated expression of IA-2β and inhibited glucose-stimulated insulin secretion in MIN6 insulinoma cells, therefore suggesting for opposite effects of IA-2 and IA-2β onto the insulin release by pancreatic islets [405].

Structural organization of the IA-2β molecule is very similar to that of IA-2 (Figure 7). The intracellular domain of IA-2β is highly conserved (over 92%) in human, mouse and rat, while the extracellular domain shows only 50-60% identity between the human sequence and the murine and rat sequences. Comparison of human IA-2 and IA-2β revealed 74% similarity within the extracellular domain, but only 27% homology within the extracellular domain [400].

A limited trypsinolysis cleaves the IA-2β molecule at position 679 resolves a 37 kD fragment, a major islet autoantigen for diabetes-related autoantibodies (Figure 7) [406]. Approximately 30-50% of patients with new-onset diabetes have autoantibodies against IA-2β [398]. Specificity of IA-2β antibodies is high and exceeds 99%. 95% of the T1D sera that react with IA-2β also react with IA-2, but only 50-80% of the diabetic sera that react with IA-2 also react with IA-2β [407]. Similarly to IA-2 antibodies, IA-2β antibodies occur more frequently in children than in adults [380] and are associated with HLA-DRB*04 alleles [408,409].

IA-2β-specific CD4+ T cells generated from NOD mice could destroy islet cell transplants and initiate diabetes in a disease recurrence model [410]. Mapping T-cell reactivity to the phogrin cytosolic domain revealed two distinct peptide epitopes designated peptide 2 (amino acids 640-659) and peptide 7 (amino acids 755-776) [411]. Both epitopes are highly conserved in human, rat and mouse and targeted by multiple diabetogenic autoreactive T-cell clones [412]. Transgenic NOD mice, expressing a susceptibility allele HLA-DQ8 as a sole class II molecule, developed a robust T cell-proliferative response when immunized with peptides 2 and 7 [412]. These results underline the potential role of the HLA-DQ8 molecule in immunogenic presentation of processed phogrin peptides, although not solely restricted to it. Since disease-related T cell-proliferative responces to peptides 2 and 7 were observed in a group of prediabetic patients and included both HLA-DQ8- and HLA-DR-restricted reactivity, at least one HLA-DR molecule in addition to HLA-DQ8 should participate in the immune recognition of these peptides. The involvement of the HLA-DR molecule into the immune presentation of the peptide 7 of IA-2β was confirmed by blocking studies with monomorphic murine autoantibodies [412]. The experiments in HLA-DQ8-transgenic NOD mice indicated that common phogrin peptides are targeted by self-reactive T lymphocytes in human and murine T1D, and that the responces may in part be associated with the similar peptide-binding specificities of human HLA-DQ8 and its ortholog I-A^{g7} in the NOD mice.

Minor Ilset Cell-Related Antigens

CD38

Antibodies against type II transmembrane glycoprotein CD38 (ADP-ribosyl cyclase/cyclic ADP-ribose hydrolase) are reported to occur in 3-5% of individuals with newly diagnosed disease and in 15-20% of long-term T1D patients [413,414]. Anti-CD38 autoantibodies are also detected in type 2 diabetic patients [415,416]. CD38 mediates Ca^{2+} release in the target cells, including pancreatic islets, and inhibits insulin secretion by β cells, since CD38-specific autoantibodies showed an agonistic activity associated with raising intracellular Ca^{2+} and insulin release by Langerhans' islets [417]. The significance of CD38 self-antibodies as an immune marker for diabetes remains to be further evaluated, but increased frequency of these antibodies in patients with long-standing disease could be useful as a marker of latent diabetes (LADA) as well as in the identification of subgroups of diabetic individuals with higher residual β-cell function [414,418].

ICA69

A novel pancreatic islet cell autoantigen of 69 kD designated ICA69 was detected by screening a human islet cDNA expression library with cytoplasmic islet cell antibody positive sera from relatives of patients with overt T1D [419]. The predicted protein sequence of ICA69 consisted of 482 amino acid residues with some homology to BSA, a possible dietary trigger of autoimmune diabetes [107,419]. However, the cross-reactivity between antibodies to BSA and ICA69 initially reported by Martin et al. [107] was not further confirmed [420].

ICA69 is not β-cell specific antigen, because its expression is found in a variety of other tissues, including brain, heart, thyroid, stomach mucosa and kidney [419]. In the human pancreas, a preferential expression of ICA-69 was found in insulin-produced cells compared to the exocrine pancreas [421]. Experiments with ric-19, a homologue of ICA69 in Caenorhabditis elegans, revealed its expression in neurons and specialized secretory cells, suggesting on the evolutionary conservation of this protein participated in the process of neuroendocrine secretion via association with certain secretory vesicles [422]. Cytological observations in mouse brain showed that most of the ICA69 pool is cytosolic and soluble and a membrane-bound ICA69 subpopulation is coenriched with synaptic vesicles. In murine pancreatic islets, ICA69 localizes in a punctate manner distinct from the insulin granules, suggesting an association with the synaptic-like microvesicles found in these cells [422]. The N-terminal region of ICA69 was shown to exhibit significant similarity to the region of arfaptins that interacts with ARF1, a small GTPase involved in vesicle budding at the Golgi complex and immature secretory granules. In insulinoma INS-1 cells, displaing a neuroendocrine phenotype, ICA69 is associated with the Golgi complex. This therefore characterizes ICA69 as an arfaptin-related protein that is likely to play a role in membrane trafficking at the Golgi complex and immature secretory granules in neurosecretory cells [423]. An exact function of ICA69 is still unknown and requires additional investigations.

Two alternative core promoters, regulating a tissue-specific transcription of ICA-69, have been found at the 5'regulatory region of the ICA69 gene. One of those is more active in the islet cell line, while a second promoter more efficiently activates transcription in neuronal cells [424]. The expression of ICA69 is likely to be under control of cAMP-responsive element-binding protein (CREB), because mutation within the CREB-binding site at the second promoter of ICA69 significantly inhanced transcriprional activity in both cell lines [424]. Reduced levels of the ICA69 expression were observed in the thymus of NOD mice compared to control B6 mice that may be of importance in regulating self-tolerance in T1D [425].

Antibodies to ICA69 are detected in prediabetic individuals and in 4-20% of patients with recent-onset diabetes [310,419]. These antibodies are independent of other islet antibodies, such as ICA and IAA. However, only 1-5% of newly diagnosed T1D patients immunoprecipitated in vitro translated ICA69 [310,426]. In addition, ICA69 antibodies could be frequently found in 30-40% of patients with other autoimmune disorders, such as rheumatoid arthrithis and Sjogren's syndrome [427,428]. The utility of ICA69 as a humoral marker for T1D is therefore controversial. The Ica-1 gene, an ortholog of human ICA69, was mapped in NOD mice, and Ica1 cDNA was isolated and characterized [429]. Both rodent and murine orthologs of human ICA69 contain an immunodominant T-cell epitope designated Ter69 and recognized by autoreactive T cells from T1D patients. In human ICA69, this epitope localized to amino acids 36-67 [430]. Injection with Ter69 peptide induced an immunodominant T cell-mediated response in the NOD mouse [430]. The ICA69-knockout NOD mouse had no obvious phenotype and developed diabetes like a wild-type NOD mose, suggesting that ICA69 is a facultative, non-obligate self-antigen in diabetes [431].

In humans, an inverse correlation between T-cell and autoantibody reactivity to ICA69 was observed [432]. The increased T cell reactivity to ICA69 in the absence of antibody reactivity at onset of T1D was shown to be associated with the susceptible HLA-DR3 allele, suggesting for a genetically controlled selective activation of T helper subsets to a specific autoantigen in diabetic patients. Analysis of overlapping 20-mer peptides, covering the entire ICA69 molecule, revealed that ICA69 peptides displayed relatively higher binding affinities for HLA-DR molecules neutral (HLA-DR1) or protective to T1D (HLA–DR2) compared with the predisposing HLA-DR3 and –DR4 molecules [433]. ICA69 peptide (amino acids 36-47) that is represented a part of the immunodominant Ter69 epitope and is recognized by T cells from T1D patients [434] demonstrated strong binding properties to HLA-DR1 and –DR2, but not to the susceptible DR3 and DR4 molecules. These findings imply that high-affinity binding of self-peptide triggers T-cell anergy, whereas low-affinity binding by diabetogenic DR3 and DR4 molecules triggers proliferative expansion of autoreactive T cells.

Imogen 38

Arden et al. [435] reported the isolation of a 1,267-bp long cDNA, encoding islet mitochondrial antigen 38 (imogen 38), which caused proliferative response of a human diabetic T-cell clone to a recombinant antigen epitope library. The predictive amino acid sequence of imogen 38 contains 365 amino acids. The antigen precursor is synthesized as a 44-kD protein, which then undergoes proteolytic cleavage to be converted into the 38-kD mature protein with removing of the 54-amino acid N-terminal mitochondrial targeting sequence. In the imogen 38 molecule, amino acids 55-70 represent T-cell binding site [436]. The function of imogen 38 is unknown. Since imogen 38 is widely distributed in many tissues, this mitochondrial protein is rather a target for bystander autoimmune attack than a primary autoantigen [435]. Further studies are needed to characterize a role of this mitochondrial antigen in β –cell mediated autoimmunity and diabetes.

Carboxypeptidase H

As a prediabetic autoantigen, carboxypeptidase H (CPH) was identified after screening a recombinant antigen epitope library from rat islets with serum from a prediabetic patient [437]. This enzyme is expressed in islet and neuroendocrine cells [437,438]. Carboxypeptidase H removes C-terminal basic amino acids from insulin and many other peptide hormone intermediates in endocrine and neural tissues. The enzyme is synthesized as a 56-kD precursor that is rapidly processed into a mature 54-kD form [438]. In human, the sequences of human brain and islet CPH cDNA are identical, except for the absence of a second ATG in the predicted 5'non-coding region of the brain cDNA [439]. In the insulin-producing β-cells, CPH is colocalized with insulin on the cell surface [440].

11% of Italian patients with newly diagnosed T1D were reported to have self-antibodies to CPH, but no diabetic sera strongly precipitated in vitro translated carboxypeptidase H [310]. In addition, comparative analysis of Chinese T1D patients and healthy controls revealed no differences in prevalence of CPH autoantibodies [441]. This antigen has not been subjected to autoantibody standartization.

Heat Shock Proteins

Antibodies against heat shock proteins (HSPs) are occurred in several autoimmune diseases, including diabetes, rheumatoid arthritis and autoimmune thyroid disease [442]. HSP includes a family of ubiquitous proteins expressed at stress conditions in response to oxidative stress, increased temperature, toxic chemicals and other harmful influences. Antibodies against a variety of HSPs, including those to HSP60, HSP65, HSP70 and HSP90, are occured in 5-20% of T1D patients [443-448]. Except for T1D, HSP-autoantibodies could be detected in subjects affected with type 2 diabetes and different autoimmune disorders, such as autoimmune thyroid disease, multiple sclerosis and rheumatoid arthritis [449,450]. For HSP60, high titres of antibodies against two epitopes (amino acids 393-413 and 435-454) have been detected in T1D patients [446]. The HSP60 epitope 394-413 shares significant identity with the antigenic epitope of GAD65, an established islet self-antigen, whereas the epitope 435-454 is similar to the immunogenic peptide p277 of Mycobacterium bovis, a tuberculosis pathogen. Additionally, a homology between an immunogenic determinant of human HSP60 (residues 443-459) and two regions of enteroviral capsid proteins VP1 and VP0 is reported [451]. A cross-reactivity between antibodies against the enteroviral antigens and recombinant hybrid protein HSP60/65 was shown, suggesting for a possible involvement of enteroviruses, particularly CBV, into the induction of β-cell autoimmunity through cross-reacting immune responses to viral and self-antigens, including HSP expressed in the islet cells [451]. However, studies on NOD mice infected with pathogenic strain CVB3/M, causing severe pancreatitis, did not support the hypothesis that CVB are causative agents of T1D. To the contrary, CVB infections provide significant protection from T1D onset in NOD mice [452]. The diabetogenicity of HSP self-antigens is needed to be be further elucidated. Compared to islet-specific antigens, such as insulin, IA-2, IA-2β and GAD-65, HSPs seem to play a secondary role in inducing T1D due to the ubiquitous distribution of these proteins in the body.

Glima 38

In 1996, a new islet-specific antigen named 38-kD glycated islet cell membrane-associated protein (glima 38) was isolated and characterized [453]. This antigen is specifically expressed in islet and neuroendocrine cells. Glima 38 represents an amphiphilic membrane glycoprotein, whose N-terminus is heavily enriched with carbohydrates (up to 40% of the molecular weight). The autoreactive epitopes in glima 38 recognized by T1D sera were shown to be conformational and independent of the carbohydrate moiety [454]. Antibodies to this antigen were reported to occur in 14-35% of prediabetic patients and 19-38% patients with recent-onset T1D [453, 455]. Glima antibodies were strongly associated with type 1 diabetes and antibody markers of rapid progression to clinical onset but have a lower diagnostic sensitivity for the disease than IAA, ICA, GADA or IA-2 antibodies [455].

Nuclear Antigens

Diabetes-related antibodies against nucleoproteins are identified in T1D patients. There are self-antibodies to the early-response nuclear transcription factor jun-B (38 kD) [456] and DNA topoisomerase II [457]. In topoisomerase II, epitopes recognized by IDDM sera resided mostly in three distinct domains. One resided in amino acid residues 1-147, another in amino acid residues 286-472, and the third in the COOH-terminal one-third of the molecule. These epitopes shared similarity (up to 36% identity and 63.6% homology) to previously identified epitopes of IDDM autoantigens [457]. In Taiwanese T1D patients, antibodies against topoisomerase II occurred in at prevalence of over 50% that even exceeds the frequency of GADA (40-50%) and IA-2 self-antibodies (24%) [457-459]. Due to the higher frequency, topoisomerase II antibodies were suggested to be useful for prediction of T1D in Taiwanese population.

AUTOANTIBODIES AS PREDICTORS OF T1D

The predictive value of self-antibodies for T1D is varied in different populations and strongly depends on the prevalence of antibodies in prediabetic patients and sensitivity of antibody-detecting assays. The current prediction of T1D is mainly based on the detection of antibodies to four major islet autoantigens, such as GAD65, insulin, IA-2/ICA512 and IA-2β [460]. Various minor islet-cell related antigens have been also identified but were enable to contribute significantly to the prediction of disease in addition to the major antibodies. The presense of major autoantibodies in prediabetic stage allows the identification of subjects at risk of T1D, and this risk can be stratisfied according to the titers of specific antibodies, the presense of multiple antibodies and association with certain HLA genotypes [460, 461].

Predictive values of prediabetic immune changes will be different in twin, family and population studies. In familial and non-familial T1D, genetic and immune markers of susceptibility may prove to have a different significance within families as compared to the general population. Since only 8-10% of all cases of type 1 diabetes have a familial history and the remaining 90% of cases occur sporadically, it is therefore important to examine the prevalence of islet-cell antibodies in the general population [462].

For example, a prevalence of major islet-cell antibodies in general population varies from 0.4 to 5%. In first-degree relatives of a diabetic patient, these antibodies are usually 5-20 times more frequent than in general population [463].

In identical twins, all major islet-cell antibodies show the highest specificity, sensitivity and positive predictive value for developing diabetes. For instance, a predictive value of IA-2 self-antibodies is greater than 90% in identical twins [381] and varies between 25 and 80% in first-degree relatives [362, 464,465]. However, the best predictive marker for the development of T1D is turning out to be not the presense of single autoantibody, but the presense of two or more autoantibodies. In first-degree relatives, a combination of any two major antibodies provides a predictive value, ranging from 37% up to 100%, whereas a combined predictive value for three presenting self-antibodies is 55-100%

[362,460,465,466]. Usually, the presense of any three of four major antibodies is enough to predict T1D with probability close to 100%.

Titers of self-antibodies also influence their predictive values. For example, low levels of ICA (10-19 JDF units) provided a predictive value of 34% for identifying first-degree relatives and normal children, who develop T1D within the next 5 years, whereas the presence of these antibodies at high titres (over 80 JDF units) increased this value up to 63% [460]. Positivity for GADA in Japanese patients yielded an overall predictive value of 34% for insulin requirement, which rose to 75% in the presense of high-titer GADA (> 10 units), and to 100% when GADA were present in combination with IAA [467].

Due to the common prevalence in T1D and high sensitivity and reproducibility of the detection assay, ICA antibodies have been chosen to screen 84,821 eligible subjects recruited in 1998-2000 for Diabetes Prevention Trial-Type 1 (DPT-1). The DPT-1 screened first- and second-degree relatives of a person with T1D (defined as onset of diabetes before age 40 years and on insulin therapy within 1 year of diagnosis). Potential subjects were screened for the presense of ICA titers greater than or equal to 10 JDF units). Subjects, who had normal production of endogenous insulin, but exhibited two autoantibodies (ICA and IAA), were considered at moderate risk of developing diabetes (25-50% over 5 years). These subjects were eligible for the oral test. Subjects were randomly assigned to receive either oral insulin or a placebo in a blinded fashion. Subjects in both the parenteral and oral arms of the study were monitored for the development of diabetes at frequent intervals. Of 84,821 individuals, a total of 293 subjects have been selected for the oral study and 339 subjects have been randomized into the parenteral study.

The DPT-1 provides one of the largest natural history studies of T1D, with evaluation of genetic and immunologic risk factors and of islet cell function. Because half of the study subjects did not receive active treatment, the data obtained from these patients should significantly improve diabetes prediction. One of the interesting subgroups defined by the DPT are those with the protective HLA allele (DQA1*0102, DQB1*0602 referred to as DQB1*0602), which is thought to confer protection from the onset of diabetes. Understanding of protective function of this allele may lead to future therapies in preventing T1D. 7.3% of 1,376 ICA-positive subjects are reported to have a protective HLA allele, and there was a higher frequency of HLA-DQ1*0102 and DQB1*0602 in blacks (4.4 times more frequent compared to Caucasians) [468]. When compared with ICA-positive DQB1*0602-negative subjects, DQB1*0602-positive individuals had lower titers of ICA (40 vs. 80 JDF units), a lower incidence of IAA (20% vs. 47%), fewer had additional self-antibodies (7% vs. 23%), and fewer had a low insulin production (13% vs. 28%). However, 2% of patients with the protective HLA genotype developed diabetes with a mean follow-up of 2 years, demonstrating that protection from of the allele is relative and not absolute.

One of the goals of the DPT was to define a group at high risk of developing diabetes. After an individual is found to be ICA-positive, it may take several months to complete the testing necessary for staging and to confirm a normal oral glucose tolerance test (OGTT). In this interval, 11% of ICA-positive relatives have developed T1D [469]. 42% developed clinical symptoms of diabetes, and 58% had hyperglycemia during staging. Almost a half of the hypeglycemic group had a normal fasting glucose, but an elevated 2-hour glucose (over 200 mg/dL) on their OGTT, but had no clinical symptoms of diabetes. This state of 'silent' diabetes may last for up to 2 years to onset of clinical disease [470], but is not associated with insulin resistance [471].

The DPT-1 has also confirmed the predictive value of insulin production. Measuring insulin production in ICA-positive 1,622 patients revealed lower insulin production rates in subjects with an impaired or diabetic OGTT, in subjects, who had multiple antibodies, and in subjects with higher titers of IAA and ICA, confirming that low insulin production rate strongly correlates with risk factors of developing T1D [472].

The DPT-1 trial demonstrates the larger number of individuals at high risk of T1D required to directly test the efficacy of any intervention with sufficient statistical power. Intensive and expensive efforts are required to identify and recruit these high-risk subjects. The DPT-1 is a good example that showed a successful usage of the ICA assay in combination with other approaches to identify those patients. The additional approaches that have a significant predictive value included the genetic analysis (i.e. HLA genotyping) and metabolic control assays (OGTT and FRIP - first phase insulin release) that strengthened the prediction of T1D. Future studies may not rely on the classical immunofluorescent ICA detection, but will likely to use antibodies to biochemical markers, such as GAD65, IA-2/ICA512 and insulin. Among the ilset-related antibodies, IAA appear to be the most suitable candidate for more stringent prediction of diabetes. IAA are the only self-antibodies so far identified that bind an antigen specific to the β cell, and are the first to appear during the prediabetic phase [463, 473].

Pathogenic Events in Prediabetic and Early Diabetic Stages

Role of Macrophages and B Cells

The major population of cells, infiltrating the islets during the early stage of insulitis in BB rats and NOD mice are macrophages and dendritic cells [474]. These cells appear in the islets before the infiltration by T lymphocytes, NKT cells and B cells. During the destruction of Langerhans' insulin-producing cells, macrophages are shown to cooperate and collaborate with T lymphocytes [474]. Macrophages are necessary for the development and activation of cytotoxic effector T cells, participating in the depletion of β-cell population. This resulted from the studies in the macrophage-depleted NOD mouse, in which T cells were unable to destroy NOD islet transplants [475]. The depletion of macrophages shifts the immune balance towards Th2-type of immune response due to the decreased expression of the macrophage-derived cytokine IL-12 and causes the reduction in production of β-cell destructing molecules, such as Fas ligand, CD40 ligand and perforin [475]. Since these molecules produced by cytotoxic CD8+ T cells, macrophages have therefore an essential role for the activation of this T-cell population that leads to the induction of diabetes in NOD mice [476]. In addition, macrophages may assist in maximizing the activation of β cell-specific CD8+ T cells through the secretion of IL-12, which induces proliferation of Th1-type CD4+ T lymphocytes, and subsequently, IL-12 and IFN-γ produced by the activated CD4+ T cells stimulate cytotoxic CD8+ T cells.

Macrophages could directly contribute to the destruction of β cells via releasing free oxygen radicals (superoxide anion radical and hydrogen peroxide) and cytokines (IL-1β, TNF-α and IFN-γ) (Figure 8) [477]. Free oxygen radicals itself are especially toxic for β cells because of the low content of free oxygen radical-scavenging enzymes in the islets. Macrophage-derived cytokines may contribute to β-cell damage by inducing the production of free oxygen radicals in the islets [478].

In NOD mice, a primary role of B lymphocytes is to present islet self-antigens on early stages of T1D. B cell-mediated production of self-antibodies is secondary phenomenon in β-cell depletion [479]. T cells from diabetic NOD mice transfer diabetes to neonatal recipients in the absence of B lymphocytes, indicating that B cells are not needed in the destruction of islet cells when diabetogenic effector T cells are generated [480]. In NOD BCIID mice, containing I-A^{g7}-deficient B cells, non-B cells (macrophages and dendritic cells) have normal expression of the diabetogenic I-A^{g7} molecule and are capable to activate autoantigen-reactive T cells [481]. However, NOD BCIID mice were resistant to the development of autoimmune diabetes. These mice showed non-invasive peri-insulitis that could be intentionally converted into a destructive process upon treatment with cyclophosphamide. This observation suggests that I-A^{g7}–mediated β-cell self-antigen presentation by β cells is crucial in overcoming a checkpoint in T-cell tolerance to pancreatic islet cells after their initial targeting has occurred [481].

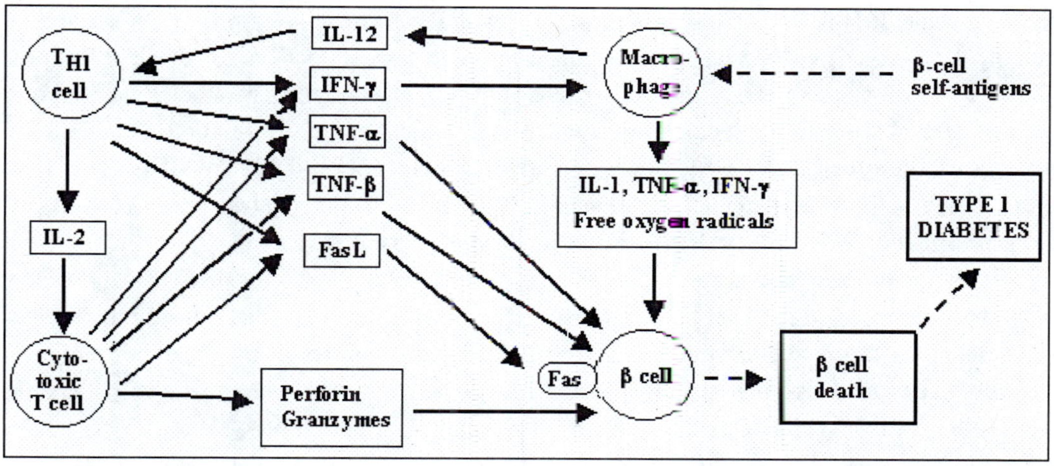

Figure 8. Cooperation between macrophages and T lymphocytes in the depletion of ilset β cells. Macrophages process β-cell self-antigens and present them to T helper (Th1) cells in conjunction with MHC class II molecules. In addition, macrophages secrete IL-12, which stimulates Th1 cells. Activated Th1 cells produce a variety of cytokines, including IFN-γ, IL-2, TNF-α and TNF-β. IL-2 stimulates differentiation and proliferation of cytotoxic T cells. These cells release large amounts of β-cell-toxic cytokines (IFN-γ, TNF-α and TNF-β) and molecules (perforin and granzymes), causing the destruction and lysis of islet cells. T lymphocytes may also induce β cell apoptosis through the secreion of Fas ligand (FasL) and induction of the expression of Fas on pancreatic β cells. Macrophages additionally release free oxygen radicals, to which β cells are highly sensitive.

Role of Autoreactive Effector T Cells

Since T1D is a T cell-mediated autoimmune disorder, self-reactive T lymphocytes play a primary role in diabetic pathogenesis. Significance of T cells in inducing autoimmune diabetes was established from early studies in animal models. BB rats treated with monoclonal antibodies against the antigens expressed on the surface of all T cells did not develop diabetes [482]. Neonatally thymectomized BB rats, NOD and NOD.Scid mice were also unable to develop spontaneous disease [483,484]. Transfer of NOD splenic cells into NOD mice showed that both CD4+ and CD8+ T lymphocytes are needed for the induction of diabetes in the recipients [485]. Islet-specific autoreactive T cell clones have been isolated from both diabetic and prediabetic NOD mice. Some CD4+ β-cell-specific T cell clones accelerate the development of diabetes in young NOD mice and destroy islet transplants in CD8+ T cell-depleted diabetes-resistant mice [486].

In addition to the involvement of CD4+ T helper cells in islet-cell destruction, CD8+ T lymphocytes also contribute into the depletion of pancreatic islets in the NOD mouse and play a role of effector cells. Some CD8+ cytotoxic T cell clones need help of CD4+ T cells to destroy islet grafts [487], some CD8+ T cell clones are able to destruct β cells without the help of CD4+ T lymphocytes [488]. All CD4+ T cell clones derived from the islets of NOD mice were restricted to the MHC class II I-A^{g7} allele. These clones showed a proliferative response to both islet cells and spleen cells from NOD mice only, but not from any other tested murine strains, indicating that these clones are I-A^{g7}-reactive clones (autoreactive T cells) [487]. None of these CD4+ clones had any cytotoxic effect on NOD islets in vitro. CD8+ T cell clones also exhibit no cytotoxicity to NOD islets in vitro. Monoclonal antinbody against MHC class I D^b molecule almost completely blocked the proliferation and cytotoxic activity of some of these CD8+ clones, whereas monoclonal antibody to MHC class I K^d blocked the activity of other CD8+ clones [487]. These results suggest that CD8+ T cell clones respond to islet cells with the restriction to MHC class I.

Cytological observations revealed different patterns of the behavior of CD4+ and CD8+ cells when attached to the islet cells. Islet-specific CD4+ T cells attached closely to the islet cells did not destroy them, whereas CD8+ T cells demonstrate visible cytotoxic activity, showing pseudopod-like protrusions into the β cells, but not into α or σ cells of pancreatic islets [487]. CD4+ cells secrete cytokines, including IL-2 and IFN-γ, which in turn help maximally activate CD8+ cytotoxic T cells. CD8+ cells may act as final effector cells directly involved into the destruction of β cells. However, both CD4+ and CD8+ cells, secreting cytotoxic cytokines (TNF-α, TNF-β and IFN-γ) and Fas ligand, could induce death of β cells via Fas-mediated apoptosis (Figure 8). Fas-deficient NOD mice was free of diabetes and isulitis, suggesting for the involvement of FasL/Fas-mediated apoptosis in the disease pathogenesis [489].

Among CD4+ T cell clones isolated from the islets of NOD mice, an H-2^{g7}-restricted clone, NY4.1, was islet-specific, recognizing the islet antigen with unique I-A^{nod} molecule on the islet cell or the intrinsic APCs [487]. From the diabetogenic H-$2K^d$-restricted CD8+ T-cell clone, NY8.3, rearranged TCR-α- and -β genes were derived to generate TCR-transgenic NOD mice, expressing the rearranged TCR-α- and/or -β genes. The TCR-β-transgenic mouse showed a 10-fold increase in the peripheral precursor frequency of β-cell specific T cells and a selective acceleration of the recruitment of CD8+ T cells to the pancreatic islets of prediabetic NOD mice [490], while the TCR-αβ-transgenic NOD (8.3-NOD) mice showed a 400-fold increase in that [491]. These mice demonstrated an earlier onset of spontaneous autoimmune diabetes and a more rapid progression in β-cell destruction compared to nontransgenic animals. In addition, TCR-transgenic mice expressing the TCR α- and β-chains of the CD4+ T cell clone NY4.1 also showed an accelerated onset of diabetes [491].

Cytokines produced by self-reactive T cells play an important role in T1D pathogenesis. Generally, Th1 cytokines (IL-2, IFN-γ) facilitate the development of diabetes, while Th2 cytokines (IL-4, IL-10, TGF-β) prevent from that. However, the role of cytokines in the pathology of autoimmune diabetes is complex. For example, genetic absense of IFN-γ in NOD mice delays, but does not prevent the development of diabetes. Systemic treatment of NOD mice with IL-10 and IL-4 prevents T1D. Meanwhile, IL-10 locally expressed in the NOD islets accelerates the development of disease, and IL-4-deficient mice do not exhibit an early T1D onset [492]. Therefore, interactions between cytokines in the immune system are complicated, and the development of T1D may depend upon which way the finely tuned balance of cytokines is tipped.

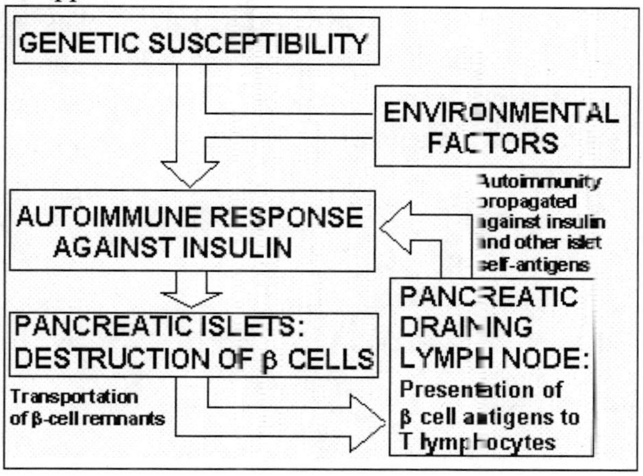

Figure 9. Induction of β-cell autoimmunity and type 1 diabetes, envolving insulin as a primary autoantigen. The interaction between genetic and environmental risk factors may result in the induction of autoimmune reactivity directed against insulin prodcuced by pancreatic islet β cells. This leads to the death of β cells in the pancreas, whose remnants are transferred into the pancreatic lymph node, where antigen-presenting cells process and display β-cell self-antigens on their surface to T cells. The immune recognition of self-antigens by T cells initiates the enchanced autoimmune attack against insulin and other ilset-specific autoantigens, causing dramatic loss in β-cell mass.

Insulin as a Trigger for Diabetes

Insulin was recently suggested to play an unique role in T1D as a primary trigger for disease [493,494]. The idea was supported by results of studies of Nakayama et al. [345] and Kent et al. [353], showing insulin as an essential autoimmune target in inducing diabetes in both mice and humans. In addition, IAA were found in the blood of NOD mice and human diabetic patients before the clinical symptoms of the disease appear [350]. Clinical diabetes starts from when 90% of insulin-secreting pancreatic islet cells are destroyed, but IAA arise from a small fraction of β-cells have been attacked, providing a useful early marker for the occurence of autoimmunity.

The β-cell targeted immune self-reactivity may occur in genetically predisposing individuals under the harmful treatment by environmental triggers, of which nutrition and infections are likely to have a major contribution on whether T1D manifests itself clinically. The debris of β cells is transferred to the pancreatic draining lymph node, where β-cell self-antigens are processed and presented by APCs to immune cells (Figure 9). Insulin serves as a primary antigen recognized by autoreactive T cells, which initiate the immune response against insulin-producing islet cells. The destruction of β cells generates new islet-specific antigenic targets for autoantibodies associated with the propagation of autoimmunity and development of diabetes [493].

Arif and colleagues [259] analyzed a repertoire of molecules, secreting by insulin-reacting T lymphocytes in diabetic and healthy individuals. They found that insulin-reacting T lymphocytes in diabetic patients have an aggressive state, producing molecules that display a harmful effect on the host β cells. Insulin-reacting T cells from healthy subjects mostly have a regulatory function, given the signaling molecules that they secrete [259]. This therefore suggests that a type of self-antigen recognized by autoreactive T cells is not only important in the induction of diabetes, but whether this recognition elecits a regulatory or a destructive state. Dysregulation of such responses might ultimately lead to autoimmune diseases, such as T1D, if lymphocytes switch from a regulatory to an aggressive state.

Chapter 6

EVIDENCE FOR THE ROLE OF GENETIC FACTORS IN THE ETIOLOGY OF TYPE 1 DIABETES FROM FAMILY AND TWIN STUDIES

FAMILY STUDIES

Evidence for a genetic susceptibility to T1D comes from family studies. The frequency of the disorder is higher in close relatives of diabetic patients than in the general population. Approximately 6% of siblings of persons with T1D also develop diabetes, whereas a prevalence of disease in the general population is only up to 0.4% [11]. The sibling risk ratio (λs), which is the ratio of the prevalence of disease in siblings to the prevalence in the general population, can be used as a quantitative measure of the genetic contribution to a disease. A λs of >5 usually indicate a significant genetic contribution to disease pathogenesis. In T1D, the value of λs is approximately 15 (6/0.4), i.e. T1D is 15 times more common in siblings of diabetic patients than in the general population. Children of T1D patients also have a higher frequency of diabetes, approximately 3–6%, compared with the 0.4% prevalence in the general population [11]. Interestingly, the gender of the diabetic parent may affect disease transmission. Offspring of T1D fathers are at much higher risk for T1D than are the offspring of T1D mothers. By 20 years of age, up to 9% of the offspring of diabetic fathers will be affected compared with only 3% of the offspring of diabetic mothers [66]. Familial clustering may be evident even before overt disease development. Islet cell antibodies, which often precede the development of T1D, are more common in first-degree relatives of patients with T1D (13-40%) than in the general population (0.4–5%) [365]. Antibody development is also influenced by the gender of the affected parent. Children of diabetic fathers are positive for autoantibodies more often than children of diabetic mothers.

TWIN STUDIES

The most powerful method of evaluating genetic predisposition to complex diseases involves twin studies. Monozygotic (MZ) twin pairs are suggested to be genetically identical, while dizygotic (DZ) twins have no more genetic similarity than other sublings. If both twins in a pair have the same disease or trait, they are said to be concordant, while a single affected twin is one of a discordant pair [495].

There are three main approaches in twin studies. Classical twin method consists in comparing concordance rates in MZ and DZ twins with population prevalence rates for a given disease. When the MZ concordance rate is significantly higher than DZ, this indicates that genetic factors are important in etiology. Approximately equal MZ and DZ concordance infers a largely environmental cause, particularly if the concordance rates are not higher than the population rate would allow by chance. In co-twin control method, MZ twins discordant for a disease are examined. The healthy co-twin provides a perfect matched-pair control. A third approach includes biometrical genetic methods to study, for example, risk factors, metabolits, behavior, physical and psychological characteristics. They may indicate an underlying liability to disease or to disease categories, if twin samples are of sufficient size [496].

Population-based twin studies refer to a national twin register cross-linked with a disease register. The advantages are that the largest possible number of twins is recruited. However, these studies are expensive, needing the resources of national registers and systematic recording of data over long periods.

Volunteer-based ascertainment is a popular but less systematic method, in which researchers scrutinize disease indices and hospital records, and adverstise through twin clubs or societies related to the disease. In general, such methods inherently biased and may lead to the overidentification of MZ and high rates of MZ concordance [497]. A more systematic approach is a prospective registration of twins through routine hospital or clinic attendance, where every patient is asked at initial registration whether he/she was born a twin, providing an unbiased sample.

Etiological clues may be derived by case studies of discordant twin pairs. Case studies of MZ twins reared apart (MZA) are of particular value, because the twins share only their genes, not a common upbringing. If series of MZA twins were found to be concordant for a disorder and more frequently than chance would dictate, then this would provide the strongest evidence of all for genetic factors in etiology. However, separated MZ twins are very rare [496].

Early twin studies in T1D were volunteer-based (Table 6). They showed a significantly higher concordance rates between MZ twins than between DZ twins, suggesting for a strong genetic contibution in T1D. However, none of these studies indicate whether concordance is measured probandwise or pairwise, making therefore the volunteer studies less conclusive.

Table 6. Volunteer twin studies in T1D

Country	Monozygotic twins			Dizygotic twins			Reference
	n	C	P	n	C	P	
USA	30	9	0.3	60	2	0.03	[498]
UK*	178	86	0.48				[499]
Japan*	11	5	0.45	10	0	0	[500]
Japan	19	9	0.47	14	1	0.08	[501]

* Like-sex study; n, sample size; C, number of concordant pairs; P, pairwise concordant rate.

Table 7. Population-based twin studies in T1D

Country	Monozygotic twins			Dizygotic twins			Reference
	n	C	CR	n	C	CR	
Sweden*	53	32	0.6 (p)	76	10	0.13 (p)	[502]
Finland*	33	3	0.231	81	2	0.048	[503]
Denmark	26	10	0.53	69	4	0.11	[504]
UK	31	11	0.35	18	1	0.06	[381]
USA*	53	12	0.23	30	0	0	[505]

In the first study [502], concordance rates are expressed pairwise; in the other four studies, probandwise.

* Like-sex study; n, sample size; C, number of concordant pairs; CR, concordance rate; p, pairwise concordant rate

Later investigations have been population-based (Table 7). A Swedish study [502] showed high MZ:DZ concordance ratio, implying significant genetic factors in T1D. This study was performed on self-reported diagnosis, a factor that might overestimate concordance. A study from Finland [503] was based on their national twin registry, except their diabetic patients are derived from hospital discharge records and the National Drug Register. Kaprio et al. [503] used the WHO guidelines for T1D diagnosis. Any ambigous cases were reviewed independently. Zygosity was determined by validated questionnaire. The concordance rate was much higher in MZ than in DZ twins, giving a correlation liability for T1D of 0.727, which favors genetic factors. Model-fitting, using the MX package gave the best fit to a simple model for type 1 diabetes with additive genetic effects and unshared environmental effects.

The Danish study [504] also used a national twin registry and collected 95 twin pairs by postal questionnaire, where one or both had disease. Kyvik and coauthors [504] used WHO criteria to classify diabetes. Most cotwins were evaluated by glucose tolerance test, and zygosity was evaluated by 11 blood and enzyme type systems. There were significantly more concordant MZ twins than DZ, giving a heritabiloity index of 0.72, which implies a strong genetic component for T1D. Kyvik et al. [504] showed the model of T1D that includes additive genetic effects, shared (i.e. family) and unshared environmental effects fitted the data best. The Danish study pointed out gene-environment interactions that may be important in T1D. This makes difficult the interpretation of hereditary estimation based on genetic modilling techniques. The authors assume the highest prevalence of T1D in Finland, which is unlikely to result from a strong environmental component, but might be due to the effect of higher penetrance.

Studies in UK showed a high correlation between the age at T1D diagnosis in concordant MZ twin pairs (n=116) [506]. In addition, the age at diagnosis significantly more closely correlated in 12 concordant MZ twins than in 12 concordant DZ twins. This shows that much of the variability of the age at diagnosis of T1D is genetically determined. The risk for T1D was higher in Finnish cotwins diagnosed at a very young age, providing the best fitting with a disease model with additive genetic and individual environmental effects and with 88% of phenotypic variance due to genetic factors and the remaining variance due to unshared environmental factors [507].

A number of twin studies have been focused on the evaluation whether β-cell autoimmunity is genetically determined. In Denmark, Petersen et al. [508] also found no significant difference in prevalence of islet antibodies between non-diabetic MZ and DZ twins, indicating that islet cell immune self-reactivity in prediabetes is environmentally rather then genetically determined. However, when discordant MZ and DZ twin pairs have been examined, a concordance rate for presence of diabetes-related antibodies was substantially higher in MZ twins, reflecting an important role of genetic factors in determining islet autoimmunity [381,505]. Gale et al. [509] discussed these conflicting findings, explaining discrepancies in the concordance rate for presence of islet self-antibodies due to the different study design (the Danish study was population-based and cross-sectional [508], while the American study was clinic-based and longitudinal [505]), differed recruitment criteria (the Danish study included all twin pairs regardless of diabetes status, whereas the American study included those, who initially was discordant for T1D and did not analyze samples drawn after the development of diabetes) and other reasons. The Danish twin cohort was reanalyzed, but still no difference in the prevalence of islet autoantibodies between MZ and DZ twins was revealed [509]. However, the observation from the American study that non-diabetic discordant twins are no more likely than singleton infants to carry islet self-antibodies favors the genetic view [510].

A high penetrance of islet cell autoreactivity was observed in MZ twins heterozygous for DQ2/DQ8, i.e. HLA alleles associated with high risk of diabetes [505]. This suggests that HLA-DQ2 and –DQ8 may determine genetic susceptibility to production of islet-specific antibodies. Studies on non-diabetic MZ twin siblings of T1D parents from UK (n=134) and USA (n=53) showed that diabetes risk was higher in twins, who was heterozygous for DR3-DQ2 and DR4-DQ8, than in twins with neither DR3-DQ2 nor DR4-DQ8, indicating a sufficient role of these HLA variants in determining genetic predisposition to family disease [511]. Non-HLA genes can also have an impact on the disease penetrance of T1D. Metcalfe et al. [512] found that the possession of the high-risk Hph I homozygous +/+ genotype of the insulin gene increased the likelihood of identical twins being concordant for T1D. On the other hand, insulin secretion or sensitivity showed no significant concordance in low-risk non-diabetic MZ twins, providing an evidence for mainly non-genetic determination of these metabolic parameters [513].

Chapter 7

TOOLS TO MAP AND IDENTIFY SUSCEPTIBILITY GENES FOR COMPLEX DISEASES

Apart from monogenic diseases (where only one gene intervenes in etiology), there is a set of complex diseases, in which genetic and environmental factors interact. Characteristically, many genes interact in complex ways with multiple environmental factors and with each other [514]. T1D is a typical example of such multifactorial and complex disorders.

CHOICE OF AN APPROPRIATE STRATEGY TO FIND A DISEASE-ASSOCIATED GENE

In a multifactorial disease, the major obstacle is that the various components of the phenotypes result from the interaction between multiple genes and others factors. The difficulty is to correlate the various components of the phenotype to each individual factor. Each gene has a weak effect, thus studies require large sample size. Studies generally lack statistical power, and the complexity of interactions between environmental factors and phenotypes are difficult to take into account. Thus the study of complex diseases genetics remains difficult and presents many additional challenges for genetic epidemiology.

The parameters to consider for designing a genetic study of a complex disease are at different levels:

1) The knowledge of pathophysiological process:

- If known or if specific hypotheses on the role of particular genes are available, the *candidate gene* approach is applied. It consists in choosing markers near the candidate gene.
- If unknown, a *genome scan* approach may be set up using markers distributed over the genome.

2) The methodological strategy most suitable according to the kind of genetic information available:

- *Linkage studies*, which consist in finding a physical linkage between a marker and a gene. These studies deal with family design.
- *Association studies*, which consist in finding a correlation between several factors and the disease. In general, these studies imply unrelated individuals or a population.

Genetic Linkage Analysis

Genetic linkage refers to co-transmission of polymorphic genetic markers or traits, physically linked on the same chromosome. Linkage studies are focused on the co-segregation of genes, or markers, situated at different loci. One tests the independence of their transmission. Their level of independence is reflected in the recombination fraction, θ, the percentage of meiotic recombination of the gametes transmitted by the parents and that exhibit a recombination between the genetic markers studied. If two factors are independent (not linked), the recombination fraction θ is maximum and equal to 0.5. The closer and/or the tighter linked the factor studied and the gene involved, the lowest the recombination fraction. There is "linkage" between the two loci [515].

Such studies usually imply a family design and focus on related individuals, who may be affected or not, by the disorder under study. The parameter of interest is designated by identity by descent (IBD). Two individuals are identical by descent at a genetic locus, if they share the same gene copy at that locus due to inheritance from a recent common ancestor. Large families with several generations are particularly informative as they give access to numerous comparable meiotic events. When co-transmission is observed in families, marker and trait (or marker and gene, or marker and marker) are said to be linked. A genomic region tagged by the markers linked together includes a factor (gene) involved in the disease and thus a candidate genomic region has been identified. Once such a region is known, it can be refined by using a number of markers located between those initially investigated. This strategy called "positional cloning" is usually laborious. After a positive result from a first linkage analysis, the region of the genome potentially implicated is often very large in terms of DNA length to be explored.

Whole genome scan is usually performed in family studies for linkage analysis. This method can provide evidence for linkage to a particular region of the genome, using genetics markers, such as microsatellites distributed over the genome. Genome-wide searches require a large number of families with individuals affected by the disease. Historically, sets of microsatellites were used to tag the genome at regular intervals. Microsatellite maps were increasingly dense. Presently, Single Nucleotide Polymorphisms (SNPs) are more and more used [516].

Several methods have been proposed for the linkage analysis of complex traits, including maximum likelihood-based methods (LOD-scores) and nonparametric approaches, such as affected sib pair (ASP) methods and the non-parametric linkage (NPL) statistic [517].

LOD-Score

The LOD-score method is based on studies of families with several generations. The aim is to estimate recombination fraction θ between a disease gene and a marker *m*. Each analysis aims to test the null hypothesis of independence, H0: $\theta = ½$, versus the alternative hypothesis of linkage, H1: $\theta < ½$, where θ is the recombination fraction as defined before. *L* represents the likelihood, corresponding to the assumption.

$$\text{LOD} - \text{score } Z(\theta) = \Sigma\log_{10}[\text{L(family if } \theta = X)/\text{L(family if } \theta = 1/2)]$$

The value of a LOD-score is the log (base 10) of the odds in favour of linkage. So a LOD-score value of 3 corresponds to odds of 1000:1 in favor of linkage. The estimate of the recombination fraction is the value θ that maximizes the function $Z(\theta)$. This method necessitates knowing the frequency of the allele and the correspondence between genotype and phenotype (penetrance). The first recommendation, which fixed the threshold for significance of linkage when the LOD-score is ≥3 [518] and which was not proposed for the purpose of the genome scan, has been the start point of a debate still relevant today about the mapping of complex traits. The main problem is the inflation risk of type 1 error (we can also say that is the problem of false positive markers) when multiple markers are tested with the LOD-score method. Now, many studies use sets of thousands of microsatellite or SNPs markers throughout the genome. It makes more complicated the debate around multiple testing, and our capacity to interpret significance of results, coming from these studies.

For multifactorial diseases, the LOD-score method is not likely to be very powerful, because it assumes that there is a major locus, with a specific mode of inheritance, which is responsible for the majority of the genetic variance. Other methods called “model-free”, which are non-parametric approaches, fit much better with the study of complex diseases.

Affected Sib-Pair Method

The Affected Sib-Pair method proposed by Penrose in 1935 is one of those non-parametric approaches. The method consists in counting, in affected sib-pair, the number of alleles transmitted by the two parents and shared between the patients in the sibship [519,520]. This method tests whether affected sib pairs share more marker alleles identical by descent (IBD) than expected (two alleles are IBD, if they are inherited from the same ancestral source). This method does not necessitate making assumptions about the mode of inheritance but it is more powerful, when identity by descent (IBD) of marker alleles can be determined. We can see that the parental genotyping is very important and guarantees the smooth running of the method. By analogy to a LOD-score statistic, the evidence of linkage of a marker in a set of affected sib-pairs can be assessed by a maximum LOD-score (MLS) statistic *T*. The threshold of significance of linkage is fixed to 3. In the affected sib-pair approach, test for the evidence of linkage is based on the maximum likelihood estimation. Thus, it has the advantage, over methods based on direct analysis of the IBD sharing among sibs, to be more powerful and to deal correctly with partial information or missing data [521].

The IBD probabilities can also be used to reject a genomic region under a genetic model, because of the incompatibility of the IBD proportions with this model.

In multiplex families, the observed distribution z2:z1:z0 corresponds to sharing 2,1 and 0 IBD alleles in affected sib pairs (Figure 10A). If no linkage, this distribution is equal 1/4:1/2:1/4. In that case, MLS is calculated as follows:

$$\text{MLS} = \log10\ [\text{L (data if z2,z1,z0)/L (data if 1/4:1/2:1/4)}]$$

In a family, the observed distribution n2:n1:n0 corresponds to sharing 2,1 and 0 IBD alleles among sibs (Figure 10B). The null hypothesis assumes no genetic linkage between marker and disease, and the expected distribution should be n/4:n/2:n/4 under H0. The linkage between the marker and given disease is estimated by χ^2 test as $\Sigma((\text{obs-exp})^2/\text{exp}$ which follows a, χ^2 distribution with two degree of freedom under H0.

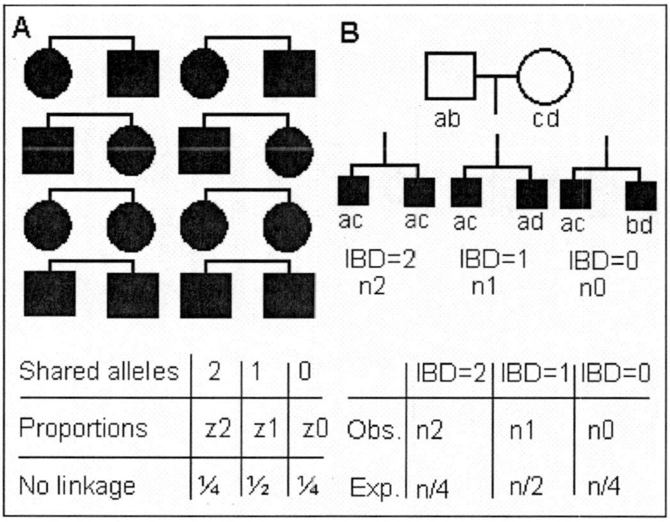

Figure 10. Affected sib-pair approach is a non-parametric method used for candidate gene and for genome-wide screen strategies. A. In multiplex families, a linkage between a given polymorphic marker and a disease is evaluated, using a maximum LOD-score (MLS) value, which represents a logarithm (base 10) of the odds in favor of linkage, i.e. how much the observed distibution z2:z1:z0 (corresponding to sharing 2,1 and 0 alleles, respectively, among IBD sibs) is differed from the random distribution 1/4:1/2:1/4 if no linkage observed. A threshold MLS value of 3.0 corresponds to odds of 1000:1 in favor of linkage. B. In a family, affected sibs could share two (IBD=2), one (IBD=1) or zero (IBD=0) marker alleles identical by descent (IBD) from their parents. To examine whether the marker is linked to the disease, the observed distribution of IBD marker alleles shared among sibs (n2:n1:n0) is compared with the expected distribution n/4:n/2:n/4 by χ^2 test (df=2).

GENETIC ASSOCIATION STUDIES

Association studies provide a complementary approach to identify new susceptibility disease genes. These analyses can be posterior to linkage analysis and confirm, or refine, the correlation between alleles of a gene in a candidate region and the disease. It is necessary to be careful about the matching of cases and controls, which have to be matched for a maximum of potential confounders, such as age and sex, and most importantly ethnicity, in addition to the status of case or control.

Such association can be highlighted if the marker is in *linkage disequilibrium* (*LD*) with a disease susceptibility locus. LD is the non-random association of alleles at two (or more) linked loci, and can offer valuable information to refine the location of disease susceptibility genes, taking advantages of few ancestral recombinations. Assessment of linkage disequilibrium is therefore important To compare marker frequencies between cases and controls, usual methods in epidemiology for case-control design can be used: contingency tables with χ^2 statistic, Fisher's exact test, odds ratios, etc. However, all these methods generate a lot of tests, and consequently emerges the problem of multiple testing. The error rate of each test made is defined by $[1 - (1 - \alpha)]^n$, n being the number of independent tests performed. For example, a number of 10 tests generate an error rate of 40%. In association studies, involving the usage of very polymorphic markers (microsatellites and minisatellites) or extremely polymorphic loci (i.e. HLA), the multiple testing has to be considered: the larger the number of tests, the larger the number of false positive results.

One solution to multiple testing can be provided by the Bonferroni correction, which consists in multiplying the *p*-value by the number of tests performed. It corresponds to decreasing the *p*-value threshold for considering a test as significant. The problem is that this method is too conservative. This correction method is used under the assumption of tests' independence, which is not adequate to genetic studies of the HLA region, because a strong disequilibrium exists in this genomic region. If the test is still significant after Bonferroni correction, the association can be considered as strong. If it is not the case, giving the two *p*-values (uncorrected and corrected) is appropriate and calls for a replication with larger sample. Other ways to try to take into account the multiple statistical tests is to decrease the number of tests by a several steps procedure: to test a limited number of patients and controls or families, to identify the polymorphisms of possible interest and then to test only those polymorphisms on an independent group of patients and controls or of families from the same population. It is very important to report also negative or borderline significant results in order that the repeated studies can take the results into account for future design of studies. Despite all these possible solutions, the repetition of studies in independent groups remains the best way to validate an association or a linkage.

Furthermore, the independence of alleles can strictly be tested with χ^2 statistics in case of Hardy–Weinberg equilibrium (HWE). This test should always be performed only in the controls. In a population of cases the Hardy–Weinberg proportions frequently deviate from the equilibrium: this is an additional indication of an association with the disease of one or more alleles at the studied locus. If there is a strong departure from HWE among controls, Pearson's χ^2 is not valid for testing the association. In this situation Armitage's test can be used to compare allele frequency distribution [522]. Because of the difficulties to collect an appropriate control group for association studies, the genetic information present in the parents of affected cases, but not transmitted to the cases may be a good source of controls because such controls are matched on genetic ancestry, and thus avoid the bias due to the population stratification (Table 8).

Table 8. Strategies for genetic analysis of complex disorders

Approach	Definition and aim	Advantages	Disadvantages
Population studies:	To find a genetic association		
1. Cohort studies	Regular monitoring of a given population with recording and monitoring of the new cases (if normal population) or of disease features (if cohort of cases)	Prospective, longitudinal; factors studied before the onset of the disease; approach going from causes to effects; permit calculation of relative risks, odds ratios and incidence	Long; misfit for rare diseases studies
2. Case-control studies	Comparison, at a given moment, of a group of patients to a group of controls	Retrospective; factors studied after the onset of the disease; approach going back from the effects to the causes; permit calculation of odds ratios only	Cases recruitment bias, controls selection
Family studies:	To find a linkage or genetic transmission		
1. Segregation studies	Study of cases distribution in pedigrees.	Retrospective; factors studied after the onset of the disease; approach going back from the effects to the causes; permit calculation of odds ratios only	Difficulties of interpretation because of families recruitment bias; no information on real identity of genes involved.
2. Linkage studies	Look for the linkage between the genetic marker and the disease	Permits to conclude to genomic region involvement; calculation of recombination fraction and LOD-score	Large number of families is needed; necessitate knowledge on disease inheritance mode, penetrance and frequency; fit much better for monogenic diseases
3. Affected sib-pair studies	Study of number of shared Identical By Descent (IBD) alleles in sibship of interest.	no assumption on inheritance mode; simple analysis	Multitest; IBD ambiguity because of parent genotype missing; family information is not always available; large number of families with 2 cases in the same sibship necessary
4. Twin studies	Concordance rates comparison between monozygotic and dizygotic twins	Estimation of environment and genetic impact on disease onset	Great difficulties of recruitment
5. Both linkage and association studies (transmission disequilibrium test, TDT)	Detecting linkage in presence of an association between a disease and alleles of a marker	designed to avoid the spurious population associations produced by ethnic stratification of a sample of affected people; power greater than Affected Sib-Pair method; no assumption on the inheritance mode	require genotypes on affected individuals and their parents; not ideally suited to the study of late-onset diseases; loss of data due to non-paternity; only heterozygous parents are informative

In genetic association studies, the distribution of a given parameter (carrier frequency, allele frequency or genotype frequency at a given gene locus) is computed in sets of unrelated individuals, differing for the phenotype of interest, and compared, using classical statistical methods. Markers must be chosen, taking into account their proximity to the candidate gene, whose function may suggest a role in the disease.

Candidate Gene Analysis

The candidate gene analysis is the most used to search an association between a gene and a disease. In this method, studies are usually based on assumptions about the role of specific known loci in the pathological process leading to disorder. Thus, this method uses knowledge about the candidate gene potential function and the disorder physiopathology to look after the most interesting candidate genes. The most important problem with this method is that there can be a very large number of potential susceptibility loci, whose role is only partially understood. A marker by marker analysis does not take into account the LD between such markers. Whole genome scan can also be used in association studies. However, the latter reach a number of statistical tests that makes it of no practical use to conclude.

Replication studies on independent samples, for linkage as well as association analyses, for multifactorial diseases are indispensable. However considering the variety of environmental exposition or ethnic backgrounds, a heterogeneity of the results is difficult to interpret.

Calculation of Genetic Risk

In human genetics and genetic epidemiology, genetic risk ratios are meaningful. These risk ratios can be defined as a measure of the association effect, reflecting the probability of disease in an individual, carrying particular alleles or genotypes as compared to the probability of disease in those, who do not have the paricular alleles or genotypes. The strength of the association depends on interactions between environmental and genetic factors or gene–gene interactions.

Let F be the risk factor (present or absent) and D the disease, then the n subjects can be classified as follows in a 2×2 contingency table:

	D+	D−	Total
Factor F+	a	c	$a + c$
Factor F−	b	d	$b + d$
Total	$a + b$	$c + d$	n

The most classical test of an association is the χ^2 test:

$$\chi^2 = n\,(ad - bc)^2/(a + b)(a + c)(c + d)(b + d)$$

There are different indexes measuring the risk:

1) *The relative risk (RR)*, which is the ratio of the probability of having the disease among the exposed individuals and the unexposed ones is estimated by:

$$RR = P(D^+/F^+)/P(D^+/F^-) = a/(a + c)/b(b + d)$$

Strictly speaking, the index RR can be calculated in cohort studies only. Keeping in mind that $z_{0.025} = 1.96$, it is possible to get for the two limits of the confidence interval (CI) estimate:

$$CI_{95\%} = [RR^{1 - (Z_{(\alpha/2)}/\sqrt{x^2}}; RR^{1 + (Z_{(\alpha/2)}/\sqrt{x^2}}]$$

If the confidence interval does not include the value 1, it can be concluded that a significant association exists between the disease *D* and the factor *F*.

2) *The odds ratio (OR)* is also derived from a multiplicative model:

$$OR = P(D^+/F^+)/Pr(D^-/F^+)/P(D^+/F^-)/Pr(D^-/F^-) = ad/bc$$

OR = 1 in the absence of an association of *F* with *D*.

For a rare disease, the relative risk is approximated by the odds ratio (OR). The advantage of OR over RR is that it can be estimated in all kinds of surveys, even in case-control studies.

3) *The attributable fraction (AF)* is the proportion of cases among the exposed, which could be avoided, if the factor was removed. This is true only if the factor is really causative. This index is also called the "etiologic fraction" by some authors.

$$AF = 1 - 1/RR$$

This index represents a measurement of the strength of the relationship between the disease and the factor. For instance, if RR = 2, half of the cases could be avoided if the factor is removed; if RR = 10, 90% of the cases could be avoided.

4) *The attributable risk (AR)* is the proportion of cases in the population, which could be avoided, if the factor was really causative. It takes into account the reduction of the risk, f the frequency of the factor F in the population, and the overall disease risk in the population:

$$AR = f(RR - 1)/f(RR - 1) + 1$$

This index is very useful for public health purposes. If the factor is widespread and the risk-elevated, any reduction in the causal factor *F* could result in a noticeable reduction of the disease. AR can be directly estimated in cohort but not in case-control studies, which do not provide RR, or *f*. If genetic information is available as a genotyped candidate gene, several methods can be used to quantify genetic risk. These include allelic, genotype and haplotype relative risks.

In case of a candidate gene with two alleles g_1 and g_2, *genotype relative risks* can be defined as:

$$RR_1 = P(D^+| g_1g_2)P(D^-| g_1g_1)$$

$$RR_1 = P(D^+| g_2g_2)P(D^-| g_1g_1)$$

And the corresponding genotype odds ratios as:

$$OR_1 = P(D^+| g_1g_2)Pr(D^-| g_1g_2)/ P(D^+| g_1g_1)Pr(D^-| g_1g_1)$$

$$OR_2 = P(D^+| g_2g_2)Pr(D^-| g_2g_2)/ P(D^+| g_1g_1)Pr(D^-| g_1g_1)$$

The haplotype relative risk (HRR) method [523] was proposed as an answer to false-positive findings in case-control studies [524]. The sampling unit of the HRR is a family with two parents and a single affected offspring. Each unit, or each trio, gives a case genotype and a control genotype, made-up of the non-transmitted alleles from the parents to the patient. The control population is thus the population of haplotypes non-transmitted. HRR considers the case and control genotypes as independent, providing an estimation of the population relative risk [525]. The formulation of a HRR thus eliminates the problems of sampling from the same homogeneous population to form both the disease sample and an appropriate control.

METHODS, TESTING ASSOCIATION AND LINKAGE AT THE SAME TIME

The most popular such method also uses the parental genotyping information and is known as the *Transmission Disequilibrium Test* (*TDT*) developed by Spielman et al. [526] in 1993. TDT tests for linkage in presence of a known association. This was first performed for the linkage studies between the insulin gene and T1D [526]

This test considers trios constituted by affected children and their two parents. This can be performed in families with one heterozygous parent at least, for the marker of interest. The TDT considers parents, who are heterozygous for an allele associated with disease and evaluates the frequency, with which that allele or its alternate is transmitted to affected offspring [527]. If results are significant, this would mean that it may exists a linkage between a marker and a disease.

In fact, this method permits searching simultaneously a disequilibrium linkage and a genetic linkage, when the association is already known. The advantages of TDT are that this method is not sensitive to the population stratification and the use of families with only one affected individual (simplex family) is possible. An unfortunate side effect of the TDT is that it effectively throws away some genotype information, owing to its exclusive use of heterozygous parents. This creates a loss of statistical power to detect genuine allelic association. In its original form, the TDT also requires parental genotypes, which are not easily accessible for late-onset disorders. Moreover, the TDT is considered as more powerful for fine mapping of susceptibility genes than the model-based analysis of linkage, when the recombination fraction is $\theta < 0.02$ [528,529]. Variants have been thought to permit the consideration of the most important quantity of information and to include different kinds of information given by other relatives [529].

Haplotypes Statistical Analysis

The haplotypes statistical analysis may be more efficient in a genomic region with strong LD to test an association between disease and multiple markers [530,531]. There are two principal methods that use the haplotype analysis in association studies: one is used to determine the exact chromosomal location, and the other to assess the association between the region and disease. The first one, as other associations studies described above, compares chromosomes from diseased subjects and from controls in order to test for heterogeneity between cases and controls. LD methods (model-based methods) or Haplotype Sharing Statistics can be performed to highlight an association. However, these methods need to prove themselves empirically; they have some disadvantages in the marker identification, particularly with multiple markers in perfect LD. Therefore, the other use of haplotype information in genetic association, and which is considered as more realistic, is to search for certain chromosomal regions associated with traits. To evaluate associations between haplotypes and phenotypes, the simplest method is the regression analysis. The null hypothesis is that any association between genomic region and traits of interest (i.e. presence or absence of disease) does not exist. If there is no statistical association, one can conclude that all haplotypes have the same effect on the risk to develop the disease of interest. There are two major pitfalls with haplotype regression analysis: haplotype uncertainty (when estimated from the population data), which has to be taken into account in the analysis, and once again the multitest problem generated by great number of haplotypes that can be tested. Although great progress is being done in the haplotype analysis, further studies still remain necessary to clarify the haplotype blocks and LD patterns throughout the genome.

THE IDENTIFICATION OF A "POSITIONAL CANDIDATE GENE"

Both methods, the linkage analysis and association study, are usually considered as complementary approaches for a given disease. The identification of a disease gene proceeds through 5 steps.

1) *SAMPLING*: Families are "collected" and the clinical investigation is repeated to ensure that there are no misdiagnoses of individuals. Here the questions are: Are diagnosis criteria well defined? What is the optimal sample size?

2) *INITIAL SCREENING (EXCLUSION MAP)*: When there are enough families to give a chance of a significant positive LOD-score, a linkage analysis is performed. The DNA is amplified by PCR for at least 200 polymorphic marker loci spread throughout the genome. This whole genomic anonymous screening should ensure that one locus is within about 7.5 cM of the disease gene. Here the most important question is about the good choice of the set of markers.

3) *FINE DEFINITION OF CANDIDATE REGION (REFINED MAP)*: When that initial linkage is found, a more dense set of markers from the same region is also tested in the same families.

4) *GENE IDENTIFICATION*: Most areas of the human genome have now been sequenced. Clones, covering the minimum area, are identified and used to find all the genes in the area. Among those are identified, those being most probably good candidate genes.

5) *MUTATION DEFINITION IN THE PATIENTS*: Mutations or polymorphisms in these genes are sought in the affected patients. At this step, association studies may be performed.

Since all the genome is already sequenced, several of these steps may be bypassed or simplified. In terms of experimental strategy, it may be possible to jump directly from the definition of the candidate genomic region, within which the gene must lie to the mutation screen, after a thorough analysis of the gene sequences over this interval [531]. The steps 3 and 4 may be performed with the bioinformatics tools. In the specific framework of complex disease, particular difficulties must be underlined. The definition of cases is often more difficult for complex diseases. Such an approach can generate important costs, but, in addition, there can be statistical difficulties, dealing with the power of studies. Due to the weak effect of each of the genes involved, a large sample size and a sufficient number of markers are required to overcome the low power of studies. In many cases, the necessary sample size may exceed the actual possibilities. Genetic heterogeneity occurs more often in complex disease due to the phenotypic heterogeneity. This heterogeneity results in associations with various genes, which have different impacts on the disease onset and development, and even various alleles in a locus. Analysis of affected members of large pedigrees may be helpful to resolve the genetic heterogeneity [515].

HOW TO ASSESS THE ASSOCIATION OF A SECOND FACTOR IN THE VICINITY OF AN ALREADY KNOWN ASSOCIATED FACTOR?

A great challenge in the identification of susceptibility genes in complex diseases is to distinguish primary associated factors, and secondary associations due to LD. The latter can involve factors that do not have a direct involvement in the etiology of disease. This problem has received some attention, particularly in the study of HLA-associated disease. This particular genomic region that lies on 6p21.3 contains many genes involved in autoimmunity and immune response. The identification of several candidate genes in MHC is complicated due to strong LD in the region. To distinguish between primary and secondary effects, several methods have been proposed. For example, the homozygous parent TDT [532], which compares the transmission of alleles from parents homozygous at the first identified locus and heterozygous at the locus studied, to affected offspring. An alternative method is the haplotype method [533], which compares allele frequencies at an investigated locus on haplotypes that are identical at a primary locus.

With the same goal, Svejgaard & Ryder [534] described a method to decide which HLA factor shows the strongest association. They consider two factors named A and B. The basic data for the analysis are the entries of the 2 x 4 table, giving the four phenotypic combinations of A and B in patients and controls, respectively (Table 11). These data are analyzed in various 2 x 2 tables, involving the stratification of each of the two factors against the other. The stronger increase of factor A is established if A is significantly associated with the condition both in B-positives and in B-negatives, when this is not true for B in A-positives and A-negatives (Table 9).

Table 9. A 2 x 4 table contingency, giving the four phenotypic combinations of A and B in patients and controls

	Patients	Controls
A+ B+	*a*	*b*
A+ B−	*c*	*d*
A− B+	*e*	*h*
A− B−	*f*	*g*

Software Available to Perform Linkage and Association Studies

As a rule, the use of an appropriate software can improve the data management and genetic analysis. In addition to standard statistics software (SAS, Stata, SPSS, etc.), there are some specific programs to deal with genetic data in the association or linkage studies.

A major part of them are available at http://linkage.rockefeller.edu/soft/list.html. The selection of the analysis software will primarily be determined by the study design chosen. However, there are options beyond these as there are a number of software packages that carry out the same analysis, and it is possible to analyse data in different ways. For example, if one has genotyped multi-generation families with the intention of carrying out parametric linkage analysis, then one can choose between Genehunter, Merlin, S.A.G.E., or one of several other programs that allow to carry out a single or multi-point analysis (some allow to carry out both). Alternatively, if somebody chose to carry out a TDT analysis then there are a large number of programs that are derivatives of the standard TDT test. Another common strategy (particularly for complex diseases) is the recruitment of affected sib-pair families for non-parametric linkage studies. After the initial screening (for example, with Genehunter or Merlin), it is possible to follow up any genomic area, demonstrating a significant linkage, by TDT analysis (there are certain methodological issues with doing this, but it can be useful for confirming which linkage results are true positive, although such confirmation is not an independent replication).

The choice of which software to use for analysis is therefore a complicated one, and is often a matter of a personal choice (or more accurately a choice between the packages that someone knows how to use). Briefly, there is no clear answer as to the “best” software to use. One of the major limitations will be the computing resources available, such as an access to UNIX hosts or LINUX, how powerful the computers are, and the software that is installed on them, see the summary section for such matters.

Chapter 8

UTILITY OF ANIMAL MODELS IN GENETIC ANALYSIS OF SUSCEPTIBILITY TO TYPE 1 DIABETES

_Dimitry A. Chistiakov_*

Department of Pathology, University of Pittsburgh Medical Center, Pittsburgh PA 15261, USA

Today, there are several murine and rodent animal models have been developed for studying spontaneous autoimmune diabetes. Among those, NOD mice and BB rats are the most intensively studied. In both models, T lymphocytes are shown to be both initiators and final effectors of β-cell depletion [535]. Clinical, immunopathologic and genetic differences distinguish these two models, indicating that the pathways, leading to autoimmune T1DM in humans, may also be diverse. Therefore, investigators, considering a rodent model to better understand the etiology of T1DM or for therapeutic interventions to prevent or cure autoimmune diabetes studies, should look for efficacy in more than one model with the ultimate goal to extrapolate such therapies to humans.

THE NOD MOUSE

T1D Pathogenesis

The NOD inbred strain was developed by inbreeding of Jcl:ICR progenitors at the Shionogi Research Laboratories in Aburahi, Japan [536]. T1D pathogenesis in NOD mice is female gender-biased (Table 10). In high-incidence colonies of NOD mice, female incidence

* Correspondence concerning this article should be addressed to Dr. Dimitry A. Chistiakov, Ph.D., Department of Pathology, University of Pittsburgh Medical Center, A719 Scaife Hall, 3550 Terrace st, Pittsburgh PA 15261; Phone: (412) 802 6114; Fax: (412) 6799; E-mail: dac58@pitt.edu

typically reaches 80–90% by 24 weeks of age, whereas male incidence is lower and much more variable, usually reaching >40% by 30 weeks of age. Recently, an incidence of 85% in females by 27 weeks and 75% in males by 40 weeks of age have been reported [537]. Since NOD mice are subject to protective immunomodulation when stimulated by a wide spectrum of extrintic pathogens, including viruses, bacteria or their products, the animals should be maintained at high standards of cleanliness and good care practice to achieve the diabetes frequencies mentioned above.

Table 10. Characteristics of the NOD mouse and BB rat models of T1D

Characteristics	NOD mouse	BB rat (diabetes-prone)
Sex predominance	♀ > > ♂	♀ = ♂
Diabetes incidence	♀: 70-90%; ♂: 20-70%	50-80%
Age at onset	12-30 weeks	8-16 weeks
Insulitis	Destructive	Destructive
Ketoacidosis	Very mild or moderate	Yes
Susceptibility	Recessive	Recessive
MHC risk alleles	I-Ab^{g7}, IEA^{null}, K^d, D^b	$RT1^u$
Non-MHC loci	> 23 loci	> 3 loci
Lymphopenia	No	Yes
Accumulation of T cells	Yes	No
B cells required	Yes	Unknown
NK cell number/function	Low or absent/Poor	High/High
Viral administration	Protects from diabetes	Not required
Hemolytic complement	Absent (C5)	Present
Cyclophosphatimide treatment	Induces diabetes	Inhibits diabetes
Insuline treatment after diabetes	Not required	Immeduately
Other co-existing autoimmune disorders	Thyroiditis, Sjogren's syndrome	Thyroiditis

The development of clinical symptoms in the NOD mouse is preceded by insulitis, the disruption of islet structure and function by infiltrating leukocytes. The first stages are detectable in NOD females around the time of weaning (4 weeks), at least 2–3 months before the development of overt diabetes. Insulitis begins as peri-insulitis, a pervasive leukocytic infiltrate, emanating from the pancreatic vasculature and secretory ducts. Soon after peri-insulitis initiation (usually in 3- to 5-weeks-old females and several weeks later in males), only a subset of islets observed in a microscopic field appear to be penetrated by leukocytes. However, as the mice proceed through puberty, an increasing prevalence of islets show intra-islet leukocytic infiltrates, coupled with erosion of between 25 and 90% of the insulin-stainable β-cell mass [538].

A distinguishing feature of the histological appearance of insulitis in NOD mice from that observed either in the T-lymphopenic BB-DP rat or in the humans is the unusual large number of leukocytes associated with all the pancreatic vascular spaces [539]. These intrapancreatic lympho-accumulations are primarily and mainly comprised of T lymphocytes and contain a greater number of $CD4^+$ (helper) than $CD8^+$ (cytotoxic) T cells [540]. B lymphocytes and macrophage/dendritic cells also are found in the infiltrates [541]. This lympho-accumulation is not restricted to the pancreas but is also evident as increased percentages of T lymphocytes in blood, peripheral lymphoid organs, and in other endocrine tissues. Accumulation of leukocytic infiltrates around the peri-vascular and peri-ductular regions of the pancreas and subsequent development of progressively more severe insulitis usually begins between 3 and 5 weeks in NOD females and several weeks later in males. Marked decreases in pancreatic insulin content are demonstrable in NOD/Lt females at around 12 weeks of age and several weeks later in males [542]. When more than 90% of the β-cell mass of the pancreas is destroyed, clinical symptoms of diabetes (hyperglycemia, glycosuria, polydipsia, and polyuria) appear quite abruptly [543]. Although intra-islet insulitis is evident early after weaning, some immunoregulatory mechanism apparently keeps many of the infiltrating T lymphocytes in a resting state until a later activation event allows more widespread destruction of the β-cell mass [544].

Genetic Susceptibility to T1D

A provisional nomenclature exists to describe mouse chromosomal regions, carrying genes capable of modulating T1D susceptibility termed 'insulin-dependent diabetes susceptibility' and abbreviated *Idd*. Similar loci have been mapped in the human and rat and are designated *IDDM* and *Iddm*, respectively. These genetic loci are uncovered by outcrossing NOD mice to T1D-resistant mouse strains and then performing a segregation analysis. Segregation analysis and the ever-increasing definition of the mouse genome have shown that many strains harbor potential *Idd* susceptibility contributions but that the NOD strain is unfortunate in terms of the large numbers randomly inbred into them during the generation of the strain. To date, greater than 30 loci on 17 chromosomes, including the mitochondrial chromosome [545], have been reported with some loci contributing more than one gene [546,547] (Table 10). Originally, these loci were given sequential numbers, as they were reported in the literature. More recently, the segments of chromosomes, carrying genes capable of influencing T1D, have been described by molecular markers that physically delimit the region.

As is the case in both the rat models of T1D and in the human disease, in the NOD mouse, the MHC plays a paramount role. The first genetic analysis of T1D in the NOD mice reported a recessive susceptibility for clinical disease linked to MHC [565]. Because the MHC complex contains genes essential for antigen processing and presentation as well as for immune cell function, and given evidence indicative of broad-based immune tolerance defects in NOD mice, it is not surprising that $H2^{g7}$, encompassing both common class I alleles, a unique class II A^{g7} allele, and absence of class II E [the HLA-DR homolog] provides the major component of genetic susceptibility [567-569]. Indeed, specific amino acid substitutions in the $H2\text{-}Ab^{g7}$ chain reflect similar residues present in the human HLA-DQ0302 allele linked to increased T1D susceptibility in Caucasians. These include a histidine residue at position 56 and a serine residue at position 57 of the β chain. X-ray crystallographic analysis has aided our understanding of the diabetogenic properties of the I-

A^{g7} molecule. The NOD I-A^{g7} molecule behaved very much like I-A^d, a MHC class II molecule that shares the same a chain with I-A^{g7}, but contains proline and aspartic acid at residues 56–57 of the β chain, and protects from diabetes. Binding affinities of a large collection of peptides were comparable for I-A^{g7} and I-A^d. Presence of negatively charged residues in the C-terminal region of the peptide increased binding affinity to I-A^{g7}. Exchange of the aspartic acid, as found in the protective I-A^d by a serine at position β57, increased the size of the position 9 (P9) pocket of I-A^{g7} and exposed positively charged residues. As a consequence of the increased pocket size at the amino acid residue that binds the antigen at P9, the I-A^{g7} P9 pocket can bind negatively charged residues and residues with larger side chains than does I-A^d. These two features significantly expand the peptide repertoire of I-A^{g7} in comparison with I-A^d. Immunoprecipitation studies suggested that I-A^{g7}-peptide complexes were less stable than similar MHC class II complexes from B6 [570]. This may further indicate that I-A^{g7} can bind more peptides but with lower affinities such that diabetogenic T cells were not centrally or peripherally deleted.

Table 11. Congenic chromosome regions linked to T1D susceptibility in the NOD mouse

NOD locus	Chromosome	Interval size	Number of genes	Candidate genes	Known gene function	Reference
Idd5.1	1	2.1 Mb	4	Ctla4	Negative T cell regulator	[548]
Idd5.2	1	1.52 Mb	45	Nramp1/Slc11a1	Endosomal/lysosomal acidification	[548]
Idd13	2	6 cM (H3a-Il1 interval)	NR*	B2m	Required for antigen presentation by MHC class I molecules	[549]
Idd3	3	0.78 Mb	8	Il2, Il21	T cell development and homeostasis	[550,551]
Idd17	3	1.1 cM	NR	Pdcd1?	Negative T cell costimulatory receptor	[552,553]
Idd10	3	0.95 Mb	7	Cd101	Costimulatory receptor of T cells	[554]
Idd18	3	0.7 Mb	2	Vav3	Guanine nucleotide exchange factor involved in signalling of T and B cell receptors	[555]
Idd6	6	10 cM	NR	NK complex; Lrmp, Bcat1, Kras2	Innate immune system; control cell proliferation	[556,557]
Idd9.1	4	39 cM	NR	Lck	T cell responsiveness	[558]
Idd11**	4	13 cM	NR	NR	NR	[559]
Idd9.2	4	3.7 Mb	13	Tnfr2, Cd30	Multiple inflammatory and immune responses	[558]
Idd9.3	4	1.2 Mb	13	4-1bb (Cd137)	Inducible costimulator of T cells, control of interactions between T and B cells	[558,560]
Idd4	11	5.2 cM	NR	PAF-AHIb1, Nos2, CC chemokines	Inflammatory responses	[561]
Idd14	13	>58 cM	NR	NR	NR	[562]
Idd23	17	20 Mb	NR	NR	NR	[563]
Idd16	17	3.1 Mb	37	Mapk13, Mapk14, class IK	Cell signalling, antigen presentation	[563,564]
Idd1	17	31 cM	>200	Class II A and E	Antigen presentation	[565, 566]

* NR, not reported; ** Idd9.1 and Idd11 are probably the same Idd locus.

It is not only the MHC class II region that contributes susceptibility in NOD mice but rather multiple loci in the extended haplotype. It is noteworthy that the extended haplotype analysis of human genes in linkage disequilibrium with T1D susceptibility, conferring HLA-DR and -DQ alleles, indicates additional susceptibility components toward the class I region [571]. While intra-MHC recombination is rare, two reports have explored the recombination within the MHC to map loci to both class I regions of the MHC. Analysis of NOD stocks congenic for recombinant haplotypes generated by genetic crossing-over between $H2^{g7}$ and $H2^{209}$ provide evidence of contributions of T1D susceptibility determinants centromeric to the Lmp2 recombination hotspot that both include and extend proximal to the H2-K gene [572]. Additional linkage to the H2-D end of the MHC complex has recently been reported [537]. Due to of this complexity, it is difficult to discuss whether the haplotype contributes susceptibility in a dominant or recessive fashion. Segregants heterozygous for $H2^{g7}$ may develop subclinical levels of insulitis (suggesting dominant $H2^{g7}$ contributions to this important diabetes subphenotype) and may even develop overt T1D, following a cyclophosphamide treatment [573]. However, T1D rarely develops spontaneously in such heterozygotes, especially when an Ea product is expressed by the other H2 haplotype [574]. In this regard, the NOD model diverges from humans, where certain HLA heterozygous haplotypes increase rather than suppress T1D susceptibility [575]. In summary, it may be appreciated that Idd1 is a collective descriptor for multiple disease-predisposing alleles within or linked to the MHC complex.

Similarity Between NOD Mouse and Human T1D Susceptibility Loci

Several of the diabetogenic components of $H2^{g7}$ (i.e., the class II alleles and the $H2\text{-}K^d$ allele) are also present in the related ALR and CTS strains [576,577]. As the ALR/Lt strain exhibits remarkable genetic resistance to autoimmune stress, it is clear that diabetogenic MHC alleles are not inherently diabetogenic but acquire diabetogenic potency only in the presence of high-risk alleles not linked to MHC [578]. Moreover, not all of the susceptibility alleles will derive from the NOD genome, and some admixtures can produce T2D rather than TID [547]. There are a number of reasons, why many of the known non-MHC mouse Idd loci are not matched by IDDM loci in the syntenic regions of the human genome. Important genus-specific differences distinguish mice from humans. The human IDDM2 locus has been identified in both association and linkage studies and is defined by polymorphisms in a variable no tandem repeat (VNTR) upstream of the human insulin (INS) gene [579,580]. While proinsulin/insulin represents a major T1D autoantigen in both humans and NOD mice, a NOD homolog of the human INS gene (Mouse Ins2 on distal chromosome 7) has not been detected in most segregation analyses [581]. This failure in association is most likely to be expected, because mice express two genes for insulin (the additional gene is Ins1 on chromosome 19). The Idd3 interleukin 2 (Il2) linkage is one of the strongest and the most commonly identified non-MHC loci, segregating in NOD outcrosses; the IL2 gene in the homologous 4q26–q27 region in humans has not yet been implicated as a major T1D susceptibility locus [581]. Of all the non-MHC loci identified in NOD outcrosses, the Idd5.1 region, containing the Cd152 (Ctla4 locus), may be reflected by the IDDM12 linkage to the homologous region on human 2q33 [582,583]. Despite the finding that non-MHC genes, contributing to T1D development in NOD mice, often are not reflected by the demonstration in humans of linkage to the homologous region, the value of the mouse system is to elucidate specific immunologic or endocrine dysfunctions that are entrained when sufficient numbers of Idd genes are present. While the human IL2 structural gene has not been implicated as a T1D gene, it is certainly possible that a gene in distant genetic proximity to IL2 could confer higher T1DM risk by affecting IL-2 glycosylation state as is implicated in the NOD mouse.

Recently, a C-to-A transversion has been discovered at mtDNA nucleotide position 5178 within the NADH dehydrogenase subunit 2 gene (mt-ND2). This results in a leucine-to-methionine amino acid substitution at position 237 [584]. The methionine-containing allele has been associated with increased longevity [585] and reductions in atherogenesis [586], blood pressure [587] and myocardial infarction [588]. Recently, in a population-based study of 385 Japanese patients (154 males and 231 females) with T1D and 469 age- and sex-matched controls, the methionine-containing allele showed an association with protection from T1D ($p = 0.017$) and with significantly reduced frequency ($p = 0.0046$) of the T1D-associated autoantibodies [584]. The authors proposed that the mt5178A genotype may confer protection against oxidative stress, although the article shed no light on a possible mechanism [584]. Mathews et al. [545] recently confirmed that mt-Nd2 is protective against T1D in crosses of the T1D-prone NOD with T1DM-resistant ALR mice. The mapping data with A^{g7}, Ins1/Ins2 vs. Ins-VNTR, CTLA4, and mt-ND2 are excellent examples of the ability to transpose susceptibility genes from human to mouse, even if the controlling genes are not transposable from mice to humans in a one-to-one ratio, many of the phenotypes diagnostic of high susceptibility may be common.

Research Utility of the NOD Mouse

The greater definition of the mouse genome and the use of introducing transgenes or targeted mutations (knockins or knockouts) in mice have lead the NOD mouse to become the most widely used model of T1D. Additionally, the NOD mouse is also the most highly used model for the study of autoimmunity, since the NOD mouse develops not only diabetes but also Sjögren's syndrome and autoimmune thyroditis [589]. A part of this polyautoimmunity may be because of defects in both NK and NKT-cell function in the NOD mouse. These cell types are essential for defense against pathogens, adaptive immune responses and in regulating immune responses. Alterations in the number or function of NKT cells have been associated with systemic sclerosis and T1D in humans and spontaneous autoimmune diseases in mice [589,590]. Likewise, the development of spontaneous insulin-dependent autoimmune diabetes in NOD mice correlates with defects in the numbers and function of NKT cells [591,592]. NK cells play a critical role in the early defense against infectious agents, in antiviral innate immune responses [593] and in xenograft rejection [594]. Therefore, the lack of NK-cell activity has led to the use of immunodeficient NOD, either NOD.Scid or NOD.Rag1$^{-/-}$ mice, as the standard model to study long-term xeno-engraftment. Recent work to humanize these NOD mice has lead to the generation of mice that can be engrafted with both human islets and human lymphocytes [595]. These new models will allow for the study of the interactions of lymphocytes in allograft rejection and autoreactive human lymphocytes and human-target tissues.

THE BB RAT

Development of Autoimmune Diabetes in BB Rats

BB rats were derived from outbred Wistar rats in Canada [596,597]. In 1974, rats with spontaneous T1D were discovered, and a selection for the diabetes phenotype commenced. Currently, multiple substrains of BB rats exist. T1D frequency in both the sexes of diabetes-prone BB (BB-DP) rats exceeds 90%, whereas no spontaneous T1D develops in diabetes-resistant BB-DR/Wor rats (Table 12). In contrast to the peri-weaning onset of lymphoaccumulation and peri-insulitis in NOD mice, the development of insulitis in BB rats occurs in the islets after the development of puberty and 2–3 weeks prior to the sudden onset of clinical symptoms. More than 90% of the observed diabetic rats develop the disease between 8 and 16 weeks of age. Most BB-DP rats develop insulitis whether or not they develop diabetes. The onset of hyperglycemia and the requirement for immediate insulin therapy is another factor, distinguishing the BB rats from NOD mice.

The earliest phases of the insulitis process in BB-DP rats also seem to be a stage, in which both permeability changes in the pancreatic vascular endothelium and macrophage insulitis are noted [598]. Because of a lack of mature peripheral T lymphocytes in BB-DP rats, especially those, expressing the T-cytotoxic phenotype, the cytotoxic NK cell was initially implicated as a primary effector of β-cell destruction [598]. Cells with this NK-like phenotype appeared to be the most prevalent of the islet-infiltrating leukocytes, but an NK-cell-specific monoclonal antibody failed to reduce the frequency of diabetes in BB-DP rats [599]. Pathogenic roles for rat CD4+ and CD8+ T lymphocytes were indicated by the finding that activated splenocytes from acutely diabetic BB-DP donors would adoptively transfer T1D into young prediabetic BB or athymic nude recipients. Further, depletion of T cells significantly reduced or ablated T1D development, and the synergistic contribution of CD4+ and CD8+ T lymphocytes to insulitis was shown, using manipulated T lymphocytes from the non-lymphopenic BB-DR strain [600].

The BB-DP rat shares with the NOD mice the susceptibility to subclinical thyroiditis and sialitis development [601]. Spontaneous lesions are more commonly encountered in diabetic (59%) vs. non-diabetic (11%) BB-DP/Wor rats. Six substrains of lymphopenic BB rats have been developed. Although the incidence of T1D among these substrains was relatively constant, major differences (ranging between 5 and 100%) in incidences of spontaneous or excess iodine-elicited thyroiditis has been observed [602]. The immunoregulatory defects induced by the lymphopenia (lyp) mutation are critical in this pathology, because it is rare in genetic segregation analysis between BB rats and non-lymphopenic strains to identify non-lymphopenic rats with thyroiditis [603]. Thyroiditis can be transferred into athymic rats by the same population of activated splenocytes that transfer T1D, suggesting that this autoreactive population contains cells that recognize antigens expressed by both β cells and thyrocytes [604].

Genetics of T1D in BB Rats

Segregation analysis between BB-DP crossed with other T1D-resistant strains have established that the MHC class II alleles encoded by the RT1^u haplotype of the BB rat are essential for diabetogenicity [605-608]. MHC susceptibility designated Iddm2 is permissive for insulitis in heterozygosity, but in outcrosses, most diabetic probands are homozygous for RT1^u. Analysis of insulitis and T1D development, following outcross of diabetes-prone BB/Wor rats to RT1^u congenic stocks of PVG rats, carrying recombinants in the class I vs. class II region, have established the requirement for the RT1-D^u/B^u alleles at the two class II loci [608]. Antigen-presenting cells of the BB rat do express the DR homolog (RT1-D^u). Sequence analysis of the BB rat DQ homolog (RT1-B^u) showed it differed from both the high diabetes-risk-conferring human HLA-DQβ alleles as well as the NOD H2-Ab^{g7} molecule. The BB rat allele contains an aspartic acid at residue 57 of the β chain instead of exhibiting diabetogenic non-Asp substitutions [609,610]. All RT1^u-expressing rat strains carry the requisite class II Iddm2 alleles. Class I alleles from non-RT1^u-positive rat strains apparently will substitute for the RT1-A^u, -E^u, and -C^u class I alleles [608].

A major genetic and phenotypic difference, distinguishing the DR from the various DP strains, is the presence in the DP line of a recessive mutation, lymphopenia (Lyp) on chromosome 4 [605,611,612]. Iddm1 was initially assigned to the recessive lyp mutation in BB-DP rats, in tight linkage to neuropeptide Y (Npy) on chromosome 4 [613]. Although DP rats develop a thymus of normal size, recent thymic T-lymphocyte emigrants to the periphery [phenotypically Thy1$^+$ and not expressing a cell surface adenosine diphosphate-ribosyltransferase (ART2)] are very short lived [614,615]. The consequence is a profound T lymphopenia/ lymphocytopenia. Hence, these rats are severely immunocompromised as reflected by impaired T-lymphocyte function in vitro, impaired ability to reject foreign tissue grafts, increased susceptibility to B lymphomagenesis and requirement for special husbandry procedures to protect against infections by opportunistic pathogens. Furthermore, evidence of the strong immunocompromised state of BB-DP rats is provided by their difficulty in rejecting non-islet allografted tissues. This markedly contrasts with NOD mice, whose T lymphocytes are long lived in the periphery, are present in large numbers and express a functional ortholog of ART2 [615]. In 2002, independent confirmation that Ian4 is the Lyp locus was published [616,617]. Through the use of positional cloning, two groups determined the presence of a frameshift mutation at nucleotide position 478 in the BB-DP DNA. This mutation results in a protein, in which the 215 C-terminal amino acids are replaced by 19 residues. This deletion removes the anchor that localizes the protein to the outer mitochondrial membrane [618,619]. Further proof for the candidacy of Ian4 resulted from the transgenic rescue experiments. In these experiments, T-cell development was salvaged in F344 rats congenic for the Lyp locus on chromosome 4, when the wild-type allele of Ian4 was expressed [620]. Ian4 (also known as Ian4l1 or Ian5) is an important regulator of T-cell apoptosis, although the function in T cells of this GTP-binding protein is unknown [620-624].

Although most diabetic probands in segregation analyses between BB-DP stocks and non-lymphopenic stocks, including BB-DR, have been homozygous for this mutation, the traits (lymphopenia vs. T1D) have been occasionally separated, leading to the speculation that another locus in tight linkage with the Lyp mutation was contributing [615,625]. Such a locus designated Iddm4 and proposed to be involved in insulitis initiation has been discovered in the outcross between BB-DR and an inbred WF stock followed by backcross to WF [626]. An ortholog for Iddm4 in the NOD mouse, if it exists, would be the Idd6 segment on mouse chromosome 6. Suggestive evidence for two other diabetogenic loci located on chromosome X and 3 and designated Iddm5 and Iddm6, respectively, was also obtained. The existence of Iddm3 was originally inferred based on the outcross of BB-DP to Fisher 344 rats [607]. This designation was subsequently used to describe suggestive evidence for a locus on chromosome 18, contributing to the development of spontaneous T1DM in the outcross of BB-DP/OK (a distinct line of BB rats in Germany) to the DA strain [627-630]. Additional evidence for weak linkages, following the outcross to other non-diabetic strains has been also suggested.

Research Utility of the BB Rat

Many researchers have written off the BB rat because of the lymphopenia, which is not shared by the great majority of human patients with T1D. Neverthless, the BB-DP and BB-DR rats have important potential to enlighten T1D research. Initially, it was thought that the genetics of T1DM in the BB rats was less complex than in NOD mice or humans. However, this may be more related to the level of study and not because of the true complexity. In fact, originally, diabetes in the NOD mouse was thought to be more oligogenic [566], since the outcross of NOD to 15 different inbred strains has led to the identification of 30 protective loci. Therefore, the genetics of the BB rat may increase in scope after further review.

Identification of a major diabetogenic gene, Ian4, in the BB rat may lead to different type of therapies for T1D. In the BB rat, the death of T cells because of the mutation in Ian4 includes the death of CD4+CD25+ T regs [624]. BB rats could then be utilized for strategies to promote Treg-cell survival or function to inhibit or reverse T1D. Further, as Ian4 is an important protein for mitochondrial stability, it may be determined that improvements in the lymphoid mitochondrial function could delete or anergize autoreactive T cells. As a sequence variation in IAN4 was not shown to be associated with T1D in human populations [630], mutations that affect the mitochondrial function in human populations, such as the C5178A variation in mt-ND2, may lead to common phenotypes of these two seemingly distinct mutations.

Conclusion

The selection process for animals that develop spontaneous autoimmune diabetes has generated several models that share many characteristics with the human form of the disease. Among those, a critical mass of information exists only for two of these, the NOD mouse and the BB rat. The pubertal or postpubertal onset in these two models mimics the clinical onset in humans. In addition, NOD mice and BB rats share immunological features with the human disease, such as the defective central and peripheral tolerance and impaired dendritic cell maturation and function. Further sharing with humans the paramount role of the MHC class II alleles, the two models show that the MHC alone is not sufficient, and there are significant contributions of non-MHC genes.

To date, the wealth of the research has been performed, using the NOD mouse model. Shared features of human and NOD mice are the important roles of environmental and dietary factors. The early gluten exposure has been associated with the T1D onset in human and is essential for T1D to initiate in the NOD mouse. NOD mice also have immune responses to islet self-antigens, such as GAD65, insulin, IA-2 and ICA69 [631]. The NOD mouse has also been utilized to find new autoantigens. In the islets of NOD mice, CD8+ T cells responded to peptides generated from the IGRP [islet glucose-6-phosphatase, catalytic subunit, 2 (G6pc2)] protein. These cells were shown to display cytotoxicity against human β cells, expressing class I HLA (HLA-A*0201) molecules, in a MHC-restricted fashion [632]. This suggests that the T cells potentially respond to the same peptides from human and murine ilset GRP and underlines a promising role IGRP as a new self-antigen in the development of T1D.

Chapter 9

GENETICS OF TYPE 1 DIABETES: A ROLE OF HLA

IDDM1 LOCUS

Structural Organization of the Human Leukocyte Antigens Locus

The genome screens confirmed that the IDDM1 locus (the HLA gene region) is the major genetic determinant of T1D risk (λ_S=2.5-3.6), accounting for 42% of the familial inheritance of type 1 diabetes [633-635]. The contribution of the IDDM1 region is easily detectable in genome-wide linkage analyses as indicated by a LOD-score of 65.8 reported in a consensus analysis of 767 multiplex T1D families [635], or by LOD-score of 116.3 as obtained in the recent whole-genome scanning of 1,435 multiplex diabetic families [636]. The IDDM1 susceptibility locus encompasses the HLA genes. The human MHC spans a 3.5-Mb region of chromosome 6p21 and consists of over 200 genes arranged into three subregions, class I, class II, and class III (Figure 11).

The class I genes encode α peptide chains, which associate with β_2 microglobulin to form the class I molecules (Figure 12A). These are expressed on the surface of all nucleated cells and play a crucial role in the restriction of cytotoxic T cell activity. The HLA class I molecules bind to peptide fragments derived from endogenous antigens and present them for recognition by the TCRs of CD8+ T cells.

The class II (HLA-D) loci are subdivided into at least one A and one B gene. These encode the α and β peptide chains, respectively, which combine to form the heterodimeric class II molecules (Figure 12B). The expression of these molecules is normally restricted to professional APCs, B lymphocytes and activated T cells. The HLA-DR, HLA-DQ, and HLA-DP molecules are involved in the activation of helper T cells. The α1 and β1 domains of these molecules form a cleft, into which peptide fragments derived from exogenous antigens can bind. These peptides are then presented for recognition by the TCRs of CD4+ T cells (Figure 13). The recognition process activates the responding T cells and initiates an immune response.

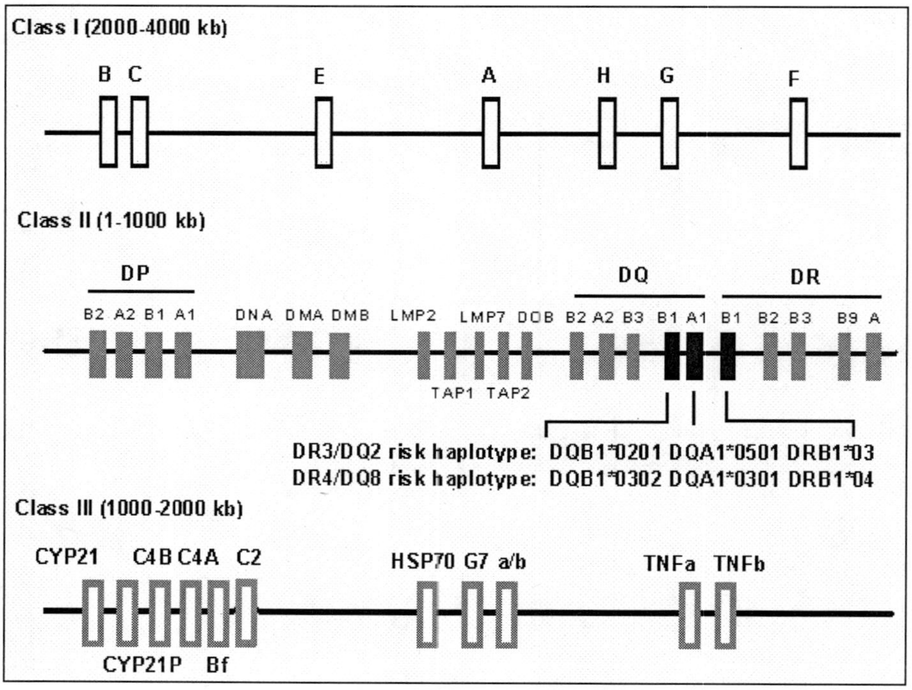

Figure 11. A simplified scheme of the genomic organization of the human HLA gene cluster. HLA class II genes, contributing to HLA-DR3/DQ2 and HLA-DR4/DQ8, two risk haplotype for T1D, are shown in solid black boxes. Abbreviations: TAP, transport associated with antigen processing; LMP, large multifunctional proteasome; HSP70, heat shock protein 70; TNF, tumor necrosis factor.

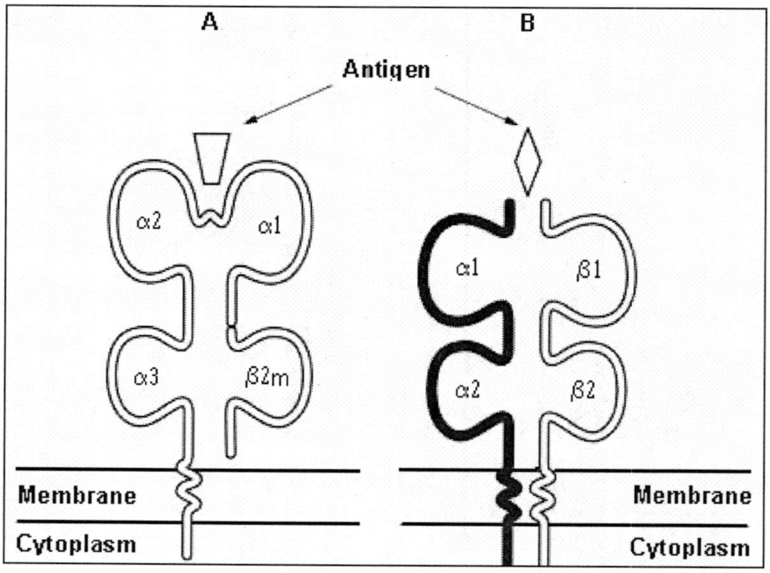

Figure 12. Schematic representation of (A) a HLA class I molecule and (B) a HLA class II molecule, showing the antigen-binding clefts. Both class I and class II molecules are membrane-bound. Class I molecule comprises α peptide chain, which associates with β2 macroglobulin (β2m). A heterodimeric class II molecule includes α and β peptide chains.

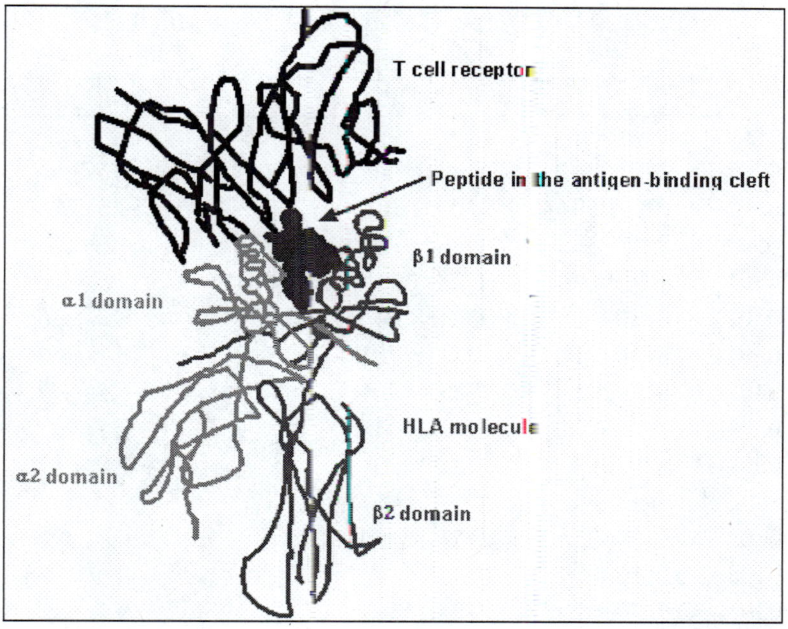

Figure 13. Antigen presentation to the T cell reseptor of CD4+ T helper cell by a HLA class II molecule.

The class III genes encode a range of molecules with a variety of functions, including complement components (C2, C4, and Bf), tumour necrosis factor, and heat shock protein, Hsp70 [637].

HLA-Linked Susceptibility to T1D

Many of the HLA genes are highly polymorphic. The class I and class II molecules encoded by these allelic variants show great variability in their three-dimensional structure, particularly in the antigen-binding regions of the molecules. This has important functional consequences, because the structure of the antigen-binding site determines the way, in which the molecule interacts with a particular antigenic peptide and T cell receptor.

Because the HLA class I and class II molecules play a pivotal role in the activation of T-cell responses, the genes, encoding these molecules, have been implicated in susceptibility to several T cell-mediated autoimmune diseases, including T1D. However, the identification of the primary disease susceptibility determinants within the MHC region is confounded by strong linkage disequilibrium between the genes—that is, particular alleles at distinct loci are inherited together more frequently than expected by chance. The combination of alleles inherited together on the same chromosome is known as a haplotype. It is difficult to distinguish the primary associations with disease susceptibility from associations, occurring secondary to linkage disequilibrium. Despite this complication, recent fine mapping studies in Caucasian populations suggested that the HLA class II genes, DRB1 and DQB1, are the major determinants of IDDM1 encoded susceptibility to type 1 diabetes [637-640].

Table 12. HLA class II alleles associated with T1D

HLA-DQ alleles	HLA-DR alleles	*RR*
Predisposing haplotypes:		
DQA1*0301-DQB*1*0302	DRB1*04	2.5-9.5
DQA1*0501-DQB*1*0201	DR1*0301	2.5-5.0
DQA1*0501-DQB*1*0302	DR1*0301/ DRB1*04	12.0-32.0
DQA1*0301- DQB*1*0201	DR1*0301/ DRB1*04	
DQA1*0301-DQB1*0402	DRB1*04/DRB1*801	4.0-15.0
DQA1*0301-DQB1*0201	DRB1*701	8.0-13.0
DQA1*0301-DQB1*0201	DRB1*901	5.5
DQA1*0301-DQB1*0401	DRB1*04	3.5-4.5
DQA1*0301-DQB1*0303	DRB1*901	2.0-4.5
Protective haplotypes:		
DQA1*0102-DQB1*0602	DRB1*1501	0.03-0.2
DQA1*0103-DQB1*0603	DRB1*1301	0.05-0.25
DQA1*0301-DQB1*0301	DRB1*04	0.2-0.5
DQA1*0501-DQB1*0301	DRB1*1101	0.05-0.5

It is clear that some combinations of *HLA-DQ* genes, i.e. those, encoding DQ8 (i.e. DQA1*03-DQB1*0302) and DQ2 (i.e. DQA1*05-DQB1*02), and particularly those present in HLA-DQ2/DQ8 heterozygotes are associated with susceptibility to T1D (Table 12). Approximately 30% of T1D patients are *HLA*-DQ2/DQ8 heterozygotes [641]. By contrast, a particular DQ6 molecule encoded by HLA-DQA1*0102-DQB1*0602 is associated with a strong protection from the disease, even in the presence of T1D-associated autoantibodies and/or of high-risk HLA alleles [642] (Table 12). The HLA-DQB*0602 allele allele is very rare (has been reported in less than 1% of patients in most populations studied and appears to confer dominant protection [642-644].

Table 13. Critical amino acid residues in the HLA-DRB1*04 β-chain associated with susceptibility to T1D

DRB1*04 allele	Amino acid positions							Strength of the disease predisposition*
	37	57	67	70	71	74	86	
0401	Tyr	Asp	Leu	Gln	Lys	Ala	Gly	++
0402	Tyr	Asp	Ile	Asp	Glu	Ala	Val	+/-
0403	Tyr	Asp	Leu	Gln	Arg	Glu	Val	--
0404	Tyr	Asp	Leu	Gln	Arg	Ala	Val	+/-
0405	Tyr	Ser	Leu	Gln	Arg	Ala	Gly	++
0406	Ser	Asp	Leu	Gln	Arg	Glu	Val	--
0407	Tyr	Asp	Leu	Gln	Arg	Glu	Gly	--

* '+/-', neutral allele; '++', strong predisposition; '- -', strong protection.

It has been more difficult to ascertain the roles of separate HLA-DR genes [645,646]. Analysis of the linkage between HLA-DQ and DR alleles on DQ8-haplotypes, demonstrated that the frequencies of only certain HLA-DR4-associated DRB1 alleles are increased among T1D patients [646]. This has since been confirmed in larger population studies [647-649]. The varying risk conferred by different HLA-DR4 haplotypes is illustrated in Table 13. There is an evidence that the different risk categories are determined by the predicted structure and action of the peptide-binding pockets, P1 and P4, of the DRB1 molecule [650].

The fact that several different class II HLA alleles and combinations of alleles may be associated with T1D can be reconciled by a hypothesis, implicating a factor common to all these alleles that is central to disease susceptibility, i.e. the presence of specific amino acid residues. Indeed, certain amino acids of the HLA-DQB1 and DRB1 chains correlate well with the disease susceptibility and resistance. These residues are known to be critical for the peptide-binding function of the class II molecule [650-654]. In particular, aspartic acid (Asp) at residue 57, which is in pocket P9 of the HLA-DQB1 molecule, is encoded by a HLA-DQB protective allele, while an alanine, valine or serine residue at the same position characterises predisposing alleles. In the absence of aspartic acid the charge at the 'right hand' end of the peptide-binding pocket becomes more positive [655]. Nevertheless, and despite the fact that residue 57 has therefore a pronounced role in the function of class II molecules with respect to peptide binding, it cannot completely account for all the complexity of HLA and T1D associations [656,657]. For example, Asp 57 is not associated with T1D in Japanese [658,659]. Interestingly, the major DQB1 allele associated with T1D in Japan, *0401, has a different residue 56 than other Asp57, bearing allotypes, and it was recently suggested that the residue 56, which is also in pocket P9, may influence the structure and function of this pocket in peptide binding and T1D susceptibility.

The disease risk conferred by HLA-DQ and DR genes may be modified by other MHC class II loci, including the class II HLA-DPB1 gene [660]. An independent association with HLA-DPB1*0301 has been observed [660-662], although this may not be the case on DR4-positive haplotypes [663]. Also, HLA-DPB1*0402 may be associated with protection on HLA-DR4 negative haplotypes [664]. Additional susceptibility loci in the class II region include the antigen-processing genes (TAP1, TAP2, LMP2, and LMP7), although a current evidence suggests that these are not directly involved in T1D [665-667].

A number of observations indicate that class II genes cannot explain all of the MHC associations with T1D. A role for MHC complex genes other than class II genes was first suggested by Thomsen et al. [668] and Pociot et al. [669] by studying HLA-DR3/4 heterozygous individuals, and by Robinson et al [670], using a family study design, which to some degree eliminated the LD effects, involving HLA-DQ/DR loci. However, in all these studies the number of subjects/families was small. Subsequently, several studies have supported a role for both MHC HLA class IV and class I genes in T1D predisposition. The most studied class IV genes are tumor necrosis factor and lymphotoxin (TNFA and TNFB) [669,671-673]. The strongest evidence for susceptibility genes in the class I region comes from the systematic assessment of microsatellite markers, spanning this region [674-680].

Functional Evidence for the Role of HLA Molecules in Disease Pathogenesis: HLA-Transgenic Mice

A direct role for HLA-DR and HLA-DQ molecules in the pathogenesis of type 1 diabetes was demonstrated in studies of HLA-transgenic mice. Most murine starins express the MHC class II molecules I-A and I-E, which are the human homologues of DQ and DR, respectively. In the NOD mice, the only MHC class II molecule (I-A^{g7}) very similar to HLA-DQA1*0301/DQB1*0302 (DQ8), which predisposes to T1D in humans, is expressed [566]. However, other HLA class II molecules (DR3, DR4 and DQ2) are also predispose to diabetes. HLA-transgenic mice allow to study a role of these HLA molecules with or without the presence of other potentially predisposing genes [681]. HLA-transgenic mice have been generated based on crosses between the NOD mouse and murine strains (C57BL/6 and C57/BL10) not-susceptible to diabetes.

One of the potential factors that could hamper the study of a role of human MHC molecules in HLA-transgenic mice is the presense of endogeneous mouse MHC class II molecules, which might interefere with and predominate over interactions with the transgenic HLA molecules. This pitfall was avoided by creating HLA transgenic mice that is deficient for mouse MHC class II (designated I-$A^{b-/-}$ or mII^{-}). Originally, this mutation was specifically targeted to the I-A^{b} molecule on the B6 genetic background [682].

HLA-transgenic animals that have been studied in the presence/absence of endogeneous murine MHC class II did not spontaneously develop insulitis and autoimmune diabetes [683,684]. This is not surprisingly, suggesting that although HLA class II molecules play a key role in susceptibilioty to disease, other factors clearly play a role. This is also true, when the HLA transgene is expressed on the NOD background in the absence of the predisposing I-A^{g7} [685]. Both HLA class I and II molecules are important in determining T1D susceptibility due to the strong LD between those. In knock-out NOD mice deficient for the endogeneous I-A^{g7} allele, MHC class I is also different because of LD with the mutated class II region. In that case, removal of the NOD I-A^{g7} leads to the removal of an important predisposing factor, MHC class I (K^{d}), and this may contribute to the disease resistance found in HLA-transgenic mice.

HLA-transgenic mice are very helpful for the study of peptide binding to the HLA molecules. These mice develop strong immune responces after immunization with GAD and proinsulin, or peptides devrived from these antigens. This facilitated mapping peptide epitopes of GAD65 for HLA-DR4 [330,686], HLA-DQ8 [685,687,688] and HLA-DR3 [689,690]. DQ8-transgenic mice also recognized proinsulin and IA-2 epitopes [691-693].

Although the HLA-transgenic mouse does not develop spontaneous diabetes, both DR3- and DQ8-trangenic mice have insulitis. When both these alleles are present together in a mixed genetic background, insulitis increases [684]. Abraham and coauthors [684] also demonstrated a spontaneous GAD reactivity in DR3/DQ8-transgenic mice, despite the fact that the self-reactive responses in DR3- or DQ8-transgenic mice alone are very week (all in the mixed genetic background). In addition, T-cell lines recognized GAD peptides 247-266 and 509-528 and restricted by HLA-DQ8 have been generated [683].

The presense of autoreactive T cells is unsufficient to develop diabetes in HLA-transgenic mice. For example, DQ8-restricted T cell lines generated in the DQ8-transgenic mouse and specific for GAD peptides 247-266 and 509-528 failed to induce detectable ilset cytotoxicity when transferred into DQ8-transgenic mice [683]. This is not surprising, since murine islets have low contents of GAD and the islet inflammation does not normally occur in HLA-transgenic mice.

Low-dose streptozotocin treatment could be used to cause a limited apoptosis and damage of islet β cells in order to increase the expression of islet antigens in mice [694]. GAD peptide-reactive T cell clones from the DQ8-transgenic mouse induced severe insulitis but did not precipitated diabetes in the recipient animals treated with a very low dose of streptozotocin [683]. In this situation, streptozotocin stimulated the expression of mouse MHC class I molecules (K^b and D^b), human class II (DQ8) molecules and T cell-specific markers (CD3 and CD8) on splenocytes and adhesion molecules ICAM-1 and VCAM-1 on the pancreatic islets, facilitating the homing of GAD peptide-reactive T cells to their target tissue.

Full T cell activation requires both stimulation through the TCR and co-stimulatory sugnal via the interaction of B7.1 or B7.2 molecules with CD28 on the surface of T cells. To evaluate whether the activation of ilset-specific CD8− T cells would stimulate the development of diabetes, DQ8-transgenic mice, lacking endogeneous murine MHC class II (mII^-) and expressing a costimulatory B7.1 molecule under control of the rat insulin promoter (RIP), were generated [695]. These mice were designated DQ8+/RIP-B7.1. Substitution of human HLA-DQ8 molecules for the murine MHC class II caused RIP-B7.1 mice to develop spontaneous insulitis and a high incidence of diabetes, with equal frequency in both sexes like in humans [696]. When murine the MHC class II $I-A^b$ molecules were replaced with human HLA-DR4 alleles in the presence of the RIP-B7.1 transgene, mice also developed spontaneous disease. No diabetes occured in the mouse, when murine MHC class II molecules were substituted by human HLA alleles protective to diabetes [697]. Thus, in this HLA-transgenic model, the induction of T1D specifically requires the presense of diabetogenic HLA alleles, such as DQ8 and DR4. High expression of DQ8 in the thymus resulted in the early onset and 100% incidence of diabetes in DQ8+/RIP-B7.1 mice [698]. In summary, expression of the RIP-B7.1 molecule is likely to have an effect on CD8+ T lymphocytes. The RIP-B7.1-mediated costimulatory effect together with an appropriative stimulus for self-reactive CD4+ T cells selected on diabetes-predisposing MHC class II molecules, is sufficient to facilitate the development of T1D.

HLA-transgenic mouse models, lacked mouse MHC class II molecules and expressed either TNF-α or INF-α (both areproinflammatory cytokines) under control of RIP as transgenes in the islets, were created. When RIP-TNF-α or INF-α was expressed on a B6 background, none of transgenic mice developed diabetes. However, in the presence pf the DQ8 transgene, 60% of DQ8+/RIP-TNF-α and 30% of DQ8+/RIP-INF-αmice developed disease [695,699]. These observations suggest that neither either TNF-α or INF-α are able to induce diabetes alone, while the development of spontaneous T1D is dependent on the presence of DQ8. The presence of the HLA molecule alone is not sufficient to inititiate diabetes, and an environmental stimulus is needed to precipitate the disease.

HLA-DR4/DQ8 and HLA-DR3/DQ2 are the commonest susceptibility haplotypes in T1D. A strong LD between DR4 and DQ8 and between DR3 and DQ2 was shown. The heterozygous combination of DR3/DQ2 and DR4/DQ8 promotes diabetes more strongly than the DR4/DQ8 homoyzgous genotype. This phenomenon was attributed to the transcomplementation of the class II molecules. For example, the α chain encoded by DQA1*0301 (DQ8 α chain) can pair only with the β chain encoded by DQ*0201 (DQ2 β chain), whereas the αchain of DQA1*0501 (DQ2 α chain) pairs with the β chain of DQB1*0302 (DQ8 β chain) [700]. In the HLA-transgenic mouse, it is possible to study a role of individual HLA alleles as well as a role of their combinations. Using this approach, Abraham et al. [684] observed that DQ8/DR3 double transgenic mice developed more insulitis than either DQ8 or DR3 single transgenic mice. In the mouse, coexpressing DQ8 and DR4, a primary role of DQ8 and putative regulatory role of DR4 in the development of spontaneous diabetes was suggested [697]. A severity of insulitis in DQ8/NOD mice was stronger than that in DR3/NOD mice, while the insulitis severity in DQ8/DR3 double transgenic NOD mice was similar to that seen in DR3/NOD mice [701]. It seems that the expression of DR3 transgene decreased severity of insulitis in DQ8/NOD mice, as in the DR4/RIP-B7.1 system on the B6 genetic background [697]. Similar phenomen was observed in humans: DR4 subtypes conferred varying degrees of protection that modify the risk mediated by DQ8 [702,703]. Thus, HLA-transgenic mice provide insight into the way, in which some HLA genes may regulate the effects of others.

In recent years, an important role of CD8+ T cells restricted by MHC class I in the pathogenesis of T1D was suggested. Once the contribution of HLA class I to T1D susceptibility is not so strong as that of the class II molecules, diabetic patients commonly express a number of HLA class I alleles [704,705]. Several HLA class I transgenic murine models have been developed. Among those, HLA-A2.1 and HLA-B27 mice are the most studied [706]. When coexpressed with mouse MHC class I (K^dD^b) and class II (I-A^{g7}) molecules, the HLA-A2.1 transgene accelerated diabetes on NOD genetic background [707]. Reverse immunological studies revealed seven peptides, including those three with the sequence identical to murine proinsulin, which were immunogenic in the HLA-A2 transgenic mouse [708]. Moreover, six of tested proinsulin peptides were processed and presented by insulin-expressing cells, suggesting the property of HLA-A2 molecules to present naturally processed epitopes derived from proinsulin, a primary T1D self-antigen.

Studies, involving HLA class I transgenic mice, are clearly an area of importance and the effects of such transgenes should be examinated in the absence of mouse MHC class I molecules (particularly K^d) known to predispose to diabetes. The development of a such transgenic murine model was recently reported [632]. In the HLA-A*0201 class I transgenic NOD mouse, lacking murine class I molecules, three immunogenic peptides derived from IGRP, a novel potential islet self-antigen, were identified as targets of diabetogenic HLA-A*0201-restricted T cells [632]. These investigations demonstrate a sufficient role of MHC class I genes to the development of autoreactive CD4+ and CD8+ T cell responses against pancreatic β cells that cause type 1 diabetes.

EFFECT OF MOLECULAR STRUCTURE ON THE FUNCTION OF HLA-DR AND HLA-DQ

The influence of the HLA-DR and HLA-DQ molecules on the risk of type 1 diabetes is probably related to their central role in the antigen presentation and activation of a helper T cell-mediated immune response. This function is largely determined by the precise three dimensional structure of the antigen-binding clefts of the molecules, formed by the α1 and β1 domains of the peptide chains. This dictates the way, in which each molecule interacts with antigenic peptides and the TCRs of responding T cells. Studies using X-ray crystallography and computer modelling have suggested that HLA molecules associated with susceptibility to type 1 diabetes share similar chemical and geometric properties in their antigen-binding clefts. These characteristics are strikingly different from those of protective HLA molecules, which again are similar to each other [650,654]. The structural differences between the predisposing and protective molecules are reflected by functional differences in (1) peptide selectivity and binding affinity, (2) the interaction with TCRs, and (3) molecular stability on the surface of the APC.

Peptide Binding

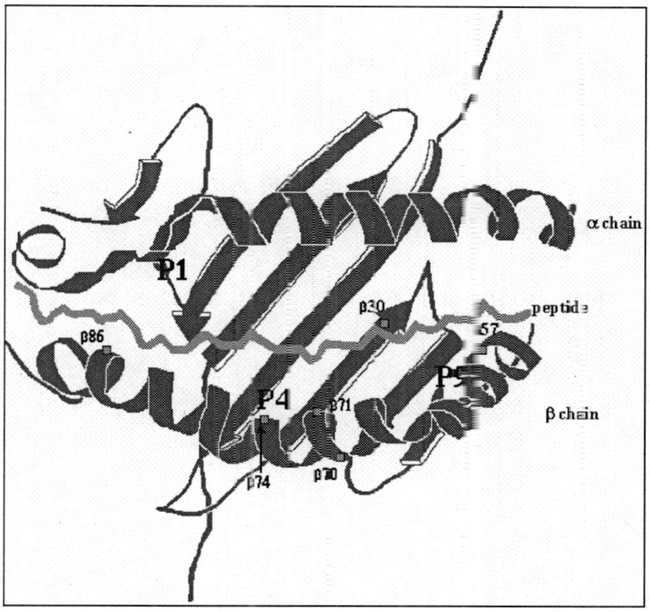

Figure 14. The antigen-binding cleft of a human leukocyte antigen class II molecule, showing the binding pockets (P1, P4 and P9) and the amono acid residues implicated in peptide binding and T cell activation.

The architecture of the antigen-binding clefts of the DR and DQ molecules is very similar (Figure 14). Both molecules bind to peptides of 12–25 amino acids in length, using conserved residues distributed throughout the binding sites. These form hydrogen bonds with the NH_2- and COOH-groups along the backbone of the peptide [709]. Amino acid side chains of the peptide also slot into a series of deep cavities within the binding cleft termed "pockets". These pockets are highly polymorphic and their structure provides the basis for the "peptide-binding motif" of the molecule; that is, the preference for particular amino acid residues at crucial anchor points along the peptide. Structurally distinct HLA molecules favor different peptide-binding motifs dictated by the shape and size of the pockets, and may therefore interact differently with a given antigenic peptide [710-712]. The key determinants of the binding motif are pockets 1, 4, and 9 (P1, P4, and P9, respectively) [650,654].

P1 Pocket

In the HLA molecules that predispose to type 1 diabetes, the P1 pocket is generally much deeper compared with that seen in the protective molecules. For example, P1 in the predisposing DR4 molecules (encoded by DRB1*0401 or DRB1*0405) contains a glycine residue at position 86 of the β chain (β86), which confers a preference for binding to large aromatic side chains in the peptide [650]. Controversy, the valine residue encoded at position β86 in the protective DR4 molecule (encoded by DRB1*0403) creates a preference for small- or medium-sized hydrophobic residues in the peptide. The P1 pockets of the predisposing DQ2 and DQ8 molecules are similarly much deeper than that of the protective DQ6.2 molecule [650].

P4 Pocket

The P4 pocket is an important determinant of peptide-binding selectivity in the DR molecule. The alanine residue at position β74 in the diabetes-permissive DR4 (DRB1*0401) molecule produces a P4 pocket with a high affinity for acidic residues. In contrast, peptides containing acidic residues at this anchor position are unable to bind to the protective DR4 molecule encoded by DRB1*0403 because of the presence of an incompatible glutamate residue at position β74 [713]. The P4 pocket in the DQ molecule is unlikely to play a crucial role in determining susceptibility to diabetes, because its predicted structure is similar in DQ2, DQ8, and DQ6.2 [650,654].

P9 Pocket

Generally, HLA class II molecules that confer the protection against type 1 diabetes carry an aspartate residue at position 57 in the β peptide chain (Aspβ57), whereas those that predispose to the disease carry an uncharged amino acid residue at this position (non-Aspβ57), although there are some exceptions to this rule [714-716]. The residue β57 is located within P9, where it plays an important role in determining the structure of this pocket. In molecules, carrying Aspβ57, a salt bridge is formed between this negatively charged residue and a conserved positively charged residue (arginine) at position α76 (in DR molecules) or α79 (in DQ molecules) [654, 717,718]. This alters the shape of P9 relative to that seen in non-Aspβ57 molecules and hence alters the preference of the molecule for particular anchor residues in the bound peptide. Several studies have suggested that the non-Aspβ57 molecules preferentially bind to peptides with an acidic (negatively charged) residue at the P9 anchor point, because this residue can form a stabilizing salt bridge with the unopposed Argα76 or Argα79 residue. [654,711,719-721]. However, this does not hold true for the DQ2 molecule, which prefers large hydrophobic residues in P9 [722]. This could be attributed to the neighbouring residues, which produce a larger P9 pocket than that found in other non-Aspβ57 molecules, for example, DQ8 [654]. This highlights the importance of the morphology of the entire pocket, rather than the influence of a single residue. Nevertheless, the amino acid residue at position β57 does have a profound impact on the peptide-binding affinity and selectivity of DR and DQ molecules [711,720,723,724]. In summary, the structural differences between the predisposing and protective HLA molecules may result in differences in their ability to bind to diabetogenic antigens. This may determine whether diabetes develops or not, although the mechanisms involved are unclear.

T Cell Interaction

Crystal structures of class II HLA-DR–peptide–αβTCR and class I HLA-A–peptide–αβTCR complexes have been elucidated [725,726]. These clearly show that different TCRs can bind in a similar orientation to different HLA molecules. The TCR presents a relatively flat surface, which is tilted at an angle to bind to the HLA–peptide complex by avoiding peaks or α-helical borders of the antigen-binding cleft (Figure 13) [726]. The activation of a particular T cell, via its receptor, is influenced by the structure of both the HLA molecule and the peptide being presented.

The T cell receptor is thought to have several docking points on the HLA class II molecule that are conserved in all DR and DQ heterodimers. In addition, it interacts with some of the polymorphic residues that distinguish one HLA molecule from another [726]. Thus, the unique combination of amino acid residues that characterises the antigen-binding cleft of a particular HLA molecule will determine, which T cell populations can respond to peptides presented by that molecule. Functional studies of DR and DQ molecules have suggested that residues β70 and β71 may be crucial contact points for T cell recognition of the HLA–peptide complex, and that residues β57 and β30 may also influence T cell activation [727-729].

Residues of the peptide presented in the antigen-binding cleft are also contacted by the TCR. The amino acid side chains of the peptide residues that bind to the P2, P5, and P8 pockets in the HLA molecule (termed p2, p5 and p8, respectively) have been suggested to be crucial for T cell activation [730]. Substitution studies have identified the central residue, p5, as the primary TCR contact point for many peptides. For example, Nepom and colleagues [731] showed that a conservative substitution at the p5 residue of a GAD peptide had little effect on binding to the DR4 (DRB1*0401) molecule, but rendered the DR–peptide complex incapable of stimulating GAD specific T cells from patients with diabetes. In contrast, De Oliveira et al. [730] showed that the TCR interaction with the p5 residue is not always essential for the antigen recognition and can be compensated by interactions with the residues at p2 and p8. Clearly, further research is necessary for detailed understanding TCR–peptide–HLA interactions.

Molecular Stability

In general, the HLA-DQ molecules associated with protection from type 1 diabetes are more stable on the cell membrane than those associated with susceptibility [732]. This could lead to an extended half-life of the "protective" DQ–peptide complexes, which might influence disease risk by altering the strength of the interaction with pathogenically relevant T cells and ultimately affecting their activation status. The stability of the DQ molecule may be determined, in part, by the amino acid residue at position 57 in the β peptide chain. The Aspβ57 residue was shown to be crucial for the stability of the protective DQ6.2 molecule [733,734]. In contrast, however, soluble DQ heterodimers encoded by DQA1*020-DQB1*0302 and DQA1*0201-DQB1*0303 were shown to have similar stability, despite differing only at residue β57 (Ala versus Asp, respectively) [724]. This suggests that other residues must also play an important role in maintaining the integrity of the class II molecule.

Possible Mechanisms, by which HLA Molecules Influence the Development of Type 1 Diabetes

Clearly, the structural differences seen between the predisposing and protective HLA molecules will affect their ability to interact with diabetogenic antigens and the TCRs of autoreactive β-cell specific T cells. Several mechanisms have been proposed to explain how this might influence the risk of developing autoimmune T1D [735].

1. Antigen binding in the periphery: predisposing HLA molecules may bind well to diabetogenic antigens in the periphery and hence activate an autoimmune T cell response, whereas protective HLA molecules may not. Alternatively, the protective molecules may bind to the autoantigens with a higher affinity, thus competing with the predisposing molecules. In this last scenario, the threshold of binding required for T cell activation restricted by the predisposing molecules may not be reached.
2. Molecular stability and thymic deletion of autoreactive T cells: protective HLA molecules may form stable complexes with self-antigens in the thymus, leading to the efficient deletion of potentially autoreactive T cells. In contrast, the less stable complexes formed by the predisposing HLA molecules may result in the inefficient T cell removal and the release of autoreactive T cells into the periphery. However, the negative selection of diabetogenic T cells by protective class II molecules has been demonstrated in one murine model [736], but not in another [737].
3. Influence on T cell phenotype: predisposing and protective HLA molecules may differently interact with the TCRs of autoreactive T cells, affecting the phenotype of the T cells (proinflammatory vs. regulatory) or their activation status (proliferative vs. anergised). This immunomodulatory hypothesis is supported by the observation that

DQ6.2 can protect against the development of diabetes, even after the onset of β-cell autoimmunity [642].

It is unclear exactly which mechanisms are involved in determining the risk of T1D. Currently, functional studies aiming to deal with this question are limited because the antigenic peptide(s) and T cell populations involved in the initiation and perpetuation of the autoimmune attack on the β cells are yet to be identified. Advances in understanding the environmental influences on disease development may be necessary before the progress can be made in identifying the crucial components of β-cell destruction. To identify pathogenically relevant T cell populations, it may be necessary to study individuals at the onset of the autoimmune attack, rather than at the time of clinical diagnosis, when such T cells may no longer be present. Suitable prediabetic subjects for these studies could be recruited from among first-degree relatives of diabetic probands, although intensive monitoring would be necessary to determine the onset of β cell autoimmunity.

Chapter 10

GENETICS OF TYPE 1 DIABETES: ROLE OF NON-HLA GENES

IDDM2: THE INSULIN GENE VNTR

The immune-mediated process, leading to development of T1D is highly specific to pancreatic insulin-producing β cells. The insulin gene, therefore, is a plausible candidate susceptibility locus, since insulin or insulin precursors may act as self-antigens. Alternatively, insulin levels could modulate the interaction between the immune system and the β cells.

Structure of IDDM2 Locus and IDDM2-Linked Predisposition to T1D

In IDDM2, the association to T1D was initially mapped within the 4.1-kb region, spanning the insulin (INS) gene on chromosome 11p15.5 (Figure 15) [738]. In overall, IDDM2 provides a sib risk (λ_S) of 1.2-1.6, accounting for approximately 10% of familial clustering of T1D. The linkage and association between IDDM2 and T1D was continiously confirmed in several genome-wide scans, including a recent whole genome screening in 1,435 multiplex affected families (OR = 1.9) [636]. A unique minisatellite (VNTR), which arises from tandem repetition of a 14-15 bp oligonucleotide sequence with the consensus ACAGGGGTSYGGGG, is located 596 bp upstream of the translational start site of the human insulin gene (INS) on chromosome 11p15.5 [579,580]. The number of tandem repeats varies from about 20 to over 200, and VNTR alleles occur in three discrete size classes: class I (20-63 repeats), class II (64-139 repeats), and class III (141-209 repeats) [580,739,740]. Class II alleles are virtually absent in Caucasians, in whom the frequencies of class I and class III alleles are 0.71 and 0.29 respectively. The class I/I homozygous genotype is associated with a two- to five-fold increase in risk of developing T1D, whereas class III alleles seem to provide dominant protection, although there are exceptions from this pattern for both class I and class III alleles [580,741-746]. Some class I alleles are not predisposing [580,747]. The class I alleles can be subdivided into three groups termed IC+, ID+ and ID-, based on a combination of variant repeat distributions and flanking haplotypes. All class I alleles are equally predisposing to diabetes except the ID- alleles that are protective when transmitted from class I ID-/class III heterozygous fathers [748]. The class III alleles can be also divided into two highly diverged lineages designated IIIA and IIIB. The class III alleles are protective against T1D, while class IIIB alleles are very protective [748]. However, a subgroup of rare class III alleles that appear to predispose to diabetes was found [749].

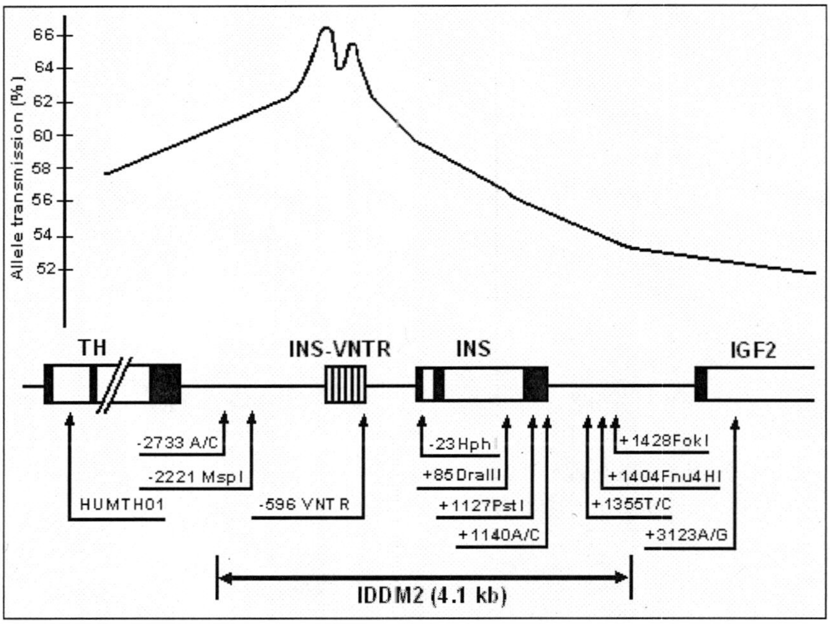

Figure 15. Structural organization of IDDM2 susceptibility locus and neighboring genes. The location of polymorphic SNPs and RFLPs is shown according to their position from the translational start of the insulin gene. Black box are exons, open bocks are introns, and the striped box is the minisatellite (VNTR). The upper curve reflects a percentage of the transmission of alleles, from heterozygous parents to type 1 diabetic offspring in sibling pairs discordant for T1D, of polymorphic markers across the insulin genomic region [742]. Disease-associated alleles should be transferred from parents to affected children with a frequency, significantly exceeding 50%. 5'INS VNTR class I alleles showed a maximum excess (66%) in transmission from parents heterozygous for class I and class III alleles to diabetic offspring, suggesting that the 5'INS VNTR exhibits the strongest linkage to T1D compared to the flanking genomic regions. Abbreviations: IGF2, insulin-like growth factor 2; INS, insulin; INS-VNTR, a variable number of tandem repeats at the 5' region of the insulin gene; TH, tyrosine hydroxylase; HUMTH01, a polymorphic tetranucleotide microsatellite in intron 1 of the tyrosine hydroxylase gene.

In the 7.8-kb region, containing IDDM2, a total of 68 SNPs have been identified [750]. Among those, only the HphI-restriction fragment length polymorphism (RFLP/HphI) and the +3213A>G SNP showed strong association with T1D (Figure 15) [738,745]. The RFLP/HphI marker represents a thymine-to-adenine nucleotide substitution at position –23 upstream the start ATG codon of the INS gene. The –23A allele is shown to be associated with higher risk of T1D [751], but this association may be explained due to the strong LD of the RFLP/HphI marker with predisposing class I alleles of the INS VNTR [750]. The +3213A>G dimorphic site is actually represents a SNP located within the IGF2 gene, encoding insulin-like growth factor 2, at position +1140 from the translation start. This dimorphism is in the strongest LD with VNTR class III alleles [743]. The class III/+3213A haplotype is more significantly associated with lower risk of T1D compared to the class I/+3213G haplotype. The −3213 G/G homozygotes showed an association with an increased risk of disease. However, this genotype is unlikely to be associated with T1D, since it could be found among both susceptible and protective haplotypes [743].

Another gene, flanking IDDM2 locus, encodes tyrosine hydroxylase (TH). A polymorphic tetranucleotide microsatellite HUMTH01 begins at base pair 1170 in intron 1of the TH gene and is located 9 kb apart from the 5'end of the INS gene [752]. The HUMTH01microsatellite consists of 5 common alleles designated Z, Z-4, Z-8, Z-12 and Z-16, which show significant LD with class III alleles of the INS VNTR [753]. The allele Z-8 is associated with a decreased risk of diabetes as a member of extended haplotypes, containing class III alleles [753]. However, the allele Z-8 is occurred in protective haplotypes as well as in predisposing haplotypes [753]. In addition, the HUMTH01 polymorphism itself showed no association with disease [754,755]. Thus, this suggests that this locus is unlikely to be a genetic marker for T1D.

Functional Relevance of the Insulin VNTR and Diabetes Susceptibility

There is some functional evidence that the INS VNTR influences the expression of insulin and other genes in the pancreas. Autopsy studies of human pancreas showed mRNA to be relatively higher for class I then class III alleles [755,756]. In vivo insulin expression was lower in class III/II than in class I/I homozygous individuals, but these results were inconsistent [757-760]. In reporter constructs, when transfected into rodent pancreatic β cells class I alleles exhibited 1.5-3-fold more expression then class III alleles [761]. Only the class I allele 698 showed lower expression than class III alleles when compared in fetal rat islet cells and in insulinoma cell lines, using native insulin and heterologous promoter constructs [579]. The allele 698 showed no association with T1D, and differences in the expression level between this allele and other class I alleles, showing increased expression, might be explained by sequence rather then length differences [580]. Such sequence heterogeneity may account for differences in binding by regulatory proteins. For example, different repeats of the INS VNTR bind Pur-1, a transcription factor, binding to the VNTR to activate transcription from the downstream promoter, with differing affinities [579]. These differences in affinity may relate to structural differences between repeats, particularly the presence of G-quartets. Pur-1 binding was shown to depend on both intra- and intermolecular G-quartet formation of the INS VNTR [762].

Since insulin represents a major autoantigen in T1D, it was postulated that insulin should normally be expressed in the thymus to indice immune self-tolerance [763]. Differential expression of INS associated with the VNTR may in turn then affect thymic selection of insulin-specific T lymphocytes and predispose to β–cell autoimmunity. In the thymus, a relative INS expression was significantly higher (2-3-fold) with class III alleles than class I [763,764]. In the pancreas, the allelic ratio was converse, suggesting for tissue-specific transcriptional effects. The higher levels of proinsulin and insulin in the thymus associated with class III VNTR alleles are postulated to promote self-tolerance through the negative selection of insulin-specific T cells in fetal development [765].

Recently, a significantly higher IL-10 release in memory T cells for the entire proinsulin and the immunodominant INS region was observed in diabetic patients carrying the class III alleles compared to that in affected individuals homozygous for class I alleles [766]. Since IL-10 is produced by CD4+CD25+ Tregs, high insulin levels in the thymus has been proposed to promote the formation of Tregs and therefore contribute to the class III allele-associated protection against the early onset of diabetes.

The IGF2 gene product may also contribute to IDDM2-associated susceptibility to diabetes. Thymic IGF2 was suggested to influence the risk of ilset autoimmunity, because it plays a role in T cell development and negative selection. It may also act as a selecting peptide for insulin-reactive T cells due to its homology to proinsulin [767]. This mechanism is unlikely to account to the disease association observed with the INS VNTR alleles, because the class I and class III alleles are associated with similar levels of IGF2 expression in the pancreas and thymus [767,768]. However, the predisposing class I alleles are associated with increased expression of IGF2 in the placenta [769]. This has been suggested to influence intrauterine growth and birth size, which are both risk factors for T1D [770].

IDDM12: Cytotoxic T Lymphocyte Antigen 4 (CTLA-4)

Structure of IDDM12 Locus and IDDM12-Linked Predisposition to T1D

The IDDM12 locus was mapped to chromosome 2q33, and the strongest evidence for linkage was obtained for D2S72-CTLA4-D2S116 region [771]. The largest family-based study, involving 1,435 affected families, confirmed the linkage of the CTLA4 (IDDM7/IDDM12) region with T1D, providing nominal LOD-score of 3.34 (nominal $P = 9.0 \times 10^5$, genome-wide $P = 0.016$), with sib risk $\lambda_S = 1.19$ and allelic $OR = 1.2$ (for CTLA-4) [636]. This genomic region contains a cluster of three candidate genes encoding T-cell costimulatory receptors CTLA-4 (or CD152), CD28 and inducible costimulator (ICOS) (Figure 16A) [772]. The most of genetic studies in various populations showed an association between T1D and different polymorphic markers within the CTLA-4 gene [773-775], but neither CD28 [776,777] nor ICOS [776]. A recent meta-analysis of 33 population case-control studies, evaluating the relation of three polymorphic markers within the CTLA-4 gene to diabetes, showed a significant association between the +49G allele and higher risk of the disease ($OR = 1.45$, $P < 0.001$) [775]. Thus, as in the case of INS, the putative causative variant at CTLA-4 has a very modest impact on T1D risk.

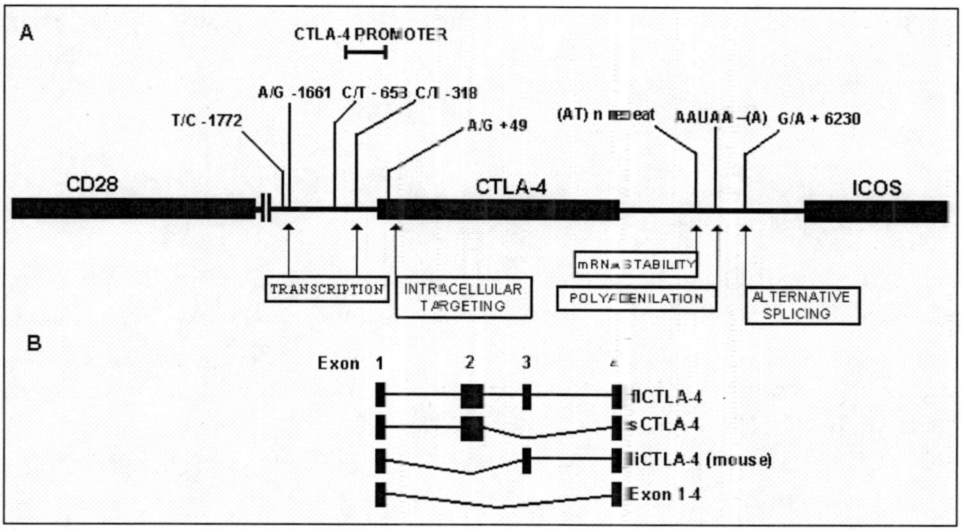

Figure 16. A. Three genes, encoding costimulatory molecules CD28, CTLA-4 (cytotoxic T lymphocyte associated antigen-4) and inducible costimulator (ICOS) located on chromosome 2q33, with positions of functional and potentially functional single nucleotide polymorphisms (SNPs) within the CTLA-4 gene. The –319 and +49 SNPs lie within a highly conserved region (approximately 400 bp), which includes a promoter of the CTLA-4 gene (marked). Potential functional roles of the SNPs are shown in open boxes. B. Various splice CTLA-4 variants. The CTLA-4 gene includes four exons. Exon 1 and 2 encode the signal peptide and ligand-binding domain, respectively. Exon 3 and 4 encode the transmembrane domain and cytoplasmic tail, respectively. Humans express full-length (flCTLA-4), soluble (sCTLA-4) and exon 1-4 splice variants of CTLA-4, whereas mice express an additional, ligand-independent (liCTLA-4) CTLA-4 isoform.

Functional and Genetic Studies of a Role of CTLA-4 Polymorphisms in Predisposing Type 1 Diabetes

A number of polymorphic markers have been identified within the human CTLA-4 gene (Figure 16A). Several SNPs are located at the 5' regulatory/promoter region of CTLA-4. There are only a few studies, evaluating an association between the CTLA-4 promoter polymorphisms and T1D, and all these stydies have been performed in a limited number of patients. In North Indians and South Moroccans, the G allele of -1661 A/G promoter polymorphism, showed association with increased susceptibility to disease [778,779]. For another promoter polymorphism, -318 C/T, the overtransmission of the C allele from parents to diabetic children (*OR* = 1.7, *P* = 0.0017) was demonstrated in a Canadian family-based study [780]. The association between the –318 C/T SNP and T1D was later confirmed in a recent case-control analysis of children, participating in the US Diabetes Autoimmunity Study in the Young (DAISY), which revealed a strong association of the C allele of the promoter polymorphism with higher T1D risk (*OR* = 3.52, *P* = 0.02), but not with persistent islet autoimmunity [781].

Among the CTLA-4 promoter polymorphisms, a nucleotide susbstitution at position –318 was found to be functionally relevant. Several studies showed an association between the -318T allele and increased level of expression both of cell-surface CTLA-4 after cellular stimulation and of CTLA-4 mRNA in non-stimulated T cells [780,782] that could be explained with higher transcriptional activity of the -318T variant of the CTLA-4 promoter [780,783,784]. This can therefore explain the association of the –318T allele with lower genetic risk of T1D.

The –318 polymorphism is located within the 400-bp highly conserved region, which includes the 335-bp promoter sequence essential for the expression of CTLA-4 [785,786]. A thymidine-to-cytosine substitution at position –318 affects the binding sequence for lymphoid enhancing factor 1 (LEF-1), a lymphocyte-specific transcription factor, and hence could mediate regulatory effects of the factor on the transcription of CTLA-4 [780,784]. Using luciferase reporter assay, a differential activation of the –318 C/T promoter variant was observed, when Jurkat T cells and HeLa cells were cotransfected with a plasmid, expressing LEF1 and various CTLA-4 promoter constructs [784]. This observation suggests that the -318 SNP modifies a putative binding site for LEF1 so that it alters the stimulating effect of LEF-1 on the expression ability of the CTLA-4 promoter. Further in vitro and in vivo analyses are necessary to confirm whether LEF-1 binds to the CTLA-4 promoter and the –318 dimorphism is able to modulate transcriptional effects of this regulatory protein.

The (-1661) dimorphism is likely to modify a potential binding site for another regulatory protein, myocyte enhancer factor 2 (MEF2). However, no significant correlation between the (-1661) SNP and MEF2 activity in cotransfection experiments was found [784], suggesting that the (-1661) promoter polymorphism is functionally inactive. Other SNPs located at the 5' regulatory region of CTLA-4 are needed to be evaluated.

The +49 A/G dimorphism situated in exon 1 and resulted in the substitution of an alanine for threonine in the signal sequence of CTLA-4, is the only polymorphism that changes the primary amino acid sequence of CTLA-4 [787]. The majority of population studies, evaluating the contribution of CTLA-4 to genetic predisposition to T1D, have considered the +49 SNP, and most of those showed a strong association between this polymorphic site and disease [774,775,788]. The +49G allele was associated with increased risk of diabetes. In vitro studies of the A49G CTLA-4 have shown that this mutant form of CTLA-4 is aberrantly processed in the endoplasmic reticulum, leading to reduced surface expression [789,790]. The defect in targeting of CTLA-4 to the cell surface can also explain quantitative differences in intracellular CTLA-4 distribution between the A/A and G/G homozygous genotypes observed by Maurer et al. [791], using confocal fluorescence microscopy. The less efficient function of CTLA-4 in G/G homozygous patients could therefore promote T-cell proliferation, leading to autoimmune disease.

There are several polymorphisms located at the 3' untranslated region (UTR) of CTLA-4. Among those, a polymorphic (AT)n repeat was mostly used in family-based studies of T1D susceptibility, such as linkage and TDT analyses [771,773,776,778,792-794]. For this microsatellite, a common allele 17 (which contains 17 (AT)n repeats and is in strong LD with the allele +49G) was associated with higher diabetes risk, whereas the allele 8 was related to reduced risk of the disease [773]. Studies in Swedish T1D patients showed a correlation between the length of the 3'UTR (AT)n repeat and diabetes risk: subjects with alleles, including 17 and more dinucleotide repeats, had significantly higher T1D risk than those, carrying alleles with 8 and less (AT)n repeats [795].

The 3'UTR CTLA-4 microsatellite seems to have functional significance, influencing a stability of CTLA-4 mRNA. Wang et al. [796] found negative correlation between the number of repeats in the 3'UTR mucrosatellite and stability of CTLA-4 mRNA. The authors observed a 1.5-fold increase in steady-state level of CTLA-4 mRNA for the 86-bp allele, containing 7 repeats, compared to the longer alleles [796] The 86-bp allele was shown to be associated with a lower risk of myasthenia gravis, an autoimmune disease. Lymphocytes from patients homozygous for this allele demonstrated the lowest level of T-cell proliferative responses upon the addition of anti-CD28 and anti-CD3 antibodies, which block stimulation of T cells, compared to cells from patients with longer microsatellite alleles [797]. The association of the long AT-repeat allele with reduced control of T-cell proliferation compared to the 86-bp allele was also showed in Japanese patients with Graves' disease, a thyroid-specific autoimmune pathology [798]. These observations could be explained by longer stability of CTLA-4 mRNA in case of the 86-bp allele, which supports elongated suppressive effect of CTLA-4 to the proliferation of T cells.

The increased mRNA stability is one of the major mechanisms, by which synergistic induction of the expression of cell surface CTLA-4 occurs in T cells after stimulation by TCR and CD28 signals [799]. The 3'UTR (AT)n repeats of CTLA-4 could play a role of AU-rich elements, which play an important role in regulating mRNA stability and degradation [800]. Long repeats might destabilize the 3'UTR of CTLA-4 mRNA, which becomes a subject of more rapid degradation compared with the mRNA molecules, containing low numbers of the (AT)n repeats.

In a large population and family-based analysis of patients from the UK, Ueda et al. [801] reported mapping a common susceptibility locus for T1D and autoimmune thyroid disease (AITD), including Graves' disease and Hashimoto's thyroiditis, within the CTLA4 region. This region lies within the noncoding 6.1-kb 3'region of CTLA-4. The susceptibility to an autoimmune disease was determined by an extended disease-associated haplotype, comprising four SNPs (CT60, JO31, JO30 and JO27-1) located within the 6.1-kb region. Among those, CT60 (+6230A/G) marker was functional showing a relationship with the efficiency of splicing and production of a soluble CTLA-4 (sCTLA-4) isoform [801]. Ueda et al. [801] observed less levels of soluble CTLA-4 in patients with the CT60G susceptibility haplotype than in individuals, carrying the CT60A haplotype, therefore suggesting that lower levels of soluble CTLA-4 mRNA are associated with the susceptible haplotype (+49G/+6230G).

A soluble CTLA-4 is a product of the alternatively spliced CTLA-4 transcript, lacking the transmembrane domain encoded by exon 3 (Figire 16B). This CTLA-4 isoform is mainly expressed in non-simulated T cells, while the full-length CTLA-4 (flCTLA-4) has the transmembrane domain and presents on the surface of activated CD4+ and CD8+ T lymphocytes [802,803]. The expression of sCTLA-4 is markedly increased in several autoimmune and allergic disease, that may reflect the dysregulation of T cell activation and should play a role in the pathogenesis of autoimmunity [804]. At present, the function of soluble CTLA-4 is poorly characterized. Since sCTLA-4 maintains the ability to bind CD80/CD86 molecules, this molecule could compete with flCTLA-4 for CD80/CD86 binding sites and cause a reduction of the inhibitory signaling. On one hand, sCTLA-4 may bind B7 expressed on APCs and, indeed, is able to interfere with the B7/CD28-mediated costimulation of T cell responses. This double-faced nature of B7 blocking by sCTLA-4 may result in different outcomes of the clinical course of disease.

Significantly elevated levels of sCTLA-4 were observed in US patients affected with T1D and prediabetic subjects with presenting islet self-antibodies, suggesting that this CTLA-4 isoform might be associated with the pathogenesis of T1D [805]. However, no correlation between the CT60 SNP and expression levels of sCTLA-4 was obtained. In principal, Ueda et al. [801] showed the strongest association between this marker and Graves'disease (OR = 1.51, P = 2.72 x 10^{-8}), while the association of the CT60 SNP with T1D in different population subsets was much less significant (OR = 1.09-1.22, P =0.15-0.018). Recently, Anjos et al. [806] functionally reanalyzed the CT60 SNP located 3' to the known polyadenylation site of CTLA-4. The authors found no effect of this SNP on the expression of either CTLA-4 or ICOS but confirmed an influence of the C/T(-318) promoter polymorphism on the transcription of both full-length and soluble CTLA-4 isoforms. In addition, no CTLA-4 transcript, containing the CT60 SNP or alternatively polyadenylated CTLA-4 mRNA was found [806]. Thus, the functional background for the association of CTLA-4 with autoimmune disease on the basis of implication of the +6230 polymorphism only remains questionable and hence needs further clarification.

Interestingly, mice have an additional CTLA-4 isoform termed ligand-independent CTLA-4 (liCTLA-4) (Figure 16B). This isoform lacks exon 2, encoding the ligand-binding domain, which contains the MYPPPY motif essential for binding to the costimulatory ligands B7.1 and B7.2 [807]. The expression of this alternatively spliced form is depemdent on a SNP at base 77 of exon 2 [801]. In diabetes-resistant mice, base 77 is adenine, whereas in diabetes-susceptible mice base 77 is a guanine. Ueda and coauthors [801] predicted that this polymorphism works by modulating alternative splicing of the CTLA-4 transcript so that the guanine favors the inclusion of exon 2 in te final transcript, whereas the adenine does not. For comparison, the human CTLA-4 base 77 in exon 2 is a thymine that also appears to favor the transcription/translation of flCTLA-4 vs. the liCTLA-4 splice variant, which may explain why liCTLA-4 has not been detected in humans [801].

In humans, a diabetes-associated etiological variant of CTLA-4 seems to be determined by an extended haplotype, which includes functionally relevant polymorphisms across the gene sequence. All polymorphic markers in the CTLA-4 gene were found to lie within the same LD block, which is 100-kb long [808, 809]. Genetic analysis, using tagging SNPs, allows cost-effective approach to reveal all major haplotypes, including those, associated with a disease, and therefore explain complex pattern of LD between adjacent markers within the same LD block [810]. Johnson et al. [808] reported finding 5 'tag' SNPs within the CTLA-4, which are a part all common haplotypes in the LD block, occurring with a frequency of over 5%. There are four promoter polymorphisms (–1722 T/C, -1661 A/G, -658 C/T and –318 C/T) plus +49 A/G marker. In North Indians, Baniasadi et al. [779] found a T1D-predisposing tag 'TGTAG' haplotype, comprising the –318T, -1661G, -1722T, +49A and +6230G alleles of CTLA-4, respectively. A susceptible tag CTLA-4 haplotype reported by Anjos et al. [780] had different composition, consisting of the –318C, -1661A, -1722T, -658C, +49G and +6230G alleles, and was occurred in 34.6% of diabetic Caucasians from the Canadian province of Quebec. The difference in haplotype constitution might be explained by population differences, since the same common risk haplotype was described in type 1diabetic Caucasian patients from the UK, occurring with a frequency of 22.4% [808].

Anjos et al. [780] showed that genetic effects of CTLA-4 promoter polymorphisms to T1D susceptibility are independent on those of markers that lie at the 3'end of this gene, since the removal of the –318T effect significantly strengthened the association with T1D at position +6230. The possibility of two independent effects at the CTLA-4 region complicates the dissection of association haplotypes. In the presence of two functional polymorphisms in the same LD block, when the predisposing allele of one is in LD with the protective allele of other, the genetic effects of individual SNPs are likely to be blunted by an increase in the frequency of haplotypes, which carry one susceptible and one protective allele. In the case of CTLA-4, under the two-effect hypothesis, the predisposing –318C/+6230G haplotype exerts its genetic effect against a background of partically predisposing -318T/+6230G and –318C/+6230A haplotypes, because the protective –318/+6230A is virtually absent due to the LD.

Another interesting thing that has to be explained is the determination of the origin and pathogenic role of increased concentrations of sCTLA-4 in autoimmunity, including T1D. Soluble CTLA-4 mRNA has a shorter half-life than full-length CTLA-4 mRNA [811]. Since both flCTLA-4 and sCTLA-4 have the same 3'UTR encoded by exon 3, the 3'-UTR microsatellite could contribute to the stability of mRNA of both CTLA-4 isoforms. It should be interesting to clarify whether the stability and half-life of the soluble isoform corellates with the length of this dinucleotide repeat. If yes, the (AT)n CTLA-4 polymorphism would represent a valuable genetic marker for the primary estimation of a role sCTLA-4 in T1D.

Immune Regulatory Function of CTLA-4

An evidence for CTLA-4 as an inhibitory immune receptor came from the phenotype of CTLA-4-deficient mice [812]. Five-six days after birth a large percentage of T cells become activated and infiltrate nonlymphoid tissues, resulting in the death of the mice by 3-4 weeks. These mice exhibited severe myocarditis and pancreatitis, lymphadenopathy and splenomegaly, and their peripheral lymphoid organs contained 5-10 times the normal amount of lymphocytes. In the CTLA-4 deficient mouse, T cells displayed phenotypic characteristics of activated T cells (CD69+, CD25+, CD44^{hi}). They were capable to spontaneous proliferation in vitro and production of large amounts of cytokines, such as IFN-γ, IL-4 and granulocyte-macrophage colony-stimulating factor (GM CSF) upon TCR engagement compared to normal mice [813]. The robust expansion of T cells in the CTLA-4 deficient mouse was not due to a defect of apoptosis, since these cells were sensitive to Fas-mediated apoptosis [814]. Together, these observations suggest a generalized and non-controlled expansion of self-reactive T cells, implying that CTLA-4 is involved in the negative regulation of T cell activation.

Experiments in TCR-transgenic mice showed that antigen-specific TCR signaling is necessary for T cell activation in CTLA-4-deficient mice [815]. In addition to TCR-mediated stimulation, these mice require costimulation. Recombinant CTLA-4-Ig can mimic biological effects of native CTLA-4 and effectively block CD28/B7 interactions to binding to both B7.1

and B7.2, therefore preventing CD28-dependent stimulation [816]. Treatment of CTLA-4 deficient mice with CTLA-4-Ig protected the animals from fatal immunoproliferation [817].

The sequence and structure of CTLA-4 is highly similar to those of CD28 [818]. Both molecules are able to bind B7.1 (CD80) and B7.2 (CD86) costimulatory ligands [819,820]. A key feature is that CTLA-4 binds B7.1 and B7.2 with significantly (approximately 10 times) greater avidity and affinity than CD28 does [821,822]. This suggests that inhibitory signals are dominant over costimulatory signals. Since CTLA-4 is primarily an intracellular molecule and is maximally expressed 30- to 50-fold less than CD28 on the surface, following the activation, the stronger CTLA-4/B7 interaction compensates for the bias towards CD28 costimulation [823].

The higher avidity of CTLA-4 for B7 is due to the structural topology of the CTLA-4 homodimer that allows for bivalent binding to B7 [823]. In contrast, CD28 is only able to bind B7 monovalently [824]. Binding of CTLA-4 and CD28 to both B7.1 and B7.2 occurs through the same MUPPPY motif located on exon 2 [818]. The increased CTLA-4 affinity is achieved via the contribution of residues outside of the MYPPPY motif that stabilize interactions with B7 molecules [825].

As mentioned above, a splice variant of CTLA-4, lacking exon 2 and thus having no B7-binding domain, exists in mice [807]. This ligand-independent CTLA-4 isoform is highly expressed in resting memory T cells and appears to be functional as an attenuator of T cell activation. The idea of B7-independent function of CTLA-4 is also suggested by data, linking liCTLA-4 both to the resistance to autoimmune diabetes [807] and to decreased T cell proliferation and IFN-γ production in response to APC/anti-CD3 stimulation [826]. The mecnanism, by which liCTLA-4 may work, is unclear, but it has been linked to decreased phosphorylation of the ζ-chain of TCR and decreased TCR signaling [807]. Ligand-independent CTLA-4 was shown to be able inhibit TCR-ζ more than full-length CTLA-4 [826]. The increased signaling capacity of liCTLA-4 is illustrated by the fact that diabetes-resistant mice display higher expression of liCTLA4 in memory/regulatory T cells than do diabetes-susceptible mice [807].

One remarkable feature of CTLA-4 expression is that most CTLA-4 molecules remain intracellular in vesicles. Only a small portion is expressed on the T cell surface [811]. Upon entering the Golgi, CTLA-4 interacts with AP-1, which mediates its traffic to the cell surface. The CTLA-4 trafficking is regulated through the phosphorylation of Tyr165 in the cytoplasmic tail of CTLA-4, which prevents binding to the AP-2 adapter and blocks endocytosis [827]. Phosphorylation of Tyr165 requires Lck-dependent and ZAP-70-dependent TCR signals and leads to retention of CTLA-4 on the cell surface [828].

T cell inhibition by CTLA-4 is achieved through two mechanisms: competetive antagonism to CD28 signals and direct negative signaling [829]. Engagement of CD28 molecules by B7 induces a costimulatory signaling cascade, which is necessary for TCR-mediated T cell activation. This coordinated signaling leads to the reorientation of intracellular CTLA-4, increasing its surface expression and clustering within lipid rafts at the immunological synapse (IS), a distinct structure observed at the surface between a T cell and an APC, interacting to each other, during the presentation of an antigenic peptide [830]. In the IS, CTLA-4 competes with CD28 for B7 engagement and reduces the amount of CD28-dependent costimulation due to greater ovidity and affinity for B7 binding compared to CD28

[829]. This mechanism does not need the obligatory envolvement of the cytoplasmic tail of CTLA-4 [831]. However, the cytoplasmic tail plays a role in proper partitioning of the CTLA-4 molecule within lipid rafts at the IS, because tailless CTLA-4 may be not able to provide properly the competitive antagonism to CD28 [832].

The second mechanism of CTLA-4-mediated T cell inactivating is the delivery of an inhibitory signal through its cytoplamic tail. In contrast to the antagonism of CD28 costimulation, this mechanism is operational, when CTLA-4 is expressed at low levels on the T cell surface [829]. There are three models proposed to explain this mechanism:

1) CTLA-4 inhibits the early events of TCR signaling
2) CTLA-4 inhibits events downstream of TCR and CD28 signaling;
3) CTLA-4 directly inhibits CD28-mediated signaling

Besides that, CTLA-4 negatively regulates cytokine production through the inhibition of accumulation of transcription factors AP-1, NK-κB and NFAT in the nucleus of activated T lymphocytes [833] and downregulates cell proliferation by inhibiting cyclin D3, cyclin-dependent kinases 4 and 6 and the degradation of cell-cycle inhibitor $p27^{kip1}$ [834]. In addition, both CTLA-4 and CD28 may control the threshold for T cell activation by regulating the expression of E3-ubiquitin ligase Cbl-b [835]. Cbl-b plays an important role in the immune regulation, since Cbl-b-deficient mice become sensitive to autoimmune disorders [836]. CD28 inhibits the expression of Cbl-b, while B7 ligation by CTLA-4 is associated with the reexpression of this ligase [836].

The cytoplamic domain of CTLA-4 lacks intrinsic enzymatic activity but contains several potential protein-protein-interacting motifs. To identify a possible role of the cytoplasmic tail of CTLA-4 in inhibiting early TCR signaling, the initial studies have been focused on the evaluation of the role of two tyrosine residues (Tyr165 and Tyr182), the location of which could provide a putative SH2-binding site. These tyrosine residues can be phosphorylated in vitro by a number of signaling thyrosine protein kinases, such as Lck, fyn, lyn, Rlk and Jak2 [837-839]. Phosphorylation of Tyr165 was suggested to cause the recruitment of SHP domain-containing tyrosine phosphatase 2 (SHP-2) and downregulate early TCR signaling via reducing tyrosine phosphorylation of TCR-ζ, LAT (linker for activation of T cells) and Ras regulator p52SHC [837]. However, mutation of Tyr165 or Tyr182 showed that neither of these residues are required for CTLA-4 T cell inhibition. In contrast, the mutation of Tyr165 accelerates the inhibitory effects of CTLA-4 as a result of higher surface expression due to inability of the mutant protein to be internalized [840]. Coimmunoprecipitation of SHP-2 with CTLA-4 failed to be reproduced in different systems, including human T lymphocytes [831,840]. These findings suggest that the negative signaling through CTLA-4 is likely mediated independently from the tyrosine phosphorylation.

Another group of studies was focused on the verification whether CTLA-4 inhibits signaling events downstream of the TCR. Schneider et al. [841] showed the differential role of B7/CTLA-4 binding in the regulation members of MAPK family by inhibiting ERK activity, while maintaining JNK activity, that finally leads to the inhibition of IL-2 production. The inhibitory effect of CTLA-4 on the activity of ERK-1/-2 is mediated through the interaction with serine/threonine phosphatase PP2A [842,843]. PP2A is a trimeric enzyme composed of a core enzyme, which comprises a catalytic subunit PP2AC and a scaffolding subunit PP2AA, and a regulatory subunit PP2AB [844]. In its interaction with CTLA-4, the A subunit of PP2A binds the lysine-rich motif located at lysine residues 152,155 and 156 of the juxtamembrane region of CTLA-4, whereas the C subunit binds the Tyr165 residue [842]. Newly synthesized CTLA-4 associates with PP2A, and the inhibitory activity of this complex is absent. Upon CTLA-4-TCR colligation, the A subunit of PP2A is tyrosine-phosphorylated, and PP2A dissociates from CTLA-4 (Figure 17) [842]. In resting T lymphocytes, PP2A is also able to associate with CD28, and their complex is likely to be inactive [843]. Upon T cell activation, CD28 is tyrosine-phosphoryalted by Lck, and this correlates with its dissociation from PP2A. Thus, PP2A acts as a negative regulator of the function of both immune receptors.

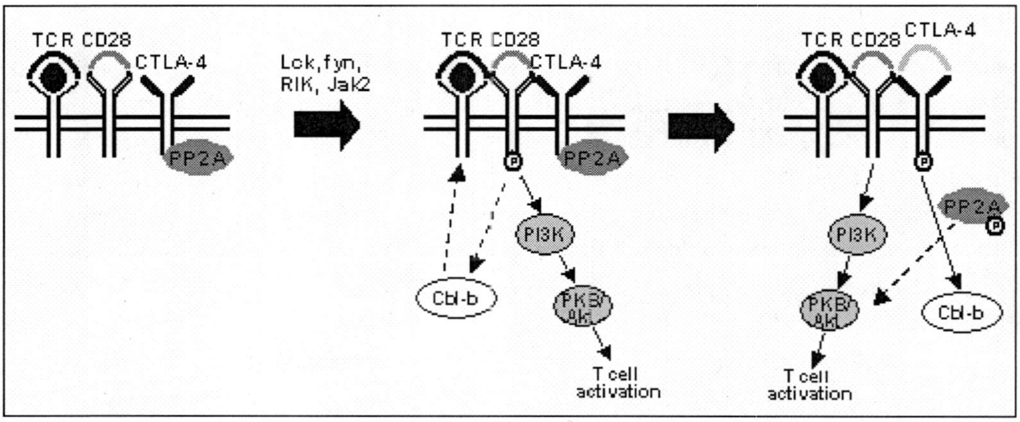

Figure 17. Mechanisms of CTLA-4-dependent T cell inactivation: crosstalk between CTLA-4 and CD28. Phosphorylation of CD28 in a Lck/ZAP-70-dependent manner by different protein kinases leads to its activation. Phosphorylated CD28 activates PKB/Akt in a PI3K-dependent manner, leading to the downregulation of the E3 ubiquitin ligase Cbl-b. Engagement of CTLA-4 with B7 leads to the phosphorylation of CTLA-4 and correlates with both the phosphorylation and dissociation of phosphatase PP2A from the cytoplasmic tail of CTLA-4. The dissociation causes the inhibition of the PKB/Akt signaling and/or enhances the activity of Cbl-B. Together, these events may mediate the inhibition of downstream signaling events. The symmetry between CD28 and CTLA-4 signaling interactions suggests that these two receptors may regulate each other via sequestration/blockage of their respective functions. Arrows denote positive regulatory events, dashed arrows denote inhibitory events, circled P denotes phosphorylation.

The precise mechanism of CTLA-4 and CD28 inhibition by PP2A is unknown. PP2A can inactivate protein kinase PKB/Akt, a major component of the CD28 signaling pathway dependent on phophatidylinositol 3-kinase (PI3K) [845]. From this, a model of the inhibitory action of CTLA-4 was suggested, in which CTLA-4 is not inhibitory when bound to PP2A and not ligated with B7.1/B7.2 ligand. This could happen in resting T cells [846]. Upon ligation of CTLA-4 with the TCR, PP2A would dissociate from CTLA-4 and be free to inactivate Akt, therefore mediating the inhibitory function of CTLA-4. Some experimental evidences favor this model. Because PP2A, PI3K and Grb2 all bind the YMNM motif of CD28, the dissociation of PP2A allows the binding of PI3K and Grb2 and further induction of CD28-dependent costimulation. Okadaic acid, an inhibitor of PP2A [847], is observed can partially inhibit IL-2 production upon TCR/CD28 ligation [843]. T cell activation through

CD28 was shown to be enhanced in T lymphocytes, lacking CTLA-4 [848]. Thus, CTLA-4 may inhibit T cell activation by downregulation of CD28 costimulatory signaling through the direct transfer of PP2A from CTLA-4 to CD28 or through phosphatase activity of PP2A on downstream steps of CD28 signaling, such as Akt.

CD28 and CTLA-4 both have the YVKM motif, to which the binding of PI3K is occured [838]. The ability of both receptors to bind PI3K suggests that CTLA-4 could potentially exchange PP2A and PI3K, sequestering PI3K and thereby reducing its ability to mediate CD28-dependent stimulation. In summary, CTLA-4 and CD28 share a set of mechanisms that regulate themselves and countregulate each other. PP2A is a very likely player of this role, inhibiting the function of the receptor when bound to it and simultaneously enhancing signaling by the other receptor through a Lck/PI3K/Akt-dependent manner.

CTLA-4 functions not only as a T cell inhibitor. Depending on the conditions of engagement, CTLA-4 could act as a positive regulator or as a negative regulator of T cell activation. In early studies, an ability of CTLA-4 to promote T cell expansion via the interaction with B7.1 was shown in CD28-deficient T cells [849]. Experiments with a recombinant ligand of CTLA-4, representing a bispecific tandem single chain Fv (ScFv) molecule directed against two different human-specific epitopes of CTLA-4, resulted in obtaining a direct evidence for the dual role of CTLA-4. The ScFv molecule is recognized by anti-CTLA-4 antibodies 24 and 26 (thus named 24/26) [850]. The 24/26 antibody effectively blocks the interaction of CTLA-4 with B7. The 24/26-mediated T cell activation is dependent on the TCR/CD3 complex formation and Lck and can be further enhanced by CD28 costimulation. This stimulating signal arises from the CTLA-4 triggering of Lck-dependent, TcR-ζ-dependent signaling cascade, following by phosphorylation of TcR-ζ and LAT and activation of ZAP-70, ERK-1/-2 and PLC-γ1 [850]. In contrast to the CTLA-4/B7 ligation, which resolves PP2A from the complex with CTLA-4, the 24/26 binding to CTLA-4 is likely to stabilize the PP2A/CTLA-4 association that then activates bystander Lck and leads to T cell activation. The above observations suggests for a role of PP2A as a critical regulator of CTLA-4 function both as an inhibitor and as an activator [842].

CTLA-4 plays an important role in maintaining the immune self-tolerance. In mice, immunoregulatory CD4+CD25+ T cells constitutively express CTLA-4 [213], although it remains to be seen whether such a specific role can be ascribed in humans. In fact, signaling via CTLA-4 is essential for the function of these cells [851]. CTLA-4 may regulate signal transduction in the thymocyte, which leads to its differentiation into the regulatory cell. CTLA-4 engagement on the effector cells may alter signal transduction and subsequent cytokine production.

The interaction between CTLA-4 and B7.1/B7.2 ligands is one of the mechanisms, by which CD4+CD25+ Tregs deliver their inhibitory signals on effector T cells. Both ligands are essential in CD25+ cell-mediated suppression in vitro, as their absence from effector T cells results in notably reduced susceptibility to suppression by CD4+CD25+ suppressor T cells compared with that of wild-type effector T cells. Based on these observations, the ligation of B7.1/B7.2 on T cells by the cell surface molecule CTLA-4 on suppressor cells was postulated to cause 'outside-in' signaling by B7.1 and/or B7.2 ligands and to result in suppression [247].

The function of CTLA4/B7 receptor-ligand pair in the T cell-T cell interaction differs from that postulated for the same receptor-ligand pair between CTLA-4 on suppressor T cell and B7.1/B7.2 ligands on DCs, resulting in the activation of indoleamine 2,3-dioxygenase (IDO). IDO is responsible for the metabolism of the essential amino acid tryptophan. Reduced amounts of free tryptophan after induction of IDO are associated with decreased activation of T cells and thus this would represent an APC-dependent mechanism of in vitro suppression [852].

In addition, CTLA-4 engagement has been shown to enhance the secretion of TGF-β by CD4+CD25+Tregs that suppress target T cells through the downregulation of the synthesis of IL-2R α chain (CD25) [853,854]. Thus, this evidence represents the indirect mechanism, by which CTLA-4 mediates the cell-to-cell suppression by Tregs. This also helps to understand why the complete inhibition of the suppressing activity exerted by human Tregs could be achieved only with the contemporaneous neutralization of both CTLA-4 and TGF-β [854].

CTLA-4 is involved in the maintainance of tolerance in autoimmune diseases. Treatment of mice with antibodies against CTLA-4 leads to the exacerbation of autoimmunity [855]. Adoptive transfer of ovalbumin-specific T cells from the DO.11 TCR-transgenic mouse into mice, expressing ovalbumin in pancreatic islets, induced acute insulitis and diabetes only if endogeneous lymphocytes, including Tregs, were removed [856]. When ovalbumin-specific CD25-negative T cells were transferred into islet-antigen-expressing mice, peripheral immunization with ovalbumin in adjuvant was needed to induce diabetes. In contrast, naïve CTLA4- and CD25-negative ovalbumin-specific T cells developed into Th1 effectors and initiated disease upon recognition of the self-antigen alone [856]. These results suggest that CTLA-4 functions to increase the activation threshold of autoreactive T cells, because in its absence self-antigen is sufficient to trigger autoimmunity without peripheral immunization. These observations also suggest that CTLA-4 and Tregs could act cooperatively to maintain tolerance, indicating that the function of CTLA-4 may be independent of regulatory cells, and deficiency of both is required to induce pathologic immune responces against the islet self-antigen. Eggena et al. [856] proposed a model, explaining the cooperativity of CTLA-4 and Tregs in maintaining self-tolerance. In this model, CTLA-4 may function at early stages of T cell development and differentiation, increasing the threshold for initial T cell activation, such that self-antigens by themselves are uncapable of activating naïve T cells [857]. Tregs may function later in T cell responces to block proliferation an differentiation at the site of self-antigen, regardless of the initiation trigger. However, more studies are required to verify and confirm the model suggested by Eggena and colleagues [856].

Lymphoid Protein Tyrosine Phosphatase (LYP) Encoded by the PTPN22 Gene: A Novel Susceptibility Locus for T1D and other Autoimmune Diseases

Recent advances in discovery of genes, conferring risk of developing diverse autoimmune disorders, include the identification and characterization of the etiological variant of human lymphoid protein phosphatase (LYP) encoded by the PTPN22 gene, which contributes to the pathogenesis of several autoimmune diseases, including T1D [858]. However, the current knowledge of LYP is mainly based on the information on its mouse homolog PEST domain enriched protein tyrosine phosphatase (PEP). The N-terminal protein phosphatase domain is highly similar in both human and murine enzymes, but the central portion is significantly differed [859]. Both enzymes are strictly expressed in lymphocytes, including T cells.

Murine and Rodent Homologs of Human PTPN22 and their Role in Autoimmunity

PEP (PEST-enriched phosphatase) is a 807 amino acid residue protein encoded by the murine orthologue of PTPN22, Ptpn8. Recent findings showed that susceptibility/ resistance to autoimmune diabetes in the Ptpn8 locus is determined by several non-coding SNPs that could alter splicing or expression of this phosphatase [860]. In addition, the Ptpn8 congenic strains differentially expressed one of the three PEP isoforms examined. A congenic interval, having the Ptpn8 gene, influenced the frequency of T1D in the NOD mouse [860]. Interestingly, a similar mechanism, by which a disease-associated genetic variation could contribute to autoimmunity, was shown for both mouse and human CTLA-4 gene [801].

PEP represents a powerful negative regulator of TCR-mediated signaling, inhibiting the activation and proliferation of T lymphocytes through the dephosphorylation of tyrosine 394 of Lck, tyrosine 417 of fyn and ZAP-70 [859,861]. For dephosphorylation of Lck and Fyn, activating protein kinases, binding the SH3 domain of Csk, an inhibitory protein kinase, to PEP is required [862]. In murine T cells, about 5% of Csk is in the complex with 25-50% of PEP, and the Sck-PEP complex exerts a synergetic inhibition of TCR signaling [863].

The Lyp-Csk interaction is crucial for normal regulation of the immune response in humans, and breakage of this interaction leads to the development of various immune defects and autoimmunity [864]. In the thymus of PEP-deficient mice, a clonal expansion of populations of memory and effector T cells was observed [865]. In the spleens, there was a spontaneous development of germinal centers, which are shown to serve as important sites for immune dysregulation in the pathogenesis of autoimmune disorders [866]. In the effector T cells from the PEP -/- mouse, the phosphorylation of both tyrosine 394 of Lck and ZAP-70 was substantially enhanced [865]. These observations suggest for a crucial role of PEP in the negative regulating of T cell development and function.

In rats, the Ptpn8 gene, a homolog of the murine Ptpn8 and human PTPN22, was found to be located in the Cia10 locus, harboring a major autoimmune arthritis-regulatory gene [867]. However, a sequence analysis of the Ptpn8 cDNA revealed no polymorphisms between the control rodent strain DA and susceptible congenic strain DA.ACI (Cia10). Other members of regulatory signaling pathways in T cells were shown to be associated with autoimmune disorders, such as diabetes and autoimmune arthritis in animal models of autoimmunity. In Komeda diabetes-prone (KDP) rats, there is the Casitas B-lineage lymphoma b (cblb) gene located within the KDP1 susceptibility locus and encoded a member of the Cbl/Sli family of ubiquitin-protein ligases, participating in the suppression of TCR-induced T cell activation [868]. A nonsence mutation, inactivating the cblb ligase, caused massive infiltration and expansion of lymphocytes into pancreatic islets, thyroid gland, kidney and other non-lymphoid organs in KDP rats [869]. A point mutation, tryptophan-to-cysteine substitution at residue 163 (W163C), in the murine gene, encoding a tyrosine kinase ctitical for TCR signaling, ZAP-70, led to the alteration of downstream signaling events, following T cell activation, hyperproliferation of antigen-specific T cells, reduced negative selection of T cells in the thymus and spontaneous autoimmune arthritis [870].

Human Lymphoid Protein Tyrosine Phosphatase (LYP) Encoded by the PTPN22 Gene is Involved in the Pathogenesis of Type 1 Diabetes

The PTPN22 gene, encoding lymphoid protein tyrosine phosphatase (LYP), a suppressor of T cell activation, is located on chromosome 1p13, spans a genomic distance of 57 kb and consists of 21 exons [871]. Human LYP is a 105-kD protein expressing in lymphocytes and containing an N-terminal catalytic tyrosine phosphatase domain, which shares a high similarity with other nonreceptor tyrosine phosphatases. Within the last N-termimal 200 amino acid residues, there are four proline-rich motifs (P1-P4), the first of each physically associates with the SH3 domain of the Csk kinase, an important suppressor of the Src family kinases Lck and Fyn, which mediate TCR signaling [862,872] (Figure 18). In addition to Sck, LYP is reported to associate with the adapter protein Grb2 [873] and the c-Cbl protooncogene [871]. LYP is among the most powerful inhibitors of T cell activation. The suppressing effect is accomplished by dephosphorylation of TCR-associated kinases, such as Lck, Fyn and ZAP-70 [859,862]. Dephosphorylation of ZAP-70 may be connected to the negative regulatory function of the c-Cbl protooncogene, as LYP forms a complex with c-Cbl [871].

A functional SNP, representing a cytosine-to-thymine substitution at nucleotide 1858 of the PTPN22 gene, was found [874]. This changes an arginine (CGC) to tryptophane (TGG) in codon 620 (R620W). Bottini et al. [874] first reported an association between the Trp620 variant with higher risk of T1D in the independent datasets from USA (OR = 1.83) and Sardinia (*OR* = 2.31) (Table 14). The finding of Bottini et al. [874] on the association between the PTPN22 R620W polymorphism and T1D was rapidly replicated in several case–control [875-881] and family-based [875-877,880,882-886] studies (Table 14 and 15). As resulted from the large-scale population study of Concannon et al. [875], the PTPN22 R620W molecular variant provides an average *OR* of about 1.7 for T1D, a value that is higher than *OR* showed by disease-associated polymorphisms of CTLA-4 (1.2-1.5). However, the estimated sib risk (λs) for the PTPN22 R620W is small and does not exceed 1.05 [875]. Based on the observed *OR*, the contribution of *PTPN22* to type 1 diabetes is approximately 2%, much lower than HLA (40–50%). Nevertheless, the knowledge that *PTPN22* may be involved in risk to type 1 diabetes, as well as in other autoimmune diseases, is significant and could provide insight into modulating T cell activity for disease prevention.

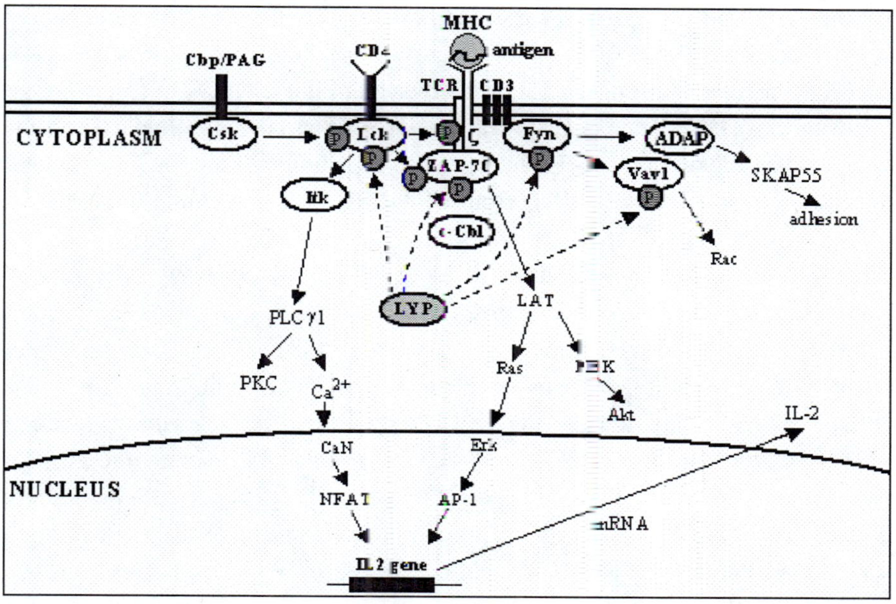

Figure 18. A known and putative role of lymphoid tyrosine phosphatase (LYP) in T cell receptor (TCR) signaling. LYP could negatively regulate TCR-induced T cell activation through the dephosphorylation of Lck, Fyn, Vav1, TCR-ζ and ZAP-70, i.e. signaling molecules that play a critical role in TCR signaling. The dephosphorylation of ZAP-70 could be mediated via the association with the c-Cbl protooncogene. Suppression of the activity of Lck and ZAP-70 leads to decreasing mobilization of intracellular Ca^{2+} and inhibition of downstream events in the LAT/Ras/Erk-dependent signaling pathway that regulates the expression of IL-2, a cytokine, whose main function is to stimulate the growth and cytotoxic response of activated T lymphocytes. Arrows denote positive regulatory events, dashed arrows denote inhibitory events, circled P denotes phosphorylation.

Table 14. Population case-control studies of the association between the R620W polymorphism of the PTPN22 gene and T1D

Population	Cases, *n*	Controls, *n*	*OR* (genetic marker)	*P*	Reference
US Caucasians	294	395	1.83 (+1858T)	5.99×10^{-4}	[874]
Sardinia (Italy)	174	214	2.31 (+1858T)	0.047	[874]
UK Caucasians	1,599	1,718	1.78 (+1858T)	1.17×10^{-14}	[875]
US Caucasians (Florida)	396	1,178	3.4 (+1858T/T)	0.008	[876]
Dutch	334	528	2.3 (+1858T)	2.0×10^{-7}	[877]
Colombian	110	308	1.83 (+1858T)	0.06	[878]
German	220	239	1.88 (+1858T)	0.0009	[879]
Finnish	546	538	4.6 (−1858T/T)	1.3×10^{-5}	[880]*
Ukranian	296	242	1.6 (−1858T)	0.0036	[881]

* OR and P-values are given for association with the appearance of islet autoimmunity (insulin antibodies).

Since the contribution of PTPN22 into the familial clustering of diabetes is very low, the detection of linkage at $P < 0.001$ with 50% power for loci, displaying so modest genetic effect ($\lambda s < 1.1$) needs at least 8,000 affected sib pair families [875]. Thus, it is not surprising that no linkage to T1D was detected for marker D1S206 at chromosome 1p13 in the largest genome-wide scan, envolving 1,435 affected families. Similar results have been obtained in screening 406 affected sib pair families from USA ($LOD = 0.75$), with the predicted sib risk of 1.23 [882].

A large population study of Smith et al [875] revealed no significant sex-specific association of this marker with disease in the UK Caucasian, US Caucasian and Romanian family datasets [875]. However, Ladner and coauthors [883] observed a more preferential transmission of the +1856T allele from parents to female diabetic siblings (P = 0.036) then to male siblings (P = 0.061) in the independent US Caucasian family dataset. In contrast, the transmission rate to affected boys (67.1%, $P = 0.0004$) was higher than that to girls (55.3%, $P = 0.317$) in Finnish diabetic families [880]. Kahles et al. [879] reported a higher strength of the association of the +1856 SNP with T1D in German females (for the +1856T allele, $OR = 3.21$ and $P = 0.0001$) than in males ($OR = 1.27$; $P > 0.05$). These results could suggest for the existence of the diabetes-related sex-specific mechanism, by which PTPN22 could drive immunity in females. For HLA-DR3/non DR4 patients, the male/female bias was shown [887]. These sex-specific differences have been explained by a T1D susceptibility locus on chromosome X, which is also interacts with the HLA region in T1D [888]. For PTPN22, the sex-specific mechanism has to be elucidated, as well as more population studies are required to support this phenomenon.

Table 15. Family-based studies of the association between the R620W polymorphism of the PTPN22 gene and T1D

Population	Families, *n* (subjects, *n*)	*RR* (genetic marker)	*P*	Reference
UK Caucasians	791 UK (1,087 trios)	1.66 (+1858T)	8.6×10^{-9}	[875]
US Caucasians	391 (636 trios)	1.73 (+1858T)	1.0×10^{-5}	[875]
Romanian	261 (233 trios)	1.54 (+1858T)	0.04	[875]
US Caucasians	406 (1960)		0.5×10^{-5}*	[882]
US Caucasians	341 (1711)		0.005*	[883]
US Caucasians	249 (746)**	*OR* = 2.49 (+1858T)***		[884]
US Caucasians (Florida)	410		< 0.003*	[876]
Dutch	218	*OR* = 3.3 (+1858T)	9.0×10^{-9}	[877]
Canadian (Montreal)	588		1.7×10^{-5}*	[885]
UK Caucasians	89 (472)	*OR* = 1.46 (+1858T)	0.046	[886]
Finnish	245		0.001*	[880]

* for the +1858 T allele; ** families with multiple autoimmune disorders, including 61 T1D cases; *** *OR* was calculated on the basis of frequency of the +1858T allele in 2,064 control subjects.

Some data suggest that the +1856 polymorphism of PTPN22 could be associated with anti-islet autoimmunity and its progression to T1D. In the US DAISY Study, 81 relatives of T1D patients, who had the highest risk haplotype DR3/DR4-DQ8, have been selected and genotyped for the +1856 SNP, but no relationship between this marker and diabetes progression have been revealed [889]. However, in this study, only one of the 81 individuals analyzed had the T/T genotype and only 12 had the C/T genotype that makes the conclusion on the absence of association between the codon 620 PTPN22 dimorphism and progression to T1D to be doubtful. In the much large population sample from Finland, a strong association between the +1856T variant of PTPN22 and the appearance of insulin antibodies was shown [880]. The highest risk of the appearance of IAA (OR = 4.5, P = 0.000013) was observed in individuals, carrying the predisposing T/T genotype. The effect of PTPN22 on the appearance of IAA was more pronounced in the high-risk HLA DR3-DQ2/DR4-DQ8, which could be explained by the higher number of disease-predisposing HLA heterodimer molecules, that promotes the autoimmune process in the former individuals. In addition, the +1856T allele of PTPN22 conferred an increased risk of developing additional autoantibodies or progression to T1D (*OR* = 4.1, *P* = 0.003) [880]. These data suggest that the R620W polymorphism of PTPN22 may be directly involved in the control of insulin-specific humoral autoimmunity and an overall progress of β-cell autoimmunity to clinical diabetes. Since the Finnish population is characterized with the highest incidence of T1D, the above observations should be evaluated in other high-risk and low-risk populations to conclude whether the observed evidences are only specific for Finland or could be shared with other ethnic backgrounds.

The codon 620 PTPN22 dimorphism was not found in Asian (Japanese and Korean) poulations [886,890]. Kawasaki et al. [886] sequenced regulatory and coding regions within the PTPN22 gene and identified five novel SNPs. Among those, the new –1123 G/C promoter polymorphism showed association with T1D in the Japanese (*OR* = 1.42, *P* = 0.015) and Korean (*OR* = 1.41; *P* = 0.0105) populations [886]. This polymorphic site is in strong LD with the +1856 C/T SNP. Furthermore, the +1858 T allele is in near-perfect LD with the G allele at position -1123. The new promoter polymorphism of PTPN22 is reported to alter the putative consensus sequence for binding transcription factor AP-4 and indeed might be functionally active. The minor –1123C allele contains a mutated binding site for AP-4 and hence is expected to display a decreased affinity for binding this regulatory protein. This needs to be evaluated functionally.

Qu et al. [885] found that the PTPN22 R620W SNP is located within a LD block, spanning 293 kb. This block includes 6 genes and more than 600 SNPs available in NCBI dbSNP database (January 2005 release; (http://www.ncbi.nlm.nih.gov/SNP/). Among those 600, a number of SNPs alter a sequence of potential regulatory elements that assumes a possibility for their finctional relevance. One of the SNPs, rs6679677, is a cytosine-to-adenine substitution, which is situated 1496 bp downstream of the R620W marker (dbSNP ID rs2476601) at the 5' end of the RSBN1 gene. The PSBN1 gene encodes for the round spermatid basic protein 1, or rosbin [891]. The minor allele disrupts a sequence of promoter CCATT-binding factors and enhancer CCATT-binding factors, such as Pax-4, Pax-5, Nrf-1 and c-Myb, and creates a putative binding site for the transcription factor Sox-5[885]. The rs6679677 SNP is in complete LD with the +1858 PTPN22 SNP, and its allele frequencies are identical to those of the codon 620 marker of PTPN22. This makes it impossible to distinguish the effects of these two SNPs on the basis of genetic data only. Carlton et al. [892] reported the association between this new SNP and rheumatoid arthritis.

These data suggest that the R620W SNP of PTPN22 is not the universal etiological variant, fully explaining the association of the *PTPN22* locus with an autoimmune disorder. The existence of other SNP that are potentially functional and show complete or near complete LD with the R620W SNP marker clearly shows that more studies are needed for further fine genetic and functional dissection of the genomic region, containing the PTPN22 gene.

The search and evaluation of other ethiological variant(s) is particularly necessary in Asian and African populations, where the +1858 marker seems to be non-polymorphic.

Functional Role of the R620W Molecular Variant of PTPN22 in Autoimmunity

Arg620 is a critical residue in the proline-rich motif P1 that binds the SH3 domain of Csk [863,893]. The disease-associated Trp620 variant is not able to bind Csk [874]. The PTPN22 R620W SNP actually represents a gain-of-function mutation. Vang et al. [894] reported an association between the Trp620 variant and increased intrinsic phosphatase activity. This variant is shown to dephosphorylated Lck, TCR-ζ and other signaling proteins and decreased Ca^{2+} mobilization and IL-2 expression more effectively than the wild-type Arg620 variant. After TCR/CD28-mediated stimulation, the production of IL-2 was less in T cells from T1D patients heterozygous for W620R than that in T lymphocytes taken from homozygous R/R patients. A recombinant LYP Trp620 molecule expressed in Jurkat T lymphocytes as twice more active as the wild-type Arg620 molecule of the enzyme [894]. Indeed, the mutant enzyme exhibits more strong phosphatase activity, which suppress TCR signaling better than the wild-type LYP. Sck binding seems to be not crucial for the function of LYP, but may restrict the ability of LYP to negatively regulate TCR signaling.

In resting T cells, the Trp620 form of the enzyme is located at the same places as the Arg620 LYP, i.e. mostly in cytosole, some in the nucleus and very little at the plasma membrane [894]. The function of the nuclear LYP is compeletely unknown. Since the residue 620 is not in the catalytic domain, both forms of the enzyme must have the same intrinsic specificity.

Bottini et al. [895] proposed a hypothesis, suggesting a role of LYP in autoimmunity. Since W/R heterozygous individuals have an increased incidence of T1D, the disease-associated PTPN22 Trp620 variant is dominant. In their hypothesis, Bottini et al. [895] consider that the W620 LYP predisposes to autoimmunity by more sufficient suppressing TCR signalling in thymocytes that results in the survival of self-reactive T cells that normally should be deleted by negative selection in individuals with the R/R genotype. Elevated activity of LYP may lead to increased threshold required for effective TCR signaling in developing thymocytes, resulting in a lack of negative selection of autoreactive cells. Another possibility may be attributed to the relationship between increased LYP activity in regulatory T cells and reduced regulatory function of those cells due to the reduced TCR signaling

[896]. This could alter the normal function of Tregs and breake central and/or peripheral tolerance. The altered function of Tregs and TCR signaling abnormalities are observed in several autoimmune diseases, including T1D, and animal models of these diseases, such as the NOD mouse [897,898].

VITAMIN D RECEPTOR (VDR)

VDR Mediates Suppressive Effects of Vitamin D on the Immune System

As mentioned above, vitamin D is the important nutrition factor, which protects from T1D and prevents the progression of islet-specific autoimmunity to T1D. 1α,25-dihydroxyvitamin D_3 (1,25$(OH)_2D_3$), a hormonally active form of vitamin D, acts on target tissues through binding to the vitamin D receptor (VDR). VDR is a nuclear hormone receptor that regulates transcription of target genes through vitamin D-responsive elements in the promoter regions of the target genes [899]. The immunoregulatory function of vitamin D is well characterized [900]. This vitamin is protective against a variety of autoimmune diseases, particularly against rheumatoid arthritis, multiple sclerosis, inflammatory bowel disease and T1D [901]. The evidences on the protective role of vitamin D in autoimmunity have been obtained from the corresponding animal models. For T1D, numerous reports suggest that the treatment or injection with 1,25$(OH)_2D_3$ inhibits and even prevents autoimmune insulitis and diabetes in the NOD mouse [902,903].

The preventive effect of vitamin D against experimental diabetes is likely to be explained by vitamin D-mediated suppression of Th1, since in T1D Th1 type of the autoimmune response is predominant [904]. 1,25$(OH)_2D_3$ reduces production of Th1 type cytokines, IL-2 and IFN-γ, while up-regulating production of Th2-associated cytokine IL-4 [905]. In addition, vitamin D could protect against autoimmunity through the induction of a population of CD4+CD25+ Tregs and immunosuppression of DCs, i.e. professional APCs, which play an important role in the initiation and propagation of T-cell mediated immune responces [906,907].

Many types of immune cells carry receptors for 1,25$(OH)_2D_3$, with the highest concentrations of VDR in CD8+ T lymphocytes [908]. Studies on the immune system status in VDR-deficient mouse found several immune abnormalities, such as impaired macrophage chemotaxis [909], histologically enlarged lymph nodes in the vicinity of the thyroid gland with an increase in mature DCs in the lymph nodes [910] and reduction in CD4+ and CD8+ peripheral T lymphocytes [911]. However, the immune defects observed in VDR-knockout mice can be restored by calcium homeostasis normalization suggesting for the essential role of calcium in the immune system as well as for redundancy in VDR-mediated immune function of vitamin D [909].

VDR Gene Polymorphisms and Susceptibility to Type 1 Diabetes

The involvement of vitamin D was suggested in the pathogenesis of both types of diabetes, type 1 and type 2. Vitamin D and their analogs are shown to suppress T cell activation through the binding to the VDR [912,913] and hence VDR gene polymorphoisms are likely to be related to Tcell-mediated autoimmune disease, including T1D. Vitamin D receptor is expressed in a variety of tissues, including immune cells, and its expression in macrophages and activated CD4+ and CD8+ T lymphocytes is greatly stimulated by vitamin D [908], suggesting for significant influence of this vitamin on the function of the immune cells.

The VDR gene was mapped to chromosome 12q13.1, spanning over 100 kb and consisting of 9 exons [914]. Five common polymorphic RFLP markers have been previously described in the VDR gene: the RFLP/FokI at the start codon of exon 2 (+4 T/C), RFLP/BsmI, RFLP/Tru9I, RFLP/ApaI (all three in intron 8) and RFLP/TaqI (T/C1055, exon 9) (Figure 19) [915]. Results of population case-control and family-based studies, using these RFLPs, are summarized in Tables 16 and 17.

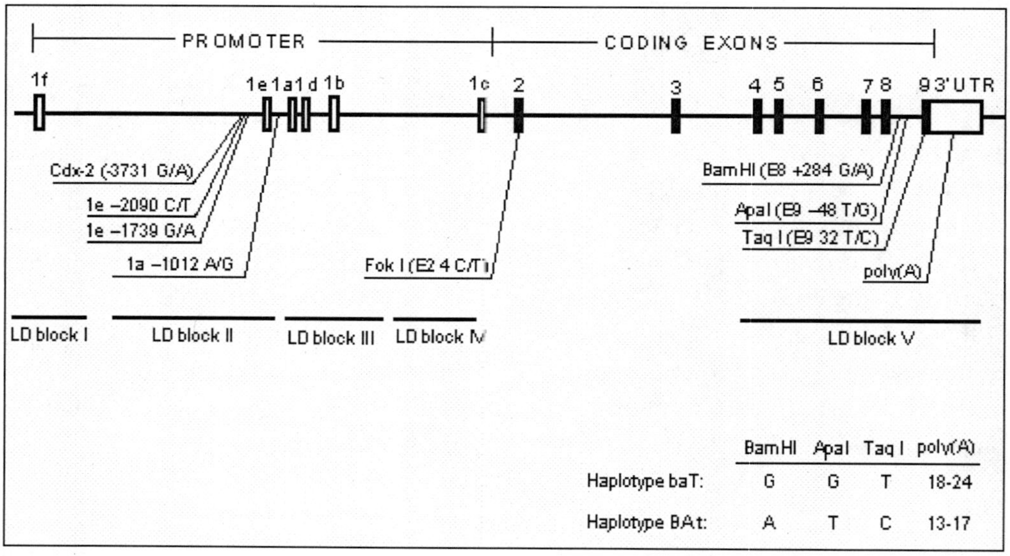

Figure 19. Exon-intron structure of the human VDR gene and positions of some polymorphic markers located within this gene. The gene spans over 100 kb on chromosome 12q13 and contains five linkage disequilibrium (LD) blocks [946]. All promoter polymorphisms shown at the picture are true or potentially functional. The designation of the –2090 C/T and –1739 G/A markers corresponds to their location upstream from the start of exon 1e. –1012 A/G SNPs denotes its location at position –1012 upstream of exon 1a. The FokI site, which is also functionally significant, corresponds to a C/T substitution at nucleotide 4 of exon 2 and lies outside of any of five LD blocks. The TaqI site represents a T/C variation at nucleotide position 32 of exon 2. In intron 8, polymorphic BamHI and ApaI are located 284 bp downstream of exon 8 and 48 bp upstream of exon 9, respectively. The BamHI, ApaI and TaqI polymorphisms are in LD with the variable poly(A) stretch at the 3'UTR as a part of the LD block 5. The G allele of the BamHI RFLP, G allele of the Apa I RFLP and C allele of the TaqI RFLP are in LD with long alleles of the poly(A) stretch, including 18-24 repeats, and constitute the baT haplotype [931]. The A-T-C allelic combination of the BamI-ApaI-TaqI is in strong LD with short poly(A) repeats (n=13-17) and corresponds to the BAt haplotype.

Morrison et al. [931] showed that RFLP/BsmI, RFLP/ApaI and RFLP/TaqI are in strong LD and form several haplotypes, from which the BAt and baT haplotypes are the most common in Caucasians (here, a capital letter denotes the presense of a cleavage site for a corresponding restriction enzyme, while a small letter denotes the absence of that). Case-control and family-based studies, evaluating VDR RFLP markers for association with T1D are inconsistent (Table 16 and 17). In studies, showing an association between the VDR RFLPs and disease, the BAt haplotype is related to a very high risk of diabetes (OR >4.0) [920,929,930]. However, these studies tested a relatively small number of patients. In Finland, three VDR RFLPs (FokI, ApaI and BsmI) were genotyped in a large population cohort, comprising around 1000 cases, more than 2000 controls and 544 affected families [922]. In the Finnish case-control study, borderline significant differences were obtained for the B allele. In the family study, a gender-specific association was observed for the faB and fAB haplotypes, which were overtransmitted and undertransmitted, respectively, from parents to sons, and for the Fab haplotype undertransmitted from parents to daughters [922]. These significant differences disappeared after correction for multiple testing. A sex-specific association of the FbaTu (FokI-BsmI-ApaI-TaqI-Tru91I) haplotype with T1D was found in Hungarian girls [919], but the size of the Hungarian sample tested was also small.

Table 16. Population case-control studies for association of RFLP markers of the VDR gene and T1D

Population	RFLPs used	Cases, *n*	Controls, *n*	*OR* (genetic risk marker)	*P* (genetic risk marker)	Reference
Brazilian	BsmI	78	94		NS	[916]
Japanese	FokI	110	250	*RR* =2.4 (F/F genotype)	0.0069 (F*allele)	[917]
German	FokI, BsmI, TaqI	75	57		NS	[918]
Hungarian	BsmI, ApaI, FokI, TaqI, Tru91I	107	109		NS	[919]
Dalmatian (South Croatia)	BsmI, ApaI, TaqI,	134	132	4.42 (BAt haplotype)	0.042 (BAt haplotype)	[920]
Japanese	BsmI	203	222	N/A	< 0.0001 (B allele)	[921]
Finnish	ApaI BsmI FokI	944 1064 985	2379 2387 2356		NS	[922]

Table 16. Population case-control studies for association of RFLP markers of the VDR gene and T1D (Continued)

Population	RFLPs used	Cases, *n*	Controls, *n*	*OR* (genetic risk marker)	*P* (genetic risk marker)	Reference
Italian	ApaI, BsmI FokI	31	36		NS	[923]
Dalmatian (South Croatia)	BsmI, ApaI, FokI, TaqI, Tru91I	134	132	N/A	<0.0388 (FbATu haplotype)	[924]

*A capital letter (F in the case of the RFLP/FokI marker) denotes an allele that is cleaved by a restriction endonuclease (FokI); a small letter (f) denotes an allele that remains indigestible. For RFLP/BsmI, alleles are designated as B and b, respectively; RFLP/ApaI: A and a, RFLP/TaqI: Tand t, RFLP/Tru91I, U and u.

Recently, Nejentsev *et al.* [932] evaluated whether the VDR gene contributes to the susceptibility for T1D in a largest family (up to 3,763 families) dataset from UK, USA, Norway, Finland and Romania. The authors developed a high dense SNP map of the VDR gene, comprising 98 nucleotide substitutions. The reconstruction of haplotypes from the subset of 55 common SNPs revealed three blocks of LD. RFLP/FokI was not in LD with any other common SNP and, therefore, was not informative for capturing information from those SNPs. The three other SNPs (BsmI, ApaI and TaqI) were localized to block B and did not capture any information about SNPs in other blocks. These common SNPs failed to show association with T1D [932]. The multiethnic family study showed a weak association with diabetes (*OR* = 1.07-1.14 for three another SNPs, rs4303288, rs12721366 and rs2544043 located in introns 2 and 6 and the 3'UTR, respectively. However, these SNPs showed no evidence for association when tested in the independent study, involving 1,587 patients and 1,827 control subjects from the UK [932].

Poon et al. [933] measured LD between 12 SNP within the VDR gene, including common FokI, TaqI, BsmI and ApaI polymorphisms, and found two LD blocks. Block 1 was 5.8-kb long and located toward the 3' end of VDR, consisting TaqI, ApaI and BsmI SNPs, whereas the 8.4-kb block 2 was situated toward the 5' end of VDR. The two blocks were separated by 10.8 kb [933]. The block 1 corresponds to the block B, while the block 2 is roughly corresponds to the block C identified by Nejentsev et al. [932].

Table 17. Family-based studies for association of RFLP markers of the VDR gene and T1D

Population	RFLPs used	Families , *n* (subjects, *n*)	*OR* (genetic risk marker)	*P* (genetic risk marker)	Reference
Southern Indians	BsmI, ApaI, TaqI	93	N/A	0.014 (BAT* haplotype) 0.0295 (bAT haplotype)	[925]
Romainian	BsmI, ApaI, TaqI	204 (756)	N/A	0.0038 (T allele)	[926]
Finnish	FokI, BsmI, ApaI	544		NS	[922]
Dutch	FokI	206 trios		NS	[927]
Chilean	BsmI, ApaI, TaqI	59 trios		NS	[928]
Basque	FokI, BsmI, ApaI, TaqI	64	4.4 (fBAt haplotype)	0.02 (fBAt haplotype)	[929]
German	FokI, BsmI, ApaI, TaqI	152 (527)	N/A	0.0106 (BAt haplotype)	[930]

*A capital letter (B in the case of the RFLP/BsmI marker) denotes an allele that is cleaved by a restriction endonuclease (BsmI); a small letter (b) denotes an allele that remains indigestible. For RFLP/FokI, alleles are designated as F and f, respectively; RFLP/ApaI: A and a, RFLP/TaqI: T and t, RFLP/Tru91I, U and u.

Results of genetic analyses of the association between VDR polymorphisms and T1D are controversial. Several studies, using relatively small numbers of patients, showed positive association between some polymorphic markers within the VDR gene and disease, whereas large-scale population- and family-based studies in Finland [922] and UK [932] failed to find a significant association between this gene and T1D. These results suggest that the VDR gene plays no major role in the etiology of T1D. In Asian populations, this gene seems to confer susceptibility for T1D more strongly than in Caucasians. Because of the complex pattern of LD, a susceptibility to T1D within the VDR region should be referred to certain extended haplotypes, consisting of allele combinations of several polymorphic markers. Among those, functional polymorphisms should play an essential role in highlighting association between the vitamin D receptor gene and disease.

Functionality of VDR Polymorphisms

The polymorphic FokI site is shown to alter binding of the transcription factor IIB and therefore affects the transcription of the VDR gene [934]. The C (or F) allele of the RFLP/FokI abolishes the start codon, and translation starts further downstream. This results in producing of the more active VDR variant, which consists of 424 amino acids and is shorter of the T allele encoded variant by 3 amino acids [935,936]. The altered VDR variant is found to modulate biological effects of vitamin D, such as inhibition of the cell growth of peripheral blood monocytes [937] and regulation of the intrabody calcium level [938], and correlates with VDR mRNA levels [939]. Since the RFLP/FokI shows no LD with any of other VDR polymorphisms, this SNP can be considered as an independent marker in the VDR gene. The FokI SNP showed association with T1D in some populations [917,924,929] as well as no association in others [918,919,922,923,927,930,932].

The BsmI, ApaI and TaqI RFLPs are located close to the 3'UTR of the VDR gene and hence are in LD with polymorphisms located at the 3'UTR. The 3'UTR is known to be involved in the regulation of mRNA stability, and therefore functional 3'UTR polymorphisms through the strong LD could explain associations of the BsmI, ApaI and TaqI with diseases. Several polymorphisms have been found at the 3'UTR of the VDR gene, including the poly(A) stretch [940]. Short poly(A) alleles, including 12-14 repeats, are shown to be in LD with the baT haplotype, while long alleles (18-22 repeats) are in LD with the BAt haplotype.

Durrin et al. [941] identified certain parts of the 3'UTR called destabilizing elements, which could be responsible for stability of the VDR mRNA. However, no functional polymorphisms at the 3'UTR of VDR linked to either the baT or BAt haplotype and influenced stability of the mRNA transcript have been found. Whitefield and coauthors [936] showed a relationship between the RFLP/FokI (F and f alleles), poly(A) repeats (long (L) and short (S) alleles) and transcription levels of VDR, testing different fibroblast cell lines with different VDR genotypes. The investigators identified the FL genotype associated with high VDR activity, whereas the fS genotype was related to low activity of the receptor [936]. Verbeek et al. [942] found no correlation between the baT and BAt haplotypes and mRNA stability, but observed 30% less of mRNA in case of the t allele. This observation also corresponded to other studies performed in vivo and in vitro [931,939,943,944].

A so called Cdx-2 polymorphism, representing a G-to-A substitution in the 1e promoter region of the VDR gene at position –3731 apart from the transcriptional start, was suggested to play an important role in intestinal-specific transcription of VDR [945]. The nucleotide substitution alters the sequence of the binding site for caudal-related homeodomain protein 2 (Cdx-2), a transcription factor. A mutated (–3731A) allele was associated with significantly higher expression of VDR mRNA compared to the G allele [945]. However, there are no data, evaluating a role of this promoter polymorphism in T1D. In a recent study, Fang et al. [946] reported finding of several new promoter polymorphisms within the VDR gene. The A/G SNP situated at position –1012 upstream of the promoter-encoding exon 1a influenced a putative GATA-binding site in the exon 1a promoter region that resulted in a markedly decreased binding of the transcription factor GATA to the G allele and a 2-fold less transcription activity of the –1012G variant of the VDR promoter [946]. Two other promoter polymorphisms, C/T and G/A, located at positions –2090 and –1739 upstream of the promoter-encoding exon 1e were found to affect potential Cdx-2 binding sites. The –2090T and –1739G alleles showed a decreased ability for binding Cdx-2 compared to their allelic wild-type counterparts [946].

Fang et al. [946] also investigated functional effects of 3'-UTR polymorphisms and found that the BAt haplotype is associated with a 15% less expression and 30% slower decay rate of of VDR mRNA compated to the baT haplotype. Thus, reduced levels of VDR expression and less stable mRNA in a case of the BAt haplotype could explain the association of this VDR haplotype with higher risk of diabetes observed in some populations.

Fang and coauthors [946] reported the existence of at least five LD blocks within the VDR gene in Caucasians (Figure 19). Four LD blocks lie in the promoter region of the VDR gene, while the 5th LD block spans across exons 4-9 and the 3'UTR. The polymorphic FokI RFLP site is independent on any of these blocks. The 5th LD block includes the BsmI, ApaI and TaqI RFLPs. The LD map of the VDR region presented by Fang et al. [946] shows that genetic effects, coming from the 3'UTR of VDR, are independent on those from the promoter region of this gene. Due to the extreme complexity of LD within the VDR locus, an association of this gene with a vitamin D-related disease could be explained by the interaction of several common extended haplotypes and their functionality. However, a large population study performed by Nejentsev et al. [932], using a high density SNP map of the VDR gene [947], revealed no major role of the sequence variation within the VDR locus in conferring T1D susceptibility. Environmental factors, such as vitamin D intake, seem to modulate risk associated with the sequence variation in the VDR gene, i.e. certain variants may only be functionally important among a subpopulation of subjects with vitamin D insufficiency. To date, a role of functionally active VDR promoter polymorphisms is underestimated in T1D and, indeed, needs more studies that should help to clarify whether the VDR gene significantly contributes to the etiology of T1D.

IDDM7 Locus

Evidence for IDDM7 (chromosome 2q33) was supported at the genome-wide level of significance (P = 0.016) by the last whole-genome scan for T1D susceptibility genes [636]. Originally, IDDM7 was mapped on the basis of evidence of allelic association of D2S152 [633,948,949]. For D2S152, an association/linkage to T1D was not replicated in some early studies, involving a dataset of diabetic families from Florida, USA [950,951]. Despite that, several later studies confirmed the existence of IDDM7 on the chromosomal region 2q33, using multiplex affected family datasets of the different ethnic origin [635,952,953]. Together with CTLA-4 (IDDM12), the 2q31-q33 region provided an estimated sib risk λ_S of 1.19, suggesting that a single common susceptibility allele would have an allelic association with *OR* of around 3.0 [636]. This effect could be identifiable in a fine mapping association study, using dense SNP maps across the region.

In IDDM7, a T1D susceptibility gene is not yet identified. Among the positional candidate genes, the GALNT3 gene that encodes UDP-GalNAc: polypeptide N-acetyl-galactosaminyltransferase-T3, an enzyme, playing a role in glycosylating antigens, was evaluated, but failed to show an association with T1D in a Danish population [953]. Another putative candidate, the NeuroD/BETA2 gene mapped to chromosome 2q32 was also tested. This gene is expressed in the endocrine pancreas and encodes a protein, participating in the regulation of tissue-specific insulin transcription in pancreatic β cells [954]. In this gene, Iwata et al. [955] identified a SNP that changes alanine to threonine at codon 45 (Ala45Thr). The Ala45Thr dimorphism showed association with T1D in Japanese [955]. This association was not found in a French population [956], but replicated in other Caucasians, including

T1D patients from Denmark [957] and Poland [958]. Although these findings need further replication in a larger population datasets, the NeuroD/BETA2 gene maintains good chances to be the T1D susceptibility gene in IDDM7 locus. A functional polymorphism within NeuroD/BETA2 should be identified, since in vitro studies of two amino acid substitutions (Ala45Thr and Pro197His) in this gene found no significant differences between different allelic variants on the regulation of the human insulin gene promoter [957].

IDDM10 Locus

IDDM10 is another non-HLA-linked T1D susceptibility region, for which a supporting evidence at the genome-wide level of significance (P = 0.021) was obtained in the largest genome screen performed by Concannon et al. [636]. IDDM10 was mapped to chromosome 10p11-q11 in UK affected families [633] and replicated by several studies mostly based on the analysis of family datasets from the UK and US [635,958-962]. However, a number of linkage studies in other populations (Scandinavians, Dutches, Sardinians and Italians) rejected an evidence for linkage to T1D on chromosome 10p11-q11 [959,963,964]. It should be noted that Concannon et al. [636] again failed to found any significant linkage for IDDM10 in the subset of families from Scandinavia, suggesting that this locus does not play a major role in etiology of T1D in North Europeans.

IDDM10 exhibits a moderate genetic effect in T1D predisposition (λ_S = 1.12 [636]). A susceptibility gene remains to be defined in IDDM10. The GAD2 gene, which maps to chromosome 10p11.23 and encodes the 65-kD isoform of GAD, a major self-antigen in T1D, was considered to be a most likely positional and functional candidate for gene, predisposing to disease in IDDM10. However, linkage and association studies failed to find a significant support for the relation between GAD2 and T1D [633,962,965-967]. Another putative candidate gene, CREM, encoding cAMP-responsive element modulator that is involved in the regulation of IL-2 production, was also evaluated, but no evidence for the association of the promoter –11 C/T polymorphism of CREM and T1D was obtained [962]. Studies on association between the SDF-1 gene, a product (stromal cell-derived factor-1) of which is responsible for stimulating migration and activation of T cells, and T1D showed controversial results [968-970]. A polymorphic marker located in intron 4 of the TCF-8 gene, coding for transcription factor, a negative regulator of the expression of CD4 and IL-2 in T lymphocytes, showed association with T1D in a subset of Russian T1D families, carrying a high risk HLA-DR4 haplotype [862]. This finding was observed in a small population sample (42 simplex families) and therefore needs to be independently supported by investigations, using much larger population samples.

Since Concannon et al. [636] obtained a genome-wide significant evidence for linkage on chromosome 10p14-q11, the CD25 gene mapped to chromosome 10p15-p14 [971] could be also considered as a strong candidate for susceptibility to T1D within IDDM10 locus. This gene encodes a receptor for IL-2, which is vitally essential for normal function of T cells, including Tregs. Using a dence SNP map, Vella et al. [972] found a highly significant association of this gene with disease in a large population sample of 3,521 cases and 3,930 controls from UK ($P = 6.5 \times 10^{-8}$) as well as in a large family collection of 472 British and

268 US multiplex families (P = 7.3 x 10^{-3}). Results of Vella et al. [972] strongly support an evidence for CD25 as a gene, defining susceptibility to T1D within IDDM10, but are also required the replication by independent genetic analyses in other populations. Interestingly, in NOD mice, IL-2 represents a major candidate gene for Idd3 [550,973]. Mice, carrying susceptibility alleles at Idd3 produced less levels of IL-2 compared to murine strains with resistant alleles at Idd3 [974]. Congenic mice, having resistant alleles at Idd3, is protected against diabetes and more sensitive to tolerance induction to islet allografs [975]. These data suggest for the important role of IL2/CD25 patway in maintaining immune tolerance.

IDDM15 Locus

Concannon et al. [636] also replicated evidence for the existence of IDDM15 locus on chromosome 6q21. In the presence of strong linkage due to IDDM1, determining the support for IDDM15 is difficult because of the positive correlation among the idenrtical-by-descent proportions in the linked loci. Using 1,401 informative pedigrees, Concannon et al. [636] obtained at position of 37 cM apart of IDDM1 the Pearson 's correlation coefficient r = 0.3132 (empirical $P < 1.0 \times 10^{-4}$) that significantly exceeded the expected value of 0.2276, suggesting for an HLA-independent effect in IDDM15 region.

IDDM15 was mapped to chromosome 6q21 at position in several Caucasian populations [960,975] and continuosly confirmed in further genome-wide scans [635,963,976]. Using a novel multimarker-based test of linkage for affected sib pairs that takes into account the effect of a known linked disease locus (i.e. IDDM1), Barber et al. [978] reanalyzed a set of 1,056 diabetic families. They found only a marginal evidence for IDDM15 (P = 0.03 to 0.02, using different methods) with a peak of linkage located 15 cM centromeric (i.e. closer to IDDM1) from D6S283 [977] that was used as a marker of IDDM15. The discrepancy between the results of Barber et al. [978] and previous studies [977] could be attributed to the quality and density of genetic maps used in that region (6q21) and different numbers of affected families tested. Using high-dense maps of highly polymorphic markers across the region should greatly benefit fine mapping and identification of disease-associated gene the IDDM locus.

The 16q22-q24 Region

For susceptibility locus located on chromosome 16q22-q24, a linkage at the level close to the genowe-wide level of significance (P = 0.075) was reported by Concannon et al. [636]. For the 16q22-q24 region, an evidence for linkage to T1D was obtained and further replicated in the UK- and US-based family datasets [635,960]. Linkage studies in other populations failed to find significant linkage to disease in this region [963,964,979] probably due to the genetic heterogeneity of T1D [963], genetic isolation [964] and non-sufficient size of the population sample tested [979]. To date, no T1D susceptibility gene is known in that region. Several positional candidate genes located at 16q22-q24 have been evaluated. For the ICSBP1 gene, encoding interferon concensus sequence binding protein 1, a member of the family of interferon-like transcription factors, no association with T1D was found [979]. Association studies of NQO1, encoding NADP(H)-quinone oxydoreductase 1, which could protect against enhanced oxidative stress in T1D, showed inconsistent results [979-982]. Interestingly, the T1D susceptibility locus on chromosome 16q22-q24 partially overlaps with the susceptibility loci mapped for other autoimmune disorders, such as celiac disease [983], asthma [984] and rheumatoid arthritis [985], suggesting that this genomic region could harbor a common but still unknown susceptibility gene for autoimmunity.

Other Loci

In the study of Concannon et al. [636], a little evidence for linkage to T1D was obtained for IDDM4 (11q13), IDDM6 (18q12-q21), IDDM9 (3q22-q25), IDDM11 (14q24-q31), IDDM16 (14q32), IDDM17 (10q25) and IDDM18 (5q33). These results suggest that these T1D susceptibility loci represent false-positive data or exhibit very weak genetic effects. Such loci may be more readily detected in certain populations due to the ethnic-specific differences in allele frequencies and population-specific genetic and environmental influences.

The exlusion mapping provided support for the existence of three non-HLA susceptibility loci on chromosomes 16, 19 and X, for which linkage could not be excluded [636]. Some evidence for a susceptibility locus on chromosome 19q11 (MLS = 1.8) was obtained in the second genome-wide scan for T1D susceptibility loci [635]. This is close to the 19q13 region, where a locus, conferring susceptibility for type 2 diabetes [986] and responsible for determining fasting plasma glucose levels [987,988], was recently mapped. The GYS1 gene, encoding muscle glycogen synthase 1, resides at 19q13.3 and shows association with type 2 diabetes and different metabolic abnormalities in type 2 diabetes [989-992].

An X-linked susceptibility locus for T1D was determined on chromosome Xp11.4-Xp21.1 by a sex-specific bias in transmission of alleles to male offspring [993]. Cucca et al. [887] provided evidence for linkage to T1D in the same region of chromosome X, but in the subgroup of patients with DR3/X genotype. In this subgroup, a significantly increased bias in male/female ratio (1.7) was observed compared to that in the DR4/Y category (Y is not DR3) [887]. Both the evidence of linkage and the bias in the M:F ratio were concentrated in the families with patients positive for the HLA-DR3, which is one of the two main predisposing haplotypes at the HLA/IDDM1 major locus. These data suggest the X-linked susceptibility in T1D is mediated by HLA-DR3 haplotypes, but is unlikely due to the transmission ratio distortion in allele transfer from parents to male offspring [994].

Concluding Remarks

To date, four genes (HLA, INS-VNTR, CTLA-4 and PTPN22), contributing in the etiology of T1D, are identified. CD25 gene represents a good candidate to become the 5th gene, conferring T1D susceptibility. The VDR gene remains to be another likely candidate, but a recent large-scale population study of Nejentsev et al. [932] failed to detect a strong association of polymorphic markers within this gene and T1D. In total, these genes are responsible for approximately 60-70% of familial clustering of disease. A recent genome-wide scan supported linkage to disease for 4 other non-HLA loci (IDDM7, IDDM10, IDDM15 and chromosome 16q22-q24) [636]. Some supporting evidence for putative T1D susceptibility loci was also obtained on chromosomes 19 and X.

More than 22 putative susceptibility loci for T1D have been previously mapped. It seems that most of them display modest and very modest effects (*OR* = 1.1-1.3) on genetic predisposition to T1D. Since these loci have been mapped based on a relatively small population datasets, evidence for linkage to T1D some of those might be false-positive. Such loci may exhibit ethnic-specific effects and be detectable only in certain populations.

To detect a causal disease-associated variant within a susceptibility gene (locus), developing high dense SNP maps are necessary. The Wellcome Trust Case-Control Consortium is performing a genome-wide search for susceptibility markers for several common complex disorders, including T1D. The analysis involves genotyping 500,000 SNPs across a human genome in at least 2,000 cases and 3,000 controls from the UK. These population samples provide 80% power at $\alpha = 5 \times 10^{-7}$ to detect genetic effect with *OR* = 1.5 at minor allele frequency of 0.1. Using 8,000 cases and 8,000 controls provides 80% power to find *OR* of more than 1.25 [995].

Recently, using a genome-wide SNP scan with non-synonymous 6,500 SNPs, Smyth et al. [996] reported finding a marker (rs 1990760) associated with T1D. This SNP represents an alanine-to-threonine substitution at codon 946 within the interferon induced with helicase C domain 1 (IFIH1) gene on chromosome 2q24. For the Thr946 allele, genotyping a total of 4,253 T1D patients and 5,842 controls provided *OR* of 0.85 ($P = 9.29 \times 10^{-8}$). The association was replicated in the family based study, involving 2,134 parent-child trios from 1,799 families from the UK, USA, Romania and Norway (for the Thr946 allele, *RR* = 0.88; $P = 4.63 \times 10^{-3}$) [996]. The combined risk ratio for the minor allele from both (case-control and family-based) analyses was 0.86 ($P = 1.42 \times 10^{-10}$).

The Ala/Thr946 SNP of IFIH1 is located within the haplotype block, containing four genes, fibroblast activation protein, IFIH1, grancalcin and potassium voltage-gated channel and subfamily H member 7. Among those, IFIH1 is the strongest functional candidate because this gene is involved into IFN-β-mediated antiviral immune responces [997]. A role of viruses in inducing β-cell autoimmunity and diabetes was discussed above. Thus, the IFIH1 gene could represent a 6th T1D-related gene, for which a comprehensive genetic analysis was performed and significant association was obtained.

Additionally, Smyth et al. [996], performing a genome-wide SNP screen, found an association with T1D for the rs1445898 SNP, i.e. Gln/Arg75 at the CAPSL gene on chromosome 5p13. This gene encodes calcyphosine-like protein with unknown function. However, the Gln/Arg75 SNP is in LD with the neighboring the IL7RA gene, which is likely finctional candidate for T1D. The IL7RA encodes a receptor for IL-7, a cytokine, which is shown to be highly expressed by diabetes-suppressive immunoregulatory DCs and helps to delay autoimmunity in NOD mice through the Tregs-mediated inhibition [998]. The IL7RA gene is located on chromosome region (5p14-p12), for which a suggestive linkage to multiple sclerosis was found, whereas the IL7RA polymorphism showed association with this autoimmune disease [999,1000]. Thus, the IL7RA gene might be a gene predisposing to both T1D and multiple sclerosis, but further large-scale population analyses of this association should be performed.

Chapter 11

SHARED GENETIC SUSCEPTIBILITY TO TYPE 1 DIABETES AND OTHER AUTOIMMUNE DISEASES

T1D AS A PART OF AUTOIMMUNE POLYGLANDULAR SYNDROMES

Autoimmune polyglandular syndromes (APSs) characterize by the coexistence of at least two endocrine gland insufficiencies that are based on autoimmune mechanisms. Associations with non-endocrine immune diseases may occur. Two major subtypes of APS, types I and 2, are distinguished according to age of presentation, characteristic patterns of disease combinations and different modes of inheritance [1001]. APS1 includes coexistence of hypoparathyroidism (frequency 80-85%) with mucocutaneous candidiasis (frequency 70-80%), Addison's disease (60-70%), T1D (less than 20%), hypogonadism (12%), AITD (10%) and non-endocrine autoimmune pathology, such as vitiligo, Sjogren's syndrome, myasthenia gravis, autoimmune hepatitis, autoimmune gastritis and some others [1002]. APS2 contains combinations between thyroid disease (70-75%), T1D (50-60%), Addison's disease (40-50%) and hypoparathyroidism (less than 5%), with absence of candidasiasis and non-endocrine disorders [1003]. A third subtype, APS3, was described in adults and, contrary to types 1 and 2, does not involve the adrenal cortex [1001]. Besides the absence of adrenal failure, no clinical differences between types 2 and 3 were found.

Compared to APS2 and APS3, APS type 1 (or APECED – autoimmune polyendocrinopathy-candidiasis-ectodermal dystrophy) shows no association with the HLA region [1004]. The gene for autoimmune regulator 1 (AIRE1) responsible for APS1 was mapped to chromosome 21q22.3 [1005]. The AIRE1 gene is widely expressed in lymphoid tissues, adrenal cortex and thyroid [1005]. A 13-bp deletion at nucleotide 964 in exon 8 is a common mutation that accounts for more than 70% of APECED alleles in a British population [1006]. However, of 235 UK patients with T1D, none were found to carry the mutation [1006]. In addition, a total of 224 Germans affected with T1D was screened, and none of them were shown to contain this deletion [1007]. It seems highly likely therefore the 13-bp deletion polymorphism of AIRE1 leads specifically to the development of APECED.

Since autoimmune diabetes is the most frequent component of both APS2 and APS3, it is possible to expect that genetic markers for T1D can also contribute to the susceptibility to these polyendocrinopathies. Studies on HLA showed an association of the T1D-predisposing DR3 and DR4 alleles with APS type 2 and type 3 [1008-1011]. The association of the DR4 allele with these syndromes could be attributed to its major role in conferring susceptibility to T1D, which is a significant component of both APS2 and APS3 [1010,1012]. However, a study in Norway reported the association between APS2 and DR3/DR4 independently from the presence of type 1 diabetes [1013]. A role of another general susceptibility gene for autoimmunity, CTLA-4, in polyglandular autoimmunity was discussed above, suggesting that this gene is likely to be important in the development of certain APS variants, such as combinations between Addison's disease with either GD or T1D [1014, 1015], vitiligo with either AITD or T1D [1016] and between AITD and diabetes [1017].

T1D AND AITD: COEXISTENCE AND SHARED GENETIC BACKGROUND

Coexistence of Thyroid Autoimmunity with Autoimmune Diabetes: Evidences from Population Epidemiological Studies

AITD most often accompanies T1D [1018]. AITD and T1D are the most common autoimmune disorders [1019]. Both have a similar pathogenesis, which involves T-cell infiltration into the target organ associated with subsequent self-antibody production against target antigens. In AITD, the target organ is the thyroid gland. Depending on the pathogenesis, two major alternate clinical outcomes are possible in thyroid autoimmunity. In Graves' disease (GD), stimulating effects of anti-thyrotropin receptor (TSHR) antibodies cause thyroid hyperfunction and hyperthyroidism, whereas in Hashimoto's thyroiditis (HT), massive apoptosis of thyrocytes and hypothyroidism occur [1020]. Typically, these disorders occur together as a component of APSs.

The association between thyroid autoimmunity and T1D is well established and supported by epidemiological data from numerous populations [1021-1024]. The frequency of thyroid diseases in diabetic subjects is 2-3-fold greater then in non-diabetic individuals [1025]. The prevalence of thyroid antibodies in type 1 diabetic patients usually ranges between 20-30% [1021,1023,1026,1027] and increases with the age of the patients [1021,1028]. Around a half of T1D patients with thyroid abnormalities further develop AITD [1021,1029]. Patients with newly diagnosed T1D, positive for GADA, showed significantly higher levels of anti-thyroid peroxidase (TPO) antibodies than GADA-negative diabetic subjects [1024]. On the other hand, 5-10% GD patients have anti-islet antibodies [1030,1031].

Family studies show an increased segregation of thyroid autoimmunity in diabetic families. Up to 36% of T1D probands were shown to have AITD (27% had HT and 9% had GD [1032]. The increased frequency of co-existent thyroid disease has been reported to present in 15.9% of parents with diabetes, and only 6.1% of parents without diabetes [1033]. In the UK, the prevalence of HT in diabetic probands (27%) and their first-degree relatives

(25%) was found to be sufficiently higher than in non-diabetic controls (11.5%) [1034]. The clustering of AITD in T1D families, therefore, suggests that the etiology of autoimmune diabetes and thyroiditis may involve common genetic backgrounds.

Genetic Markers of Shared Susceptibility to Type 1 Diabetes and Thyroid Autoimmunity in Humans

Since the HLA class II cluster contains genes essential for antigen processing and presentation, which are basic mechanisms of initiating immune (and autoimmune) response, it is not surprising that this gene region is involved in the pathogenesis of numerous autoimmune disorders [1035]. A role of the HLA-DR3/DR3 and DR3/DR4 genotypes as major risk factors in etiology of T1D is well established [1036]. For GD, the predisposing allele is also DR3 but its contribution to genetic susceptibility for GD is much weaker than that for T1D, providing *RR* of up to 5.7 [1037]. Data on HLA risk factors for HT are less suggestive than for GD. Several population and family-based studies showed an association of HT with DR3 (*RR* is up to 5.1) [1038-1041], which was subsequently supported by the evidence on enhanced severity of thyroglobulin-induced experimental autoimmune thyroiditis (EAT) in DR3-transgenic mice [1042,1043]. Compared to T1D predisposition, where the HLA region represents a major susceptibility locus (IDDM1), the contribution of the HLA genes in etiology of AITD is much weaker.

The etiological variant of HLA in T1D is well known, representing representing the absence of aspartic acid at position 57 (non-Asp-57) of the DQβ chain [714]. The relative risk of T1D for individuals, who is homozygous for non-Asp-57, is 107. Later, the significance of the position 52 of the DQα chain for T1D susceptibility was also shown. In Caucasians, the presence of non-Asp-57 in the DQβ chain and Arg-52 in the DQ□ chain permits a self-antigen to fit in the antigen-binding pocket inside the HLA molecule and to be recognized by the TCR [1044].

The DR3 allele, a major HLA risk factor in thyroid autoimmunity, has multiple sequence variations. In 2004, a total of 28 subtypes of the HLA-DRB1*03 allele was known [1045]. To identify, which of the DRB1 sequences actually represents a primary etiological variant, the HLA-DRB1 gene was sequenced in Caucasian GD patients. Sequence analysis revealed that the frequency of DRB1variant, encoding arginine at position 74, was significantly increased in GD patients compared to controls (*OR* = 4.6) [1046]. In DR*3*-negative individuals, DRβ1-Arg74 was still significantly associated with GD, suggesting that the primary association of GD is with DRβ1-Arg74, whereas the association with HLA-DR3 is secondary [1046]. Logistic regression analysis of each of 102 amino acid positions of the exon 2-encoded peptide-binding domain of DRB1 in the independent case-control study (871 affected and 621 control subjects from the UK) showed the strongest association with GD for codon 74 [1047]. These findings suggest that an amino acid variation at position 74 of the DRBβ1 chain could represent a primary etiological variant, which confers susceptibility to GD. Except for arginine, other amino acids, situating at position 74, include alanine and glutamine. The DRβ1-Gln74 variant is always observed on the DR7 allele, which was reported to be protective for GD in several populations [1046,1048,1049]. This suggests, that position 74 plays a critical role in the pathogenesis of GD, presenting DRBβ1-Gln74 as a protective variant and DRBβ1-Arg74 as a causative variant for GD development. As in T1D, the presence of arginine-74 allows a self-antigen peptide to fit in the antigen-binding groove of the HLA class II molecule and initiate thyroid-specific autoimmune response [1046].

Although a HLA etiological variant for HT needs to be found, the similarity of susceptibility mechanisms in T1D and GD affecting the affinity of the antigen-binding pocket of the class II molecule provides opportunity to suggest for possibility of the related mechanism of HLA-associated predisposition in Hashimoto's disease.

There are several case-control studies, presenting results on the evaluation of a role of HLA in conferring susceptibility to both T1D and AITD. In Germany, thyroid antibodies were more prevalent in the subset of patients with the predisposing DR3/DR4 genotype compared to other HLA allele variants [1021]. In Czech Republic, elevated levels of thyroid antibodies were detected in T1D patients, carrying the HLA-DQB1*0302 allele [1050]. Studies in France and Japan found no differences in the distribution of HLA class II alleles between diabetic patients with and without AITD [1051,1052]. However, another study in Japanese population showed a higher prevalence of HLA-DR9, DQA1*0301 and DPB1*0501 in T1D subjects complicated with GD [1053]. In Taiwanese, who had both diabetes and AITD, the DRB1*0405/DQA1*301/DQB1*0401 haplotype was reported to be increased [1054]. In Korea, a predisposing role of the HLA-DQB1*0401 allele for the development of thyroid autoimmunity was shown in patients with T1D [1055].

Family-based genetic analyses provided more consistent results in determining common HLA markers for susceptibility for both T1D and AITD. Santamaria et al. [1056] showed that diabetic subjects with the DQB1*0302 allele have a higher risk to develop GD. The susceptible role of the DR3 and DR4 allele was confirmed in other studies [1017,1057-1059]. Levin et al. [1059] dissected a role of these alleles, showing that DR3 is the major HLA allele that contributes to the joint genetic susceptibility to T1D and AITD, whereas other alleles (i.e. DR4) are phenotype-specific. A subsequent study in the enlarged family dataset (55 families with AITD and T1D from the US) revealed that DR3-DQB1*0201 is the major HLA haplotype, contributing to shared susceptibility, with DR3 conferring most of the shared risk [1060]. In the study of Golden et al. [1060], a *LOD* score for HLA was highest for T1D alone, and when the AITD-affected individuals were added to the analysis, the *LOD* score decreased from 7.57 to 2.2. The decrease in *LOD* score shows that HLA contributes significantly less to the inherited susceptibility to AITD in T1D families. Therefore, other non-HLA genes must contribute to strong familial clustering between T1D and AITD.

One of the non-HLA genes, which share genetic susceptibility for diabetes and thyroid autoimmunity, is CTLA-4 [788,1061]. The association of the G(+49) allele of CTLA-4 with increased risk of AITD in diabetic individuals was shown by several studies [1062-1064]. The CTLA-4 locus showed suggestive linkage with disease in the subset of US Caucasian families affected with both AITD and T1D (i.e. affected with APS1), then providing an evidence for the contribution of CTLA-4 to both diabetes and AITD in the same individual [1060]. As mentioned above, the major susceptibility region for GD, HT and T1D in the CTLA-4 locus was mapped to the 6.1-kb region 3' of the CTLA-4 gene, with the functionally relevant CT60 (+6230 A/G) SNP, associated with the eficiency of splicing and production of sCTLA-4 isoform [801]. Clinical measurements in the serum of in patients with AITD showed increased levels of sCTLA-4, suggesting for a role of this isoform in the pathogenesis of thyroid autoimmunity [1062]. However, the biological significance of elevated sCTLA-4 serum level has not been yet clarified. The association between the +6230G allele of CTLA-4 with increased risk of GD is significantly stronger (*OR* = 1.51, *P* = 2.72 x 10^{-8}) compared to T1D (*OR* = 1.09-1.22, *P* =0.15-0.013) [801]. This therefore could suggest for a more significant contribution of CTLA-4 in genetic susceptibility for AITD than for T1D.

A recently discovered PTPN22 as a gene, contributing to general autoimmunity, showed association with both T1D and AITD in several populations [875,884,1066,1067]. In Caucasians, a functionally active R620W variant of PTPN22 showed strong association with increased risk of both GD (*OR* = 1.43-1.88) and HT (*OR* = 1.63 [884]. In Polish GD patients, Skorka et al. [1067] reported a correlation between the predisposing Trp620 allele and age of GD onset, showing a 2-fold difference in the average age of disease onset between subjects homozygous for Arg/Arg (42 years) and Trp/Trp (20.8 years). However, in Asians, where the PTPN22 R620W variant is absent, no association with GD was found [1068]. A strength of genetic association of the R620W marker with AITD is very similar to that for T1D (see Tables 16 and 17). A pathogenic mechanism, by which this SNP is involved in etiology of autoimmune diabetes and thyroid autoimmunity, is likely to be very similar for both diseases [895].

Additional susceptibility loci for T1D and AITD with overlapping regions of linkage have been mapped in the human genome. These loci are likely to contain susceptibility genes that confer susceptibility to both diseases, but these genes are not defined yet. One of those was mapped on chromosome Xp11. A genetic study in the UK population revealed evidence for linkage to GD for marker DXS8083 with a maximum NPL score of 2.2 [1069]. The finding of the susceptibility locus for GD on chromosome X could reflect significant (up to 10-fold) prevalence of AITD in females compared to males [1070]. This locus is situated in the region, where a T1D susceptibility locus (IDDMX) was previously mapped [887]. The region Xp11 showed a nominal linkage (MLS of more than 1.5) with AITD in the recent largest genome-wide scan, comprising 558 AITD families [1071]. IDDMX locus was also replicated in exlusion mapping in the last whole-genome screen for T1D susceptibility [636]. There are no studies, evaluating the positional candidate genes on chromosome Xp11 for association to AITD or T1D. The TLR7 gene, encoding toll-like receptor precursor, which participates in recognizing microbial pathogens and regulating innate immunity, could be a likely positional candidate for the susceptibility gene [1072].

The recent genome-wide scan also showed a nominal linkage to AITD on chromosome 5q23. Previously, linkage to AITD on the chromosome arm 5q was reported for region 5q31-q33 in Asians [1073-1075]. This region harbors a susceptibility gene for several autoimmune diseases, including T1D (IDDM18) [1076]. However, IDDM18 has been not confirmed in the last whole-genome search for T1D susceptibility loci [636]. Therefore, to date, genetic loci shared susceptibility to both AITD and T1D include HLA, CTLA-4 and PTPN22 genes with some supporting evidence for chromosome Xp11. To find additional common loci, which are likely to display weak genetic effects, a genome-wide scan in a large number of families affected with both diseases is needed.

T1D AND CELIAC DISEASE

Celiac disease (CD) is a second frequent autoimmune disorder associated with T1D. In general population, 4-9% of type 1 diabetic patients are reported to have celiac disease [1077-1080]. In first-degree relatives of T1D patients, a prevalence of CD is shown to be up to 6% [1034,1081].

Celiac disease is resulted from the gastrointestinal self-immunity induced by dietary wheat gluten and related proteins from barley and rye. CD is described as a rare disease, affecting primarily young children with prevalence in the general population of approximately 1 in 3000 [1082]. However, CD-related antibodies could be detected more frequently, being presented in 1/133 to 1/250 adult individuals [1023]. Endomysial and anti-transglutaminase (TTG) autoantibodies represent major immunologic markers for CD diagnosis. Antibodies against TTG are sensitive and specific indicators of the gastrointestinal autoimmune process, occurring in at least 95% of patients with bipsy-proven CD [1083]. Up to 75% T1D patients have abnormalities ob biopsy in the intestine. Approximately 5-10% of individuals affected T1D are found to be positive for endomysial and TTG self-antibodies [1077-1080,1084]. Similarly, around 5% of CD patients have diabetes-related islet-specific antibodies [124].

A putative pathogenic mechanism, linking T1D and CD, suggests the envolvement of gluten and related cereal proteins for inducing autoimmune response in genetically predisposing individuals with impaired function of the galt-associated lymphoid tissue, that normally prevents potentially harmful antigens from reaching the systemic circulation and induces systemic tolerance against luminal antigens [1085,1086]. The highest risk is predicted for subjects, carrying HLA markers susceptible for both diseases, i.e. DR3-DQ2. These T1D subjects are shown to develop high titres of TTG antibodies [1084]. In the intestine, this enzyme creates antigenic neoepitopes in gluten peptides, which are more efficiently presented to the immune system in the context of HLA-DQ2 or DQ8 background. The HLA region represents the major susceptibility locus for CD, with the estimated sib risk λ_S to be between 2.3 and 5.5, a value similar to that proposed for T1D [1087].

In the HLA region, susceptibility to both diseases was shown to be associated with the MICA-A gene encoding an MHC class I -related chain A. In exon 5 of MICA-A, the allele 5.1 results in the insertion of a nucleotide, which results in a premature stop codon. The truncated MICA-A5.1 variant is enable to effectively bind to a receptor, NKG2D, which could play a role in the thymic maturation of T cells [1088]. The allele 5.1 was shown to be susceptible in T1D [1089,1090] and CD [1091,1092]. However, it is difficult to reveal whether the MIC-A gene contributes to autoimmunity independently from the HLA genes due to the strong linkage disequilibrium between MIC-A polymorphisms and certain HLA alleles [1091].

Among non-HLA genes, an association with both CD and T1D was shown for the CTLA-4 gene [1093,1094]. In a Dutch population, the association of a susceptible haplotype CTLA-4 with CD and T1D was observed only in patients with high-risk HLA genotypes, which share the DQ2 allele, that may suggest for modulating effects of this CTLA-4 variant in shared genetic susceptibility for both diseases [1094].

T1D AND ADDISON'S DISEASE

Autoimmune diabetes and Addison's disease (AD) coexist in the same individual as a part of APS2. AD affects approximately 0.5-1.5% of T1D patients [1095,1096]. AD is associated with adrenal antibodies directed against the adrenal cortex. Antibodies against 21-hydroxylase (21-OH), en enzyme that participats in the metabolism of steroid hormones, are highly specific for AD, presenting in more than 90% patients with this disease [1097]. 21-OH antibodies could be found in approximately 1.5-2.5% type 1 diabetic subjects [1095,1096,1098], while islet antibodies are detected in up to 6% of AD patients [1099]. Yu et al. [1095] reported that T1D individuals, exhibiting 21-OH antibodies and carrying the DRB1*0404 allele, have a higher risk of progression from the adrenal autoimmunity to AD.

The DQ8-DQ2 genotype, consisting of DRB1*0404/DQ8 and DRB*301/DQ2, is a strongest risk marker in etiology of AD [1095,1096,1100]. The DR3-DQ2 and DR4-DQ8 both are diabetic HLA-associated risk markers, suggesting on sharing genetic susceptibility backround between T1D and AD. However, the DRB1*0404 allele is very rare in the general population (about 0.7%), while presenting in 30% of AD patients [1095]. Of non-HLA loci, an association with AD was shown for CTLA-4 [1014,1015,1101] and PTPN22 [1066], both are general autoimmunity genes, involving in the pathogenesis of T1D and other autoimmune disorders.

Chapter 12

Current Approaches in the Treatment of Type 1 Diabetes: Pancreatic Islet B Cell Replacement

The pancreatic islet β cell replacement is focused on the treatment of patients affected by T1D and by type 2 diabetes. In T1D, β-cell mass is lost, owing to the autoimmune destruction of β-cells [1102]. In type 2 diabetes, inadequate β-cell function and low β-cell mass cannot meet the increased insulin demands generated by the resistance of peripheral tissues to insulin action [1103]. Failure of exogenous insulin treatment to restore euglycemia and to prevent the development of diabetic complications initiated the search for therapies to replace lost β-cells. Human islets display a limited proliferative capacity in tissue culture that prevents a wide use of islet cell transplantation. Forced ex vivo expansion of human islets has resulted in premature cell senescence and dedifferentiation, although modest improvements have been achieved by maintaining the islets in a three-dimensional configuration with a fibrin matrix [1104]. The clinical use of widely available xenogenic islet cells, such as porcine islets, faces the huge barriers of strong rejection reactions and the risk of undetermined zoonotic infections [1105,1106]. This emphasizes a search of islet sources to meet the needs of all T1D patients, making the generation of new insulin-secreting β-cells by genetic engineering or by the differentiation of stem cells to be a major goal of the modern diabetes research.

B Cell Therapy in Diabetes Mellitus

Currently, for β cell therapy, islet cells from cadaver donors are used [1107]. However, this source is restricted by the limited supply of cadaveric pancreas donors. The creation of genetically engineered β cells was attempted, using β cells and non-β cells as a start material. Due to the xenobiotic origin and oncogenic characteristics, rodent insulinoma cell lines are unlikely sources for human β cell therapy. The generation of human immortalized β cells by transduction with incogenes has been more challenging, because human β-cell lines are difficult to propagate and lose differentiated function [1108]. However, the possibility of impaired insulin secretion and tumorogenicity of such cell lines still remains. Attempts to remove the oncogene and telomerase gene expression through the Cre-loxP recombination system significantly reduced tumorigenicity, but not completely [1109]. Further studies are needed to reduce this potential risk. Using of non-β cells, which share some functional characteristics with β cells, such as neuroendocrine cells, hepatocytes or intestinal K cells, is associated with the introduction of the entire set of genes, encoding the glucose-sensing and insulin secretory machinery of the β-cell, into those cells [1110]. However, it is still difficult to regulate the insulin production in such surrogate cells on levels closely similar with those in native β cells.

Cultured embryonic stem (ES) cells from the mouse [1111-1113] and human [1114,1115] have been found to differentiate into insulin-producing β cells. Typically, ES are able to differentiate to a variety of cell types, among those insulin-positive cells could be selected, amplified and induced to differentiate into mature β cells. To provide this, the expression of β-cell specific transcription factors (Pdx-1, Pax-4 and others) should be induced in the ES cell [1116,1117]. Unfortunately, the current understanding of the β-cell differentiation is limited that restricts a large-scale application of ES in the islet cell therapy. Anyway, the capacity of ES cells to differentiate into β cells supports their potential use to generate unlimited amounts of insulin-producing cells in the future.

Islet regeneration, or neogenesis, was reported in many studies, envolving experimentally induced damage of the pancreas, and therefore suggests for the existence of pancreatic progenitor cells in adults [1118]. A slow turnover of β cells was shown in vivo, and new islet cells could be generated from the progenitor cells located among pancreatic duct cells [1119,1120]. Insulin-producing cells have been generated from mouse [1121] and human adult duct cells [1122]. Mechanisms, leading to the differentiation of adult duct cells into insulin-producing cells are mostly unknown and need to be resolved for successful exploration of adult pancreatic stem cells as a source for β cells.

Although bone marrow stem cells from humans and mice were used to express multiple β-cell genes, the insulin content has remained very low [1123]. However, experiments with murine bone marrow cells showed supporting evidences for a potential significance of those cells in inducing the regeneration of endogenous pancreas [1124] or differentiation into insulin-producing islet cells [1125].

The possibility to develop new sorces of β cells, particularly from stem cells, that could be used in cell therapy of diabetes offers exciting perspectives. However, there is a substantial lack of understanding of the mechanisms that rule the expansion of β cells and and the differentiation of stem cells into β cells. Strict criteria, such as the expression of specific markers of mature β cells (not insulin expression only), abequate insulin processing and content, physiologically regulated insulin expression and others, should be used to establish a true regeneration of β cells [1126]. In addition, adequate in vivo models are needed to access their function and tumorogenicity.

INSULIN GENE THERAPY

Insulin gene therapy is an approach, which might overcome the weakness of islet cell therapy in order to its vulnerability to autoimmune attack. Multiple attempts have been done to introduce insulin-producing machinery of β cells into non-β cells that are not targets of islet-specific autoimmune responces. However, a simple transfer of a system of insulin biosynthesis into non-insulin-producing cells by genetic manipulations without proper regulation is unlikely. There are several mandatory conditions required for successful insulin gene therapy. The efficient insulin gene therapy should have an effective insulin gene delivery mechanism, a system of regulation of the insulin biosynthesis that responds to glucose within extremely narrow physiological limits, a system of insulin processing into its active form and a choice of an appropriate target cells, which possess biochemical characteristics similar to β cells, but are not targets for β-cell specific self-reactivity.

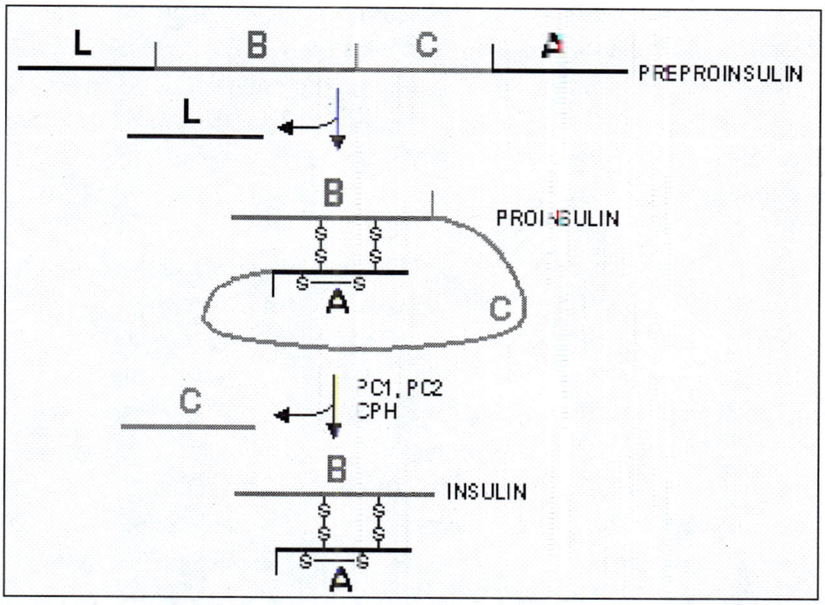

Figure 20. Scheme of the enzymatic conversion of preproinsulin into insulin. The insulin precursor, preproinsulin, is a single chain polypeptide. Removal of a 24-residue leader peptide (L) leads to the formation of proinsulin consisting of 81 amino acids. Proinsulin contains both A and B chains separated with the C-peptide. In islet β cells, proinsulin is stored in special secretory granules, where it undergoes disulfide bond formation. When serum glucose concentration is increased, three islet proteases (proconvertase PC2, proconvertase PC3 and carboxypepidase H (CPH)) subsequently cleave proinsulin resulting in formation of the C-peptide and mature insulin, which is further secreted. Mature insulin molecule includes two chains, A and B, bound by one intrachain and two interchain disulfide (-S-S-) bridges.

Mature insulin molecule includes two chains, A and B, bound by one intrachain and two interchain disulfide bridges. The insulin precursor, preproinsulin, is a sigle chain polypeptide (Figure 20). Removal of a 24-residue signal peptide results in the formation of proinsulin, consisting of 81 amino acids. Proinsulin contains both A and B chains separated with the C-peptide. Proinsulin is stored is special secretoty granules, where it undergoes disulfide bond formation. Increase in intracellular Ca^{2+} leads to the activation of two insulin-processing proteases, proconvertase PC2 and proconvertase PC3. PC2 cuts proinsulin between the B chain and the C-peptide at a Arg-Arg residues, and then PC3 cleaves between the A chain and C-peptide at a Lys-Arg residue. Carboxypepidase H removes the exposed Arg-Arg residues on the C-terminus of the B chain, and the active insulin is secreted (Figure 20).

Since islet β cells have specific characteristics, such as special proteases, secretory granules and glucose receptors, essential for proper processing and release of insulin in response to extracellular glucose levels, the ideal target cells for insulin therapy should be non-β cells possessing these characteristics [1127]. Neuroendocrine cells are likely candidates for those target cells, because they have enzymes for processing inactive precursors into active peptide hormones and a regulated secretory system. Experiments on a mouse corticotrophic cell line derived from the pituitary gland showed that cotransfection of insulin gene with genes, encoding glucose transporter 2 (GLUT2) and glucokinase resulted in glucose-responsive insulin secretion [1128,1129]. However, these cells also express adrenocorticotrophic hormone that stimulates glucocorticoid synthesis and then inhibits insulin secretion. The expression of the human insulin transgene under control of the 5'-promoter region of the glucose-dependent insulinotropic polypeptide in endocrine intestinal K cells yielded biologically active insulin and protected mise from STZ-induced diabetes [1130]. K cells have glucose-responsive exocytosis and all enzymes required for proinsulin-insulin convertion and hence are likely to reperesent an appropriate target for insulin gene therapy [1131].

Hepatocytes could be attractive target cells for insulin gene therapy due to the presence of glucose-sensing molecules (GLUT2 and glucokinase) similar to those in pancreatic islets [1132]. The limitation of hepatocytes is lack of processing enzymes and glucose-regulated insulin secretion. Hepatocytes have several glucose-responsive genes, whose promoters could be used for liver-targeted insulin gene therapy [1133]. With different outcomes, insulin was expressed in liver cells under control of promoters from the glucose-regulated genes, such as glucose-6-phosphatase [1134], pyruvate kinase [1135,1136], glucose-dependent insulinotropic polypeptide [1130] and Spot-14 [1137]. The main explanation of failure to produce insulin in rapid response to increased glucose concentrations is the absence in hepatocytes of a system that quickly reacts to blood glucose levels by insulin release, i.e. secretory granules. Thus, it is necessary to develop a system that closely mimics the rapid response to blood glucose. An example of such system is using of drug-induced protein disaggregation, which results in the release of insulin from a fusion protein, containing an aggregated domain and accumulated in the endoplasmic reticulum, when the drug was added [1138]. Additional approaches to improve the regulation of insulin secretion may include insertion of multiple copies of glucose-responsive elements or addition of insulin-sensitive elements into promoter regions, regulating insulin expression.

To overcome the absence of insulin-processing proteases in hepatocytes, an attempt to introduce a novel proteolytic site into the proinsulin gene, which could be recognized by furin, was performed. This protease is widely expressed, including liver. Thus, the introduction of furin-digestable proinsulin into hepatocytes should result in the production of functional insulin [1139-1142]. A glucose-dependent expression of the human insulin transgene directed by three glucose-inducible regulatory elements and the liver-specific albumin promoter was obtained in hepatocytes [1142]. A therapy with furin-cleavable insulin improved hyperglycaemia in STZ-treated diabetic rats [1142,1143], thereby supporting the feasibility of hepatocyte-based insulin gene-therapy for treatment of T1D.

Conclusion

The ultimate goal for T1D treatment is producing insulin in a phisiologically regulated manner withot triggering autoimmune response. Islet transplantation, regeneration of insulin-producing β cells and insulin gene therapy have been used for the cure of diabetes. However, none of these approaches separately could be fully satisfactory for clinical care to diabetic patients. Islet transplantation is limited by the source of islets and requirement for life-long immune suppression. Insulin gene therapy is limited by appropriate insulin production in response to physiological levels of glucose. β cell regeneration is complicated by persistent self-reactivity against newly generated β cells.

The ultimate goal of islet transplantation is to completely restore glucose homeostasis and prevent long-term diabetic complications without the need for maintenance immunosuppressive therapy. Unlike other solid organ transplants, islet transplantation is disadvantaged, because there is a lack of an effective predictive marker of early rejection – and for this reason the immunosuppressive regimens used in islet transplantation often cause negative side effects of over-immunosuppression. The degree of systemic immunosuppression should be reduced, ultimately towards inducing a permanent state of unresponsiveness to the allograft (tolerance). In that case, the islet transplantation could be applied in the earliest stages of diabetes, including transplantation in children.

At present, there are several experimental approaches to induce tolerance in islet transplantation. One strategy is based on the blockade of critical costimulatory molecules on the surface of T cells. This strategy showed significant promise in preclinical models. For example, in a primate model of islet transplantation, the blockage of CD154, CD28 and CD3 by specific antibodies resulted in long-term survival of islet xenografts [1144,1145] and allografts [1146,1147]. Moreover, the agent Campath-1H, a humanized antibody specific for CD52 determinants on the surface of T cells, has demonstrated considerable success in maintaining function of renal allografts in patients [1148] and is currently being explored in clinical islet transplantation [1149].

Another approach to avoid immunosuppression is the encapsulation of islets in immunoprotective devices prior to implantation. Several immunoisolation systems have been extensively studied and have been shown to enhance the survival of both allogeneic and xenogeneic islets [1150]. However, a wide use of these systems is seriously impeded by multiple limitations, including an adequate access of the encapsulated islets to blood supply and oxygen for survival. Developments in polymer biology are definitely required before this approach can be applied to patients.

It has been suggested that islet transplantation could serve as a primary test that lead for novel tolerance protocols, because failure to achieve tolerance would result in the patient's return to insulin therapy rather than potential death in the case of losing a life-sustaining heart or liver transplant. Nevertheless, limitations such as the need to overcome both alloimmune and autoimmune barriers, as well the lack of specific serological markers to detect allograft rejection, may prove to be significant challenges as new tolerance strategies are tested in islet transplantation.

In recent years, landmark advances in islet isolation and less diabetogenic immunosuppression have moved islet transplantation forward from research to clinical reality. With the introduction of the Edmonton Protocol [1151] and ongoing developments, islet transplantation has now been accepted as a safe and effective therapy for select patients with type 1 diabetes. At present, because patients receiving islet allografts must exchange insulin for life-long immunosuppressive therapy, the procedure can only be justified in patients with very unstable forms of diabetes. Development of novel immunosuppressive protocols using more specific and less toxic drugs, ultimately towards inducing tolerance, is an important step in applying islet transplantation earlier in the course of the disease, including transplantation in children.

In insulin therapy, more studies are required to achieve tight regulationin response to physiological levels of glucose and for safe delivery of the insulin gene before this strategy can be considered for clinical application to human T1D patients. Even though there are many technical difficulties to be overcome, recent advances in gene transfer technology may make possible that insulin gene therapy may play an increasing role in clinical practive in the future.

Chapter 13

PREDICTION OF TYPE 1 DIABETES

Since T1D represents a complex disorder, current prediction of this disease is based on three levels, which include the genetic predisposition, the identification of pre-diabetes by way of islet-specific self-antibodies and using metabolic tests.

ESTIMATION OF GENETIC RISK FOR THE DEVELOPMENT OF T1D

T1D arises in genetically susceptible individuals and is characterized by increased clusterization in families, suggesting on a significant role of genetic backround in etiology of T1D. The HLA region and HLA class II genes particularly is a major genetic susceptibility locus (IDDM1) for T1D. By performing HLA-DR/DQ typing in T1D patients, the general population and unaffected individuals, the absolute risk of developing diabetes can be determined (Table 18).

In Caucasians, the HLA DR3/4 (DRB1*03-DQA1*0501-DQB1*02/DRB1*04-DQA1*0301-DQB1*0302) genotype is shown to be related to the highest risk of T1D (Table 20). This risk marker could be found in approximately 20-30% of T1D patients and in up to 50% of patients with diabetes diagnosed in early childhood [1152-1154]. Whereas several genotypes of HLA contribute to increased risk of T1D, other genotypes (i.e. genotypes, containing the DRB1*1501-DQA1*01/DQB1*0602 haplotype) confer the protection. Thus, based on the HLA–DR and –DQ genotypes, the risk for T1D could be easily stratified more than 100 times. Several studies tried to rank HLA genotypes on the basis of risk they confer [1152,1154,1155,1156], and some of them suggested algorithms for preselection of newborns, who are at high risk and who will comprise a large proportion of future T1D cases [1155,1156].

Table 18. Absolute risk for T1D according to HLA-DR/DQ genotypes

HLA-DR/DQ genotype	Risk in a general population	Risk in first-degree relatives of T1D patients
DR 3/4, DQ*0201/*0302	1/15**	1/ 4-5*
DR 4/4, DQ*0300/*0302	1/20**	1/6*
DR 3/3, DQ*0201/*0201	1/45***	1/10**
DR4/X, DQ*0302/X (X is not *0602)	1/60***	1/15**
X/X	1/600****	1/125****
DR*0403 or DQ*0602	1/15,000*****	1/15,000*****

* Very high risk; ** High risk; *** Moderate risk; **** Low risk; ***** Protected.

HLA-linked susceptibility is modified by several factors, including a T1D family history. For example, a risk to develop islet autoimmunity and clinical diabetes in children, carrying DR3/4 and having a T1D first-degree relative, is more than 10-fold that of children with the DR3/4 genotype, but without a T1D first-degree relative [1157]. In addition, genes can interact with other genes or with the environment and thus the risk conferred by HLA could be modified for some genotypes. In the case of IDDM2 susceptibility locus in the insulin gene, a significant heterogeneity in the distribution of INS genotypes in patients with different HLA genotypes is observed [1158]. Combining HLA and INS genotyping, therefore, should improve T1D risk stratification [1159], but not in a manner strictly predicted from the multiplicative model. Modification of T1D risk by the environment is also could be genotype-specific [1160].

Combining family history of T1D with HLA genotype allows stratification of individuals into risks, ranging more than 1000-fold. With respect to family history, risk varies, depending on which relative(s) has T1D. In the DPT-1 study, siblings of patients with T1D more frequently developed islet-specific antibodies than offspring or parents of patients with T1D [1161]. The number of relatives with T1D also affects the risk of T1D. In the BABYDIAB study, the children's risk was significantly increased if both parents or a parent and a sibling had disease as compared with a single affected family member [1162]. Using of both criteria, i.e. T1D family history and genetic markers (i.e., HLA and INS) will be very helpful to improve the prediction of diabetes. Approximately 50% of children, carrying high risk HLA alleles and having more than one first-degree relative with T1D, develop islet self-antibodies by age 5. Moreover, for children of affected parents, the risk to develop disease could be stratified from almost 0% (offspring with protective HLA genotypes and one parent with T1D) to 20% (children with DR3/4 and two affected family members [1162].

The recent identification of two new genes (CTLA-4 and PTPN22) involved in the pathogenesis of T1D should further improve the estimation of T1D risk, although these loci exhibit a modest genetic effect to the susceptibility to T1D. Since T1D susceptibility linked to CTLA-4 and PTPN22 is associated with immune dysregulation, taking into account of those loci could potentially identify distinct subgenotypes, with different immune dysregulation pathways, leading to the common disease phenotype that may respond to different preventive interventions.

Islet-Specific Autoantibodies as Immunological Markers for Islet Autoimmunity and Clinical Diabetes

There are four major self-reacting antibodies (against glutamic acid decarboxylase 65 kD isoform, insulin and islet antigens IA-2 and IA-2β) that could be found in sera of diabetic patients with high frequency and therefore be useful for diabetes prediction. Predictive value of those antibodies in early diagnosis of T1D have been discussed above.

Since islet-specific autoantibodies may be found in the blood of prediabetic individuals, these antibodies are markers of prediabetes and are used to identify subjects with increased risk to develop T1D [1163]. Accurate and reproducible quantification assays of serum titres for diabetes-related antibodies are very important. For detection of GADA and IA-2A antibodies, high concordance was obtained between different laboratories, allowing WHO to specify a standard for worldwide comparison of levels of these antibodies [1164]. For IAA, there was a less consensus between the laboratories, particularly in cases when low titres of IAA were present.

Most studies, estimating a value of islet antibodies in predicting T1D, have been preformed in first-degree relatives of diabetic patients, i.e. individuals with increased genetic susceptibility to T1D. In those subjects, diabetes-related antibodies are occurred with higher frequency (5%-10%) [466,1165,1166]. In the US DPT-1 study, a largest screeing of first-degree relatives for the presence of four major diabetes-related antibodies was carried out. At least one of these self-antibodies was found in 8.2% of relatives, and more than one antibody in 2.3% [1166]. On the basis of population screening for islet antibodies, other disease-specific characteristics related to age, gender, genetic backround and other parameters have been also reported [1167-1169].

Compared to other antibodies, IAA have an advantage in early detection of prediabetes, because these antibodies are shown to be among the first self-antibodies to appear in children, who develop T1D [473]. Not all children, who develop IAA, progress to multiple antibody status of T1D [1170,1171]. The affinity status of IAA plays an important role in their value as markers of the progression from islet autoimmunity to clinical disease. Children, who have low titres of transient IAA with lower affinity are unlikely to develop multiple antibodies and progress to T1D. In contrast, children with high-affinity persisent IAA ($K_d > 10^9$ L/mol) develop multiple antibodies and have 50% risk to progress to T1D within 6 years [1168]. In contrast to low-affinity IAA, the recognition epitope for binding high-affinity insulin antibodies is also present on the proinsulin molecule [1168]. Based on that, the development of IAA detection assays with improved specificity is possible.

Presence of multiple islet antibodies suggests for increased risk to develop T1D. In relatives, who have only one antibody, T1D risk is about 20% but it increases in relatives with two and more antibodies up to 35% and 61% within 5 and 10 years, respectively [1167]. Multiple subclass antibodies are usually synonymous with high titer, but these features can be separate indicators of disease risk also in subjects with low titers of islet antibodies. In the BABYDIAB study, the follow-up analysis of self-antibodies in first-degree relatives during 15 years revealed significant correlation between higher-titer IAA and IA-2A self-reactivity and risk of T1D, with the appearance of antibody subclasses IgG2, IgG3 and/or IgG4 [1167]. Using different combinations of these diabetes-related antibodies, it is likely to stratify diabetes risk from less than 10% to around 90% within 5 years. Antibodies against IA-2 are associated with a higher risk of disease than GADA and IAA [1172]. In patients positive for IA-2 antibodies, those with antibodies, reacting to IA-2A and IA-2B antigens, show a higher diabetes risk than IA-2B-negative subjects [1167]. This therefore makes useful to measure not only titer, but also a number of epitope targets in predicting T1D risk.

Using genetic markers is very helpful to further stratify T1D risk in subjects who are positive for islet antibodies and in risk to progress to the development of clinical disease. In several prevention trials, such as BABYDIAB, DIPP, DAISY, DPT-1 and others, a positive correlation between the carriage of high-risk HLA genotypes and early onset (and incidence) of islet autoimmunity was shown [1157,1173]. For example, in German children (BABYDIAB study) with the high-risk DR3/4 and DR4/4 genotypes, the risk for developing diabetes-related antibodies by age 5 exceeds 20% compared to 4% in offspring without those genotypes [1159].

Multiple studies showed that individuals positive for islet antibodies and carrying high risk HLAmarkers had an increased risk to develop T1D, whereas subjects with islet antibodies, but having the protective HLA-DQ6 allele, exhibited a reduced risk to progress to clinical diabetes [642,1174]. Genetic risk factors found in children with multiple persistent antibodies were absent in children, who developed single or transient antibodies [1159,1175]. In addition, high-affinity pathogenic IAA were shown to be associated with the carriage of the high-risk HLA-DR4 allele [1168]. Thus, HLA and probably other T1D susceptibility genes may help for further stratification of diabetes risk in antibody-positive individuals, since genetic factors clearly influence the magnitude and breadth of the islet-specific autoimmune response.

METABOLIC MARKERS IN PREDICTING RISK FOR T1D

In prediabetes, insulin responces to intravenous glucose challenges are often impaired. Several studies tried to find whether combining islet antibody detection and first-phase insulin response (FPIR) in an intravenous glucose tolerance test are helpful in prediction of T1D development. In antibody-positive relatives, who have a low FPIR, a faster rate of progression to T1D was observed compared to relatives with normal FPIR [472,1176]. In the DIPP study, low FRIP was associated with some immunological characteristics, such as the presence of IAA, higher levels of ICA and multiple islet antibodies [1177]. Persistent loss of FPIR measured during intravenous glucose tolerance test in ICA-positive relatives carries at least 50% risk of progression to disease over 5 years [1178]. Changes in glucose tolerance measured during oral glucose tolerance testing typically occur later in the disease process, reflecting significant β–cell destruction. Among metabolic characteristics, FPIR seems to be useful in predicting T1D for antibody-positive subjects, who are in the preclinical phase of disease [1179].

DIABETES PREVENTION TRIALS

The ability to predict T1D, particularly in high-risk first-degree relatives, has enabled investigators worldwide to perform multicenter trials aimed at its prevention. The DPT-1 study, a multicenter US trial, characterized above was started to determine whether antigen-based (insulin) therapy of nondiabetic relatives can prevent or delay the onset of diabetes. In Finland, a trial to reduce type 1 diabetes in genetically at risk (TRIGR) was performed to verify whether the avoidance of nutritional cow's milk proteins for at least first 6 months of life will reduce diabetes in a high-risk population, such as a Finnish population. Finnish infants, who have T1D first-degree relatives, have been first genotyped to select those, carrying high-risk HLA genotypes, i.e. positive for DQB*10302 and/or DQB1*02 and negative for protective DQ*10602, *0603 or *030 alleles [1180]. After full breast-feeding, the intervention group (n = 114) received a casein hydrolysate formula, whereas the control group (n =110) received a cows' milk containing formula. After a mean observation period of 4.7 years and adjustment for duration of study formula feeding, life-table analysis showed a significant protection by the intervention from positivity for ICA (p=0.02) and at least one autoantibody (p=0.03), suggesting for a putative pathogenic role of dietary factors in inducing β-cell autoimmunity, despite a limited power of the study, and the possibility to manipulate spontaneous islet autoimmunity by dietary intervention in infancy [1181].

Two European trials have been designed to evaluate whether treatment with nicotinamide might prevent progression to diabetes in high-risk first-degree relatives. Nicotinamide could protect against the rapid onset of T1D through the inhibition of polyADP-ribosylation that depletes cellular stores of NAD^+ and ATP and through the protection from oxygen free radicals [174,1182]. In the Deutsche Nicotinamide Intervention Study (DENIS), 2,415 siblings of T1D patients were screened for ICA, and 164 siblings from 68 families, showing higher titres of ICA (greater or equal to 20 JDF units) have been selected [1183]. The intervention was consisted of oral nicotinamide (1.2 g/m^2) divided into two daily doses or placebo. However, four-year follow-up revealed no significant improvement in the incidence of T1D. In addition, at 2 year, FPIR was shown to be decreased in the nicotinamide group, while remained stable in the placebo. Thus, the DENIS study failed to show any protective effects of the nicotinamide treatment onto the development of T1D.

Another study, the European Nicotinamide Diabetes Intervention Trial (ENDIT) involved patients from 18 European countries, Canada and USA. Approximately 30,000 subjects, first-degree relatives of children with T1D, at age 5-40 years have been screened for ICA, and 552 individuals with high-titer ICA (more than 20 JDF units) were chosen and randomized [1184]. Similar to DPT-1, most of these subjects are aged under 20 years and are mainly siblings of T1D probands. The proposed 5-year observation period was designed with 90% power to observe a 35% reduction in disease incidence. The participants were randomly allocated oral modified release nicotinamide (1.2 g/m^2) or placebo. As the DENNIS study, the ENDIT study showed lack of protective effect of nicotinamide at the dose used in prevention from the early onset of diabetes [1185].

Optimal Strategies in Prediction of Type 1 Diabetes

To date, there are several genetic, immune and metabolic markers are available for prediction of T1D. These markers could be used in combination to select subject at high genetic risk of T1D, to identify subjects with islet autoimmunity and to stratify T1D in the preclinical period. Genetic selection is established to be the most useful strategy to preselect at-risk individuals. Genotyping with T1D susceptibility genetic markers, particularly those located within HLA class II genes, is very helpful in early selection of individuals with the genetic background susceptible to T1D. Family history of T1D should be taken into account, while selecting those individuals that will allow the stratification of subjects into risks, ranging more than 1000-fold.

Islet-specific antibodies are suggested to be the best predictors in identifying β-cell autoimmunity and preclinical disease. Among those, IAA take an advantage to serve as a predictor of inducing islet-specific self-reactivity due to their early appearance, islet-specific reactivity and high frequency in patients with preclinical diabetes [1186]. Further screening for IAA affinity, epitope reactivity and self-antibody persistence provides opportunity for selecting patients with high-affinity persistent IAA, associated with increased risk of progression from β-cell autoimmunity to clinical disease [1168,1170].

In ICA-positive individuals, the risk of T1D might be stratified by the identification of multiple islet-specific autoantibodies in the same individual [1166,1167]. The consideration of antibody characteristics, such as autoantibody titers and subclasses, epitope reactivity, presence of IA-2A- and IA-2B-specific self-antibodies will be helpful in the further stratification of diabetes risk [1167, 1172, 1187]. Genetic (HLA genotyping) and metabolic risk markers (low FPIR, elevated C-peptide levels) could be also useful to stratify the risk of progression to clinical diabetes [1157,1159,1176,1177,1188].

The environmental triggers also play a crucial role in inducing T1D, and the identification of environmental markers usefull for early prediction of disease is very important. Results of the Finnish TRIGR study suggested for a role of dietary factors, such as cow's milk proteins, in the induction of β-cell autoimmunity [1181]. The TEDDY (The Environmental Determinants of Diabetes in the Young) study was recently launched to evaluate a role of various environmental factors in the development of T1D. The TEDDY study proposes to newly recruit 5,940 neonates from the general population with a pre-determined type 1 diabetes risk of 3% and 1,152 neonates with first degree relatives who have type 1 diabetes and who have a pre-determined type 1 diabetes risk of 10%. Thus, we propose to study a total of 7,092 participants across six clinical centers worldwide (Finland, Germany, Sweden and three in North America). The North American Centers are expected to recruit 60% of the 7,092 participants. The participants will be followed with blood sampling every three months for islet autoantibody measurements until age 4 years and then every six months until the age of 15, for a total of 95,742 samples over the first 5 years of the study (approximately 57,445 from North America and 38,296 from Europe), and a total of 269,496 over the entire study (approximately 161,697 from North America and 107,798 from Europe). The long-term goal of the TEDDY study is the identification of infectious agents, dietary factors or other environmental agents, including psychosocial factors, which trigger T1D in genetically susceptible individuals or which protect against the disease. Identification of such factors will lead to a better understanding of disease pathogenesis and result in new strategies to prevent, delay or reverse T1D.

ACKNOWLEGMENTS

I greatly thank Inna Tyurina for her very friendly and enthusiastic support and great stimulatory influence, while writing this book. I truly appreciate this.

REFERENCES

[1] Alberti, K.G. & Zimmet, P.Z. (2001). Definition, diagnosis and classification of diabetes mellitus and its complications. Part 1: diagnosis and classification of diabetes mellitus provisional report of a WHO consultation. *Diabetic Medicine, 15*, 539-553.

[2] Seissler, J., de Sonnaville, J.J.J., Morgenthaler, N.G., Steinbrenner, H., Glawe, D., Khoo-Morgenthaler, U.Y., Lan, M.S., Notkins, A.L., Heine, R.J. & Scherbaum, W.A. (1998). Immunological heterogeneity in type 1 diabetes: presence of distinct autoantibody patterns in patients with acute onset and slowly progressive disease. *Diabetologia, 41*, 891-897.

[3] Horton, V., Stratton, I., Bottazzo, G.F., Shattock, M., Mackay. I., Zimmet. P., Manley, S., Holman, R. & Turner, R. (1999). Genetic heterogeneity of autoimmune diabetes: age of presentation in adults is influenced by HLA DRB1 and DQB1 genotypes (UKPDS 43). UK Prospective Diabetes Study (UKPDS) Group. *Diabetologia, 42*, 608-616.

[4] Turner, R., Stratton, I. Horton, V., Manley, S., Zimmet. P., Mackay. I.R., Shattock, M., Bottazzo, G.F. & Holman, R. UKPDS 25: autoantibodies to islet-cell cytoplasm and glutamic acid decarboxylase for prediction of insulin requirement in type 2 diabetes (1997). UK Prospective Diabetes Study Group. *Lancet, 350*, 1288-1293.

[5] Atkinson, M.A. & Eisenbarth, G.S. (2001). Type 1 diabetes: new perspectives on disease pathogenesis and treatment. *Lancet, 358*, 221-229.

[6] Imagawa, A., Hanafusa, T., Miyagawa, J. & Matsuzawa, Y. (2000). A novel subtype of type 1 diabetes mellitus characterized by a rapid onset and an absence of diabetes-related antibodies. Osaka IDDM Study Group. *New England Journal of Medicine, 342*, 301-317.

[7] Verge, C.F., Stenger, D., Bonifacio, E., Colman, P.G., Pilcher. C., Bingley. P.J. & Eisenbarth, G.S. (1998). Combined use of autoantibodies (autoantibody, GAD autoantibody, insulin autoantibody, cytoplasmic islet cell antibodies) in type 1 diabetes: Combinatorial islet autoantibody workshop. *Diabetes, 47*, 1857-1866.

[8] Hatziagelaki, E., Jaeger, C., Petzoldt, R., Seissler, J., Scherbaum, W.A., Federlin, K. & Bretzel, R.G. (1999). The combination of antibodies to GAD-65 and IA-2ic can replace the islet-cell antibody assay to identify subjects at risk of type 1 diabetes mellitus. *Hormone Metabolism Research, 31*, 564-569.

[9] Zimmet, P.Z., Tuomi, T., Mackay I.R., Tuomi, T., Rowley, M.J., Lcher, C.C. & Knowles, W.J. (1994). Latent autoimmune diabetes mellitus in adults (LADA): the role of antibodies to glutamic acid decarboxylase in diagnosis and prediction of insulin dependency. *Diabetic Medicine, 11*, 299-303.

[10] Ingawa, A., Hanafusa, T., Miyagawa, J.I. & Matsuzawa, Y. (2000). A novel subtype of Type 1 diabetes mellitus characterized by a rapid onset and an absence of diabetes-related antibodies. *New England Journal of Medicine, 342*, 301-307.

[11] Regan, F.M., Reiterer, E.E., Salzano, G. & Dunger, D.B. (2005). Type 1 diabetes in children: a review. *Practioner, 249*, 503-508.

[12] Umpierrez, G.E. & Kitabchi, A.E. (2003). Diabetic ketoacidosis: risk factors and management strategies. *Treatments in Endocrinology, 2*, 95-108.

[13] Kaufman, F.R., Halvorson, M., Miller, D., Mackenzie, M., Fisher, L.K. & Pitukcheewanont, P. (1999). Insulin pump therapy in type 1 pediatric patients: now and into the year 2000. *Diabetes Metabolism Research and Reviews, 15*, 338-352.

[14] Schreiber, M., Steele, A., Goguen, J., Levin, A. & Halperin, M. (1996). Can a severe degree of ketoacidosis develop overnight? *American Society for Nephrology, 7*, 192-197.

[15] Palmer, J.P. (1983) Alcoholic ketoacidosis: clinical and laboratory presentation, pathophysiology and treatment. *Clinical Endocrinology and Metabolism, 12*, 381-389.

[16] Bohn, D. & Daneman, D. (2002). Diabetic ketoacidosis and cerebral edema. *Current Opinion in Pediatrics, 14*, 287-291.

[17] Trachtenbarg, D.E. (2005) Diabetic ketoacidosis. *American Family Physician, 71*, 1705-1714.

[18] Glaser, N. & Kuppermann, N. (2004). The evaluation and management of children with diabetic ketoacidosis in the emergency department. *Pediatric Emergency Care, 20*, 477- 484.

[19] Hoffman, R.P. (2004). Practical management of type 1 diabetes mellitus in adolescent patients: challenges and goals. *Treatments in Endocrinology, 3*, 27-39.

[20] Heise, T., Koschinsky, T., Heinemann, L. & Lodwig, V.; Glucose Monitoring Study Group. (2003). Hypoglycemia warning signal and glucose sensors: requirements and concepts. *Diabetic Technology and Therapeutics, 5*, 563-571.

[21] McAulay, V., Deary, I.J. & Frier, B.M. (2001). Symptoms of hypoglycaemia in people with diabetes. *Diabetic Medicine, 18*, 690-705.

[22] Gruppuso, P.A. (2003). Achieving glycemic control in young children with type 1 diabetes: approaches, pitfalls and new technologies. *Medicine and Health, Rhode Island, 86*, 107-111.

[23] Madsbad, S. (2002). Insulin analogues: have they changed insulin treatment and improved glycaemic control? *Diabetes Metabolism Research and Reviews, 18 (Suppl 1)*, S21-S28.

[24] McEvilly, A. & Kirk, J. (2005). Twenty years of a multidisciplinary paediatric diabetes home care unit. *Archives of Disease in Childhood, 90*, 342-345.

[25] Passa, P. (2002). Diabetes trends in Europe. *Diabetes Metabolism Research and Reviews, 18 (Suppl 3)*, S3-S8.

[26] Rewers, M., Norris, J. & Dabelea, D. (2004). Epidemiology of type 1 diabetes mellitus. *Advances in Experimental Medicine and Biology, 552*, 19-26.

[27] Schranz, A.G. (1998). Trends in incidence of childhood type 1 diabetes in Malta. *Diabetes Care, 41*, 194-195.

[28] Songini, M., Bernardellini, L., Clayton, D., Montomoli, C., Pascutto, C., Chislandi, M., Fadda, D., Bottazzo, G.F. & Sardinian Study Groups. (1998). The Sardinian IDDM Study: 1. Epidemiology and geographical distribution of IDDM in Sardinia during 1989 to 1994. *Diabetologia, 41*, 221-227.

[29] Frazer de Llado, T.E., Gonzalez de Pijem, L. & Hawk, B. (1998). Incidence of IDDM in children living in Puerto Rico. Puerto Rican IDDM Coalition. *Diabetes Care, 21*, 744-746.

[30] Onkamo, P., Vaananen, S., Karvonen, M. & Tuomilehto, J. (1999). Wordwide increase in incidence of type 1 diabetes – the analysis of the data on published incidence records. *Diabetologia, 42*, 1395-1403.

[31] Tuomilehto, J., Karvonen, M., Pitkaniemi, J., Virtala, E., Kohtamaki, K., Toivanen, L. & Tuomilehto-Wolf, E. (1999). Record-high incidence of Type I (insulin-dependent) diabetes mellitus in Finnish children. The Finnish Childhood Type I Diabetes Registry Group. *Diabetologia, 42*, 655-660.

[32] Gay, E.C., Hamman, R.F., Carosone-Link, P.J., Lezotte, D.C., Cook, M., Stroheker, R., Klingensmith, G. & Chase, H.P. (1989). Colorado IDDM Registry: lower incidence of IDDM in Hispanics. Comparison of disease characteristics and care patterns in biethnic population. *Diabetes Care, 12*, 701-708.

[33] Boyle, J.P., Engelgau, M.M., Thompson, T.J., Goldschmid, M.G., Beckles, G.L., Timberlake, D.S., Herman, W.H., Ziemer, D.C. & Gallina, D.L. (1999). Estimating prevalence of type 1 and type 2 diabetes in a population of African Americans with diabetes mellitus. *American Journal of Epidemiology, 149*, 55-63.

[34] Schatz, D.A. & Bingley, P.J. (2001). Update on major trials for the prevention of type 1 diabetes mellitus: the American Diabetes Prevention Trial (DPT-1) and the European Nicotinamide Diabetes Intervention Trial (ENDIT). *Journal of Pediatric Endocrinology and Metabolism, 14 (Suppl. 1)*, 619-622.

[35] Zimmet, P.Z., Rowley, M.J., Mackay, I.R., Knowles, W.J., Chen, Q.Y., Chapman, L.H. & Serjeantson, S.W. (1993). The ethnic distribution of antibodies to glutamic acid decarboxylase: presence and levels of insulin-dependent diabetes mellitus in Europid and Asian subjects. *Journal of Diabetes Complications, 7*, 1-7.

[36] Tuomi, T., Zimmet, P., Rowley, M.J., Min, H.K., Vichayanrat, A., Lee, H.K., Rhee, B.D., Vannasaeng, S., Humphrey, A.R. & Mackay, I.R. (1995). Differing frequency of autoantibodies to glutamic acid decarboxylase among Koreans, Thais, and Australians with diabetes mellitus. *Clinical Immunology and Immunopathology, 74*, 202-206.

[37] Serrani-Rios, M., Goday, A. & Larrad, T.M. (1999). Migrant populations and the incidence of type 1 diabetes: an overview of the literature with a focus on the Spanish-heritage Countries in Latin America. *Diabetes Metabolism Research and Reviews, 15*, 113-132.

[38] Motala, A.A., Omar, M.A. & Pirie, F.J. (2003). Diabetes in Africa. Epidemiology of type 1 and type 2 diabetes in Africa. *Journal of Cardiovascular Risk, 10*, 77-83.

[39] Shamis, I., Gordon, O., Albag, Y., Goldsand, G. & Laron, Z. (1997). Ethnic differences in the incidence of childhood IDDM in Israel (1965-1993). Marked increase since 1985, especially in Yemenite Jews. *Diabetes Care, 20*, 504-508.

[40] Rewers, M., Stone, R.A., LaPorte, R.E., Drash, A.L., Becker, D.J., Walczak, M. & Kuller, L.H. (1989) Poisson regression modeling of temporal variation in incidence of childhood insulin-dependent diabetes mellitus in Allegheny County, Pennsylvania, and Wielikopolska, Poland, 1970-1985. *American Journal of Epidemiology, 129*, 569-581.

[41] Muntoni, S. & Songini, M. (1992). High rate of IDDM in Sardinia. Sardinian Collaborative Group for Epidemiology of IDDM. *Diabetes Care, 15*, 1317-1322.

[42] LaGasse, J.M., Brantley, M.S., Leech, N.J., Rowe, R.E., Monks, S., Palmer, J.P., Nepom, G.T., McCulloch, D.K. & Hagopian W.A. Washington State Diabetes Prediction Study. (2002). Successful prospective prediction of type 1 diabetes in schoolchildren through multiple defined autoantibodies: an 8-year follow-up of the Washington State Diabetes Prediction Study. *Diabetes Care, 22*, 505-511.

[43] Joner, G. & Sovik, O. (1991). The incidence of type 1 (insulin-dependent) diabetes mellitus 15-29 years in Norway 1978-1982. *Diabetologia, 34*, 271-274.

[44] Bruno, G., Merletti, F., Vuolo, A., Pisu, E., Glorio, M. & Pagano, G. (1993). Sex differences in incidence of IDDM in age group 15-29 yr. Higher risk in males in Province of Turin, Italy. *Diabetes Care, 16*, 133-136.

[45] Christau, B., Kromann, H., Andersen, O.O., Christy, M., Buschard, K., Arnung, K., Kristensen, I.H., Peitersen, B. Steinrud, J. & Nerup, J. (1977). Incidence, seasonal and geographic patterns of juvenile-onset insulin-dependent diabetes mellitus in Denmark. *Diabetologia, 13*, 281-284.

[46] Melton, L.J., III, Palumbo, P.J. & Chu, C.P. (1983). Incidence of diabetes mellitus by clinical type. *Diabetes Care, 6*, 75-86.

[47] Thivolet, C., Beaufrere, B., Betuel, H., Gebuhrer, L., Chatelain, P., Durand, A., Tourniaire, J. & Francois, R. (1988). Islet cell and insulin autoantibodies in subjects at high risk for development of type 1 (insulin-dependent) diabetes mellitus: the Lyon family study. *Diabetologia, 31*, 741-746.

[48] Karvonen, M., Pitkaniemi, J. & Tuomilehto, J (1999). The onset age of type 1 diabetes in Finland has become younger. The Finnish Childhood Diabetes Registry Group. *Diabetes Care, 22*, 1066-1070.

[49] Gardner, S.G., Bingley, P.J, Sawtell, P.A., Weeks, S. & Gale, E.A. (1997). Rising evidence of insulin-dependent diabetes in children aged under 5 years in the Oxford regions: time trend analysis. The Bart's-Oxford Study Group. *British Medical Journal, 315*, 713-717.

[50] Tuomilehto, J., Rewers, M, Reunanen, A., Lounamaa, P., Lounamaa, R., Tuomilehto-Wolf, E. & Akerblom, H.K. (1991) Increasing trend in type 1 (insulin-dependent) diabetes mellitus in childhood in Finland. Analysis of age, calendar time and birth cohort effects during 1965 to 1984. *Diabetologia, 34*, 282-287.

[51] Nystrom, L., Dahlquist, G., Rewers, M. & Wall, S. (1990). The Swedish childhood diabetes study. An analysis of the temporal variation in diabetes incidence 1978-1987. *International Journal of Epidemiology, 44*, 22-25.

[52] Bruno, G., Merletti, F., Biggeri, A., Cerutti, F., Grosso, N., De Salvia, A., Vitali, E. & Pagano, G. (2001). Increasing trend of type 1 diabetes in children and young adults in the province of Turin (Italy). Analysis of age, period and birth cohort effects from 1984 to 1996. *Diabetologia, 44*, 22-25.

[53] Green, A., Sjolie, A.K. & Eshoj, O. (1996). Trends in the epidemiology of IDDM during 1970-2020 in Fyn County, Denmark. *Diabetes Care 19*, 801-806.

[54] Laron, Z., Mansour, T., Slepon, R., Karp, M. & Shohat, T. (1994). Incidence of diabetes mellitus in various population groups in Israel (1989 and 1990). *Israel Journal of Medical Sciences, 30*, 770-774.

[55] Gale, E.A. & Gillespie, K.M. (2001). Diabetes and gender. *Diabetologia, 44*, 3-15.

[56] Blohme, G., Nystrom, L., Arnqwist, H.J., Lithner, F., Littorin, B., Olsson, P.O., Schersten, B., Wibell, L. & Ostman J. (1992). Male predominance of type 1 (insulin-dependent) diabetes mellitus in young adults: results from a 5-year prospective nationwide study of the 15-34-year age group in Sweden. *Diabetologia, 32*, 56-62.

[57] Lee, W.W., Ooi, B.C., Thai, A.C., Loke, K.Y., Tan, Y.T., Rajan, U. & Tan, C.L. (1998). The incidence of IDDM in Singapore children. *Singapore Medical Journal, 39*, 359-362.

[58] Matsuura, N., Fukuda, K., Okuno, A., Harada, S., Fukushima, N., Koike, A., Ito, Y. & Hotsubo, T. (1998). Descriptive epidemiology of IDDM in Hokkaido, Japan: the Childhood IDDM Hokkaido Registry. *Diabetes Care, 21*, 1932-1936.

[59] Huen, K.F., Low, L.C., Wong, G.W., Tse, W.W., Yu, A.C., Lam, Y.Y., Cheung, P.C., Wong, L.M., Yeung, W.K., But, B.W., Cheung, P.T., Kwan, E.Y., Karlberg, J.P. & Lee, C. (2000). Epidemiology of diabetes mellitus in children in Hong Kong: the Hong Kong childhood diabetes register. *Journal of Pediatric Endocrinology and Metabolism, 13*, 397-302.

[60] Westlund, K. (1966). Incidence of diabetes mellitus in Oslo, Norway, 1925-1954. *British Journal of Preventive and Social Medicine, 20*, 105-116.

[61] Raghupathy, R. (1997). Th1-type immunity is incompatible with successful pregnancy. *Immunology Today, 18*, 478-482.

[62] Whitacre, C.C., Reingold, S.C. & O'Looney, P.A. (1999). A sex gap in autoimmunity. *Science, 283*, 1277-1278.

[63] Kelso, A. (1995). Th1 and Th2 subsets: paradigms lost? *Immunology Today, 16*, 374-379.

[64] Krischer, J.P., Cuthbertson, D.D. & Greenbaum, C. Diabetes Prevention Trial-Type 1 Study Group. (2004) Male sex increases the risk of autoimmunity but not type 1 diabetes. *Diabetes Care, 27*, 1985-1990.

[65] Hagopian, W.A., Sanjeevi, C.B., Kockum, I., Landin-Olsson, M., Karlsen, A.E., Sundkvist, G., Dahlquist, G., Palmer, J. & Lernmark, A. (1995). Glutamate decarboxylase-, insulin-, and islet cell-antibodies in a general population-based study of Swedish children. *Journal of Clinical Investigation 95*, 1505-1511.

[66] Yu, L., Chase, H.P., Falorni, A., Rewers, M., Lernmark, A. & Eisenbarth, G.S. (1995). Sexual dimorphism in transmission of expression of islet autoantibodies to offspring. *Diabetologia, 38*, 1353-1357.

[67] Warram, J.H., Krolewski, A.S., Gottlieb, M.S. & Kahn, C.R. (1984). Differences in risk of insulin-dependent diabetes in offspring of diabetic mothers and diabetic fathers. *New England Journal of Medicine, 311*, 149-152.

[68] Bleich, D., Polak, M., Eisenbarth, G.S. & Jackson, R.A. (1993). Decreased risk of type 1 diabetes in offspring of mothers who acquire diabetes during adrenarche. *Diabetes, 42*, 1433-1439.

[69] Waldhor, T., Schrober, E., Rami, B., Tuomilehto, J. (1999). The prevalence of IDDM in the first-degree relatives of children newly diagnosed with IDDM in Austria: a population-based study. Austrian Diabetes Incidence Study Group. *Experimental and Clinical Endocrinology and Diabetes, 107*, 323-327.

[70] Soltesz, G. (2003). Diabetes in the young: a paediatric and epidemiological perspective. *Diabetologia, 46*, 447-454.

[71] Akerblom, H.K., Vaarala, O., Hyoty, H., Ilonen, J. & Knip, M. (2002). Environmental factors in the etiology of type 1 diabetes. *American journal of Medical Genetics, 115*, 18-29.

[72] Jun, H.S. & Yoon, J.W. (2001) The role of viruses in type I diabetes: two distinct cellular and molecular pathogenic mechanisms of virus-induced diabetes in animals. *Diabetologia, 44*, 271-285.

[73] Gamble, D.R., Kinsley, M.L., FitzGerald, M.G., Bolton, R. & Taylor, K.W. (1969). Viral antibodies in diabetes mellitus. *British Medical Journal, 3*, 627-630.

[74] Gamble, D.R., Taylor, K.W., Cumming, H. (1973). Coxsackie viruses and diabetes mellitus, *British Medical Journal, 4*, 260-262.

[75] Yoon, J.W., Austin, M., Onodera, T. & Notkins, A.L. (1979). Isolation of a virus from the pancreas of a child with diabetic ketoacidosis. *New England Journal of Medicine, 300*, 1173-1179.

[76] Andreoletti, L., Hober, D., Hober-Vandenberghe, C., Belaich, S., Vantyghem, M.-C., Lefebvre, J. & Wattre, P. (1997). Detection of coxsackie B virus RNA sequences in whole blood samples from adult patients at the onset of type 1 diabetes mellitus. *Journal of Medical Virology, 52*, 121-127.

[77] Nairn, C., Galbraith, D.N., Taylor, K.W. & Clemens, G.B. (1999). Enterovirus variants in the serum of children at the onset of type 1 diabetes mellitus. *Diabetic Medicine, 16*, 509-513.

[78] Chehadeh, W., Weill, J., Vantyghem, M.C., Alm, G., Lefebvre, J., Wattre, P. & Hober, D. (2000). Increased level of interferon-α in blood of patients with insulin-dependent diabetes mellitus: relationship with coxsackie virus B infection. *Journal of Infectious Diseases, 181*, 1929-1939.

[79] Chehadeh, W., Kerr-Conte, J., Pattou, F., Alm, G., Lefebvre, J., Wattre, P. & Hober, D. (2000). Persistent infection of human pancreatic islets by coxsackievirus B is associated with alpha interferon synthesis in beta cells. *Journal of Virology, 74*, 10153-10164.

[80] Devendra, D. & Eisenbarth, G.S. (2004). Interferon alpha – a potential link in the pathogenesis of viral-induced type 1 diabetes and autoimmunity. *Clinical Immunology, 111*, 225-233.

[81] Soldevilla, G., Buscema, M., Doshi, M., James, R.F., Bottazo, G.F. & Pujol-Borrell, R. (1991). Cytotoxic effect of IFN-gamma plus TNF-alpha on human islet cells. *Journal of Autoimmunity, 4*, 291-306.

[82] Kaufman, D.L., Erlander, M.G., Clare-Salzer, M., Atkinson, M., Maclaren, N.K. & Tobin, A.J. (1992). Autoimmunity to two forms of glutamate decarboxylase in insulin-dependent diabetes mellitus. *Journal of Clinical Investigations, 89*, 283-292.

[83] Hou, J., Said, C., Franchi, D., Dockstader, P., Chatterjee, N.K. (1994). Antibodies to glutamic acid decarboxylase and P2-C peptides in sera from coxsackie virus B4-infected mice and IDDM patients. *Diabetes, 43*, 1260-1266.

[84] Marttila, J., Juhela, S., Vaarala, O., Hyoty, H., Roivanien, M., Hinkkanen, A., Vilja, P., Simell, O. & Ilonen, J. (2001). Responces of coxsackievirus B4-specific T cells lines to 2C protein – characterization of epitopes with special reference to the GAD65 homology region. *Virology, 284*, 131-141.

[85] Schloot, N.C., Willemen, S.J., Duinkerken, G., Drijhout, J.W., de Vries, R.R. & Roep, B.O. (2001). Molecular mimicry in type 1 diabetes revisited: T cell clones to GAD65 peptides with sequence homology to Coxsackie or proinsulin peptidesdo not cross react with homologous counterpart. *Human Immunology, 62*, 299-309.

[86] Roep, B.O., Hiemstra, H.S., Schloot, N.C., De Vries R.R., Chaudhuri, A, Behan, P.O. & Drijfhout, J.W. (2002). Molecular mimicry in type 1 diabetes: immune cross-reactivity between islet autoantigen and human cytomegalovirus but not Coxsackie virus. *Annals of the New York Academy of Sciences, 958*, 163-165.

[87] Harkonen T., Paananen, A., Lankinen, H., Hovi, T., Vaarala, O., & Roivainen, M. Enterovirus infection may induce humoral immune response reacting with islet cell autoantigens in humans. *Journal of Medical Virology 926*, 426-440.

[88] Williams, C.H., Oikarinen, S., Tauriainen, S., Salminen, K., Hyoty, H., Stanway, G. (2006). Molecular analysis of an echovirus 3 strain isolated from an individual concurrently with appearance of islet cell and IA-2 autoantibodies. *Journal of Clinical Microbiology, 44*, 441-448.

[89] See, T.M. & Tilles, J.G. (1995). Pathogenesis of virus-induced diabetes in mice. *Journal of Infectious Diseases, 171*, 1131-1138.

[90] Horwitz, M.S., Bradley, L.M., Harbertson, J., Krahl, T., Lee, J. & Sarvetnick, N. (1998). Diabetes induced by coxsackievirus: initiation of bystander damage and not molecular mimicry. *Nature Medicine, 4*, 781-785.

[91] Serreze, D.V., Ottendorfer, E.W., Ellis, T.M., Gauntt, C.J. & Atkinson, M.A. (2000). Acceleration of type 1 diabetes by coxsackievirus infection requires preexisting critical mass of autoreactive T-cells in pancreatic islets. *Diabetes, 49*, 708-711.

[92] Yoon, J.-W. (1995) A new look at viruses in type 1 diabetes. *Diabetes Metabolism Reviews, 11*, 83-107.

[93] Jordan, G.W. & Cohen, S.H. (1987). Encephalomyocarditis virus-induced diabetes mellitus in mice: model of viral pathogenesis. *Reviews of Infectious Diseases, 9*, 917-924.

[94] White, L.L. & Smith, R.A. (1990). D variant of encephalomyocarditis virus (EMCV-D)-induced diabetes following natural killer cell depletion in diabetes-resistant male C57BL/6J mice. *Viral Immunology, 3*, 67-76.

[95] Guberski, D.L., Thomas, V.A., Shek, W.R., Like, A.A., Handler, E.S., Rossini, A.A., Wallace, J.E., Welsh, R.M. (1991). Induction of type 1 diabetes by Kilham rat virus in diabetes-resistant BB7Wor rats. *Science, 254*, 1010-1013.

[96] Taki, S. (2002). Type 1 interferons and autoimmunity: lessons from the clinic and from IRF-2-deficient mice. *Cytokine and Growth Factor Reviews, 13*, 379-391.

[97] Foulis, K., Farquaharson, M.A. & Hardman, R. (1987). Aberrant expression of class II major histocompatibility complex molecules by β cells and hyperexpression of class I major histocompatibility complex by insulin containing islets in type 1 (insulin-dependent) diabetes mellitus. *Diabetologia 30*, 333-343.

[98] Somoza N., Vargas, N., Roura-Mir, C., Vives-Pi, M., Fernandez-Figueras, M.T., Ariza, A., Gomis, R., Bragado, R., Marti, M. & Jaraquemada, D. (1994). Pancreas in recent onset of insulin-dependent diabetes mellitus. Changes in HLA, adhesion molecules and autoantigens, restricted T cell receptor V beta usage, and cytokine profile. *Journal of Immunology, 153*, 1360-1377.

[99] Chakrabarti, D., Hultgen, B. & Stewart, T.A. (1996). INF-alpha induces autoimmune T cells through the induction of intracellular adhesion molecule-1 and B7.2. *Journal of Immunology, 157*, 522-528.

[100] Conrad, B. (2003). Potential mechanisms of interferon-alpha induced autoimmunity. *Autoimmunity, 36*, 519-523.

[101] Uto, H., Matsuoka, H., Murata, M., Okamoto, T., Miyata, Y., Hori, T., Ido, A., Hirono, S., Hayashi, K. & Tsubouchi, H. (2000). A case of chronic hepatitis C developing insulin-dependent diabetes mellitus associated with various autoantibodies during interferon therapy. *Diabetes Research and Clinical Practice, 49*, 101-106.

[102] Eibl, N., Gschwantler, M., Ferenci, P., Eibl, M.M., Weiss, W. & Schernthaner, G. (2001). *European Journal of Hastroenterology and Hepatology, 13*, 295-298.

[103] Bosi, E., Minelli, R., Bazzigaluppi, E. & Salvi, M. (2001). Fulminant autoimmune Type 1 diabetes during interferon-alpha therapy: a case of Th1-mediated disease? *Diabetic Medicine, 18*, 329-332.

[104] Wesche, B., Jaeckel, E., Trautwein, C., Wedemeyer, H., Falorni, A., Frank, H., von zur Muhlen, A., Manns, M.P. & Brabant, G. (2001). Induction of autoantibodies to the adrenal cortex and pancreatic islet cells by interferon alpha therapy for chronic hepatitis C. *Gut, 48*, 378-383.

[105] Wasmuth, H.E., Stolte, C., Geier, A., Gartung, C. & Matern, S. (2001). Induction of multiple autoantibodies to islet cell antigens during treatment with interferon alpha for chronic hepatitis C. *Gut, 49*, 596-597.

[106] Scott, F.W. (1990). Cow milk and insulin-dependent diabetes mellitus: is there a relationship? *American Journal of Clinical Nutrition, 51*, 489-491.

[107] Martin, J.M., Trink, B., Daneman, D., Dosch, H.M. & Robinson, B. (1991). Milk proteins in the etiology of insulin-dependent diabetes mellitus (IDDM). *Annals of medicine, 23*, 447-452.

[108] Karges, W., Hammond-McKibben, D., Cheung, R.K., Visconti, M., Shibuya, N., Kemp, D. & Dosch, H.M. (1997). Immunological aspects of nutritional diabetes prevention in NOD mice: a pilot study for the cow's milk-based IDDM prevention trial. *Diabetes, 46*, 557-564.

[109] Gerstein, H.C. (1994). Cow's milk exposure and type 1 diabetes mellitus. A critical overview of the clinical literature. *Diabetes Care, 17* 13-19.

[110] Nigro, G., Campea, L., De Novellis, A. & Orsini, M. (1985). Breast-feeding and insulin-dependent diabetes mellitus. *Lancet, 1*, 467.

[111] Kimpimaki, T., Erkkola, M., Korhonen, S., Kupila, A., Virtanen, S.M., Ilonen, J., Simell, O. & Knip, M. (2001). Short-term exclusive breastfeeding predisposes young children with increased genetic risk to Type 1 diabetes to progressive beta-cell autoimmunity. *Diabetologia, 44*, 63-69.

[112] Virtanen, S.M., Laara, E., Hypponen, E., Reijonen, H., Rasanen, L., Aro, A., Knip, M., Ilonen, J., Akerblom, H.K. (2000). Cow's milk consumption, HLA-DQB1 genotype, and type 1 diabetes mellitus. A nested case-control study of siblings of children with diabetes. *Diabetes, 49*, 912-917.

[113] Miyazaki, I., Cheung, R.K., Gaedidk, R., Hui, M.F., Van der Meulen, J., Rajotte, R.V. & Dosch, H.M. (1995). T cell activation and anergy to islet cell antigen in type 1 diabetes. *Journal of Immunology, 154*, 1461-1469.

[114] Dahlquist, G., Savilahti, E. & Landin-Olsson, M. (1992). An increased level of antibodies to beta-lactoglobulin is a risk determinant for early-onset type 1 (insulin-dependent) diabetes mellitus independent of islet cell antibodies and early introduction of cow's milk. *Diabetologia, 35*, 92, 980-984.

[115] Savilahti, E., Saukkonen, T.T., Virtala, E.T., Tuomilehto, J., Akerblom, H.K. (1993). Increased levels of cow's milk and beta-lactoglobulin antibodies in young children with newly diagnosed IDDM. The Childhood Diabetes in Finland Study Group. *Diabetes Care, 16*, 984-989.

[116] Vaarala, O., Klemetti, P., Savilahti, E., Reijonen, H., Ilonen, J., Akerblom, H.K. (1996). Cellular immune response to cow's milk beta-lactoglobulin in patients with newly diagnosed IDDM. *Diabetes, 45*, 178-182.

[117] Lorini, R., Avanzini, M.A. & Vitali, L. (1994). Anti-beta-lactoglobulin antibodies in newly diagnosed children with IDDM and their siblings. *Diabetes Care, 17*, 780-782.

[118] Monetini, L., Cavallo, M.G., Stefanini, L., Ferrazzoli, F., Bizzarri, C., Marietti, G., Curro V, Cervoni, M. & Pozzilli, P.; IMDIAB Group. (2001). Bovine beta-casein antibodies in breast- and bottle-fed infants: their relevance in Type 1 diabetes. *Diabetes Metabolism Research and Reviews, 17*, 51-54.

[119] Banchuin, N., Boonyasrisawat, W., Vannasaeng, S., Dharakul, T., Yenchitsomanus, P.T., Deerochanawong, C., Ploybutr, S., Sriussadaporn, S. & Pasurakul, T. (2002). Cell-mediated immune responses to GAD and beta-casein in type 1 diabetes mellitus in Thailand. *Diabetes Research and Clinical Practice, 55*, 237-245.

[120] Monetini, L., Cavallo, M.G., Manfrini, S., Stefanini, L., Picarelli, A., Di Tola, M., Petrone, A, Bianchi, M., La Presa, M., Di Giulio, C., Baroni, M.G., Thorpe, R., Walker, B.K. & Pozzilli, P.; IMDIAB Group. (2002) Antibodies to bovine beta-casein in diabetes and other autoimmune diseases. *Hormone and Metabolic Research*, 2002, 34, 455-459.

[121] Hvatum, M., Scott, H. & Brandtzaeg, P. (1992). Serum IgG subclass antibodies to a variety of food antigens in patients with coeliac disease. *Gut, 33*, 632-638.

[122] Monetini, L., Barone, F., Stefanini, L., Petrone, A., Walk, T., Jung, G., Thorpe, R., Pozzilli, P. & Cavallo, M.G. (2003). Establishment of T cell lines to bovine beta-casein and beta-casein-derived epitopes in patients with type 1 diabetes. *Journal of Endocrinology, 176*, 143-150.

[123] Elliott, R.B., Martin, J.M. (1984). Dietary protein: a trigger of insulin-dependent diabetes in the BB rat? *Diabetologia, 26*, 297-299.

[124] Bonifacio, E., Ziegler, A.G., Hummel, M., Dittler, J., Lampasona, V., Pastore, M.R. & Bosi, E. (1998). Gluten: is it also a determinant of islet autoimmunity? *Diabetes Metabolism Reviews, 14*, 258-259.

[125] Funda, D.P., Kaas, A., Bock, T., Tlaskalova-Hogenova, H. & Buschard, K. (1999). Gluten-free diet prevents diabetes in NOD mice. *Diabetes Metabolism Research and Reviews, 15*, 323-327.

[126] Schmid, S., Koczwara, K., Schwinghammer, S., Lampasona, V., Ziegler, A.G., Bonifacio, E. (2004). Delayed exposure to wheat and barley proteins reduces diabetes incidence in non-obese diabetic mice. *Clinical Immunology, 111*, 108-118.

[127] Catassi, C., Guerrieri, A., Bartolotta, E., Coppa, G.V. & Giorgi, P.L. (1987). Antigliadin antibodies at onset of diabtes in children. *Lancet, 2*, 158.

[128] Klemetti, P., Savialahti, E., Ilonen, J., Akerblom, H.K. & Vaarala, O. (1998). T cell reactivity to wheat gluten in patients with insulin-dependent diabetes mellitus. *Scandinavian Journal of Immunology*, 47, 48-53.

[129] Savilahti, E., Akerblom, H.K., Tainio, V.M. & Koskimies, S. (1988). Children with newly diagnosed insulin-dependent diabetes mellitus have increased levels of cow's milk antibodies. *Diabetes Research, 7*, 137-140.

[130] Barera, G., Bianchi, C., Calisti, L., Cerutti, F., Dammacco, F., Frezza, E., Illeni, M.T., Mistura, L., Pocecco, M., Prisco, F., Sacchetti, C., Saggese, G., Stoppoloni, G., Tonini, G. & Ghiumello, G. (1991). Screening of diabetic children for coeliac disease with antigliadin antibodies and HLA typing. *Archives of disease in childhood, 66*, 491-494.

[131] Karagiozoglou-Lampoudi, T., Nousia-Arvanitaki, S., Augostidou-Savopoulou, P., Salem, N., Polymenidis, Z. & Kanakoudi-Tsakalidou, F. (1996). Insulin secretion decline unrelated to jejunal morphology or exocrine pancreatic function in children with celiac disease. *Journal of Pediatric Endocrinology and Metabolism, 9*, 595-591.

[132] Not, T., Tomassini, A., Tonini, G., Buratti, E., Pocecco, M., Tortul, C., Valussi, M., Crichiutti, G., Berti, I., Trevisiol, C., Azzoni, E., Neri, E., Torre, G., Martelossi, S., Soban, M., Lenhardt, A., Cattin, L. & Ventura, A. (2001). Undiagnosed celiac disease and risk of autoimmune disorders in subjects with type 1 diabetes. *Diabetologia, 44*, 151-155.

[133] Van Etten, E., Decallonne, B., Verlinden, L., Verstuyf, A., Bouillon, R. & Mathieu, C. (2005). Analogs of 1alpha,25-dihydroxyvitamin D3 as pluripotent immunomodulators. *Journal of Cellular Biochemistry, 88*, 223-226.

[134] Mathieu C, Gysemans C, Giulietti A, Bouillon R. (2005) Vitamin D and diabetes. *Diabetologia, 48*, 1257-1267.

[135] The EURODIAB Substudy 2 Study Group. (1999). Vitamin D supplement in early childhood and risk for Type I (insulin-dependent) diabetes mellitus. *Diabetologia, 42*, 51-54.

[136] Hypponen, E., Laara, E., Reunanen, A., Jarvelin, M.R. & Virtanen, S.M. (2001). Intake of vitamin D and risk of type 1 diabetes: a birth-cohort study. *Lancet, 358*, 1500-1503.

[137] Stene, L.C. & Joner, G. (2003). Use of cod liver oil during the first year of life is associated with lower risk of childhood-onsettype 1 diabetes: a large, population-based, case-control study. *American Journal of Clinical Nutrition, 78*, 1128-1134.

[138] Fronczak, C.M., Baron, A.E., Chase, H.P., Ross, C., Brady, H.L., Hoffman, M., Eisenbarth, G.S., Rewers, M. & Norris, J.M. (2003). In utero dietary exposures and risk of islet autoimmunity in children. *Diabetes Care 26*, 3237-3242

[139] Cantorna, M.T., Zhu, Y., Froicu, M., Wittke, A. (2001). Vitamin D status, 1,25-dihydroxyvitamin D3, and the immune system *American Journal of Clinical Nutrition, 80 (Suppl. 6)*, 1717S-1720S.

[140] Sandler, S., Buschard, K. & Bendtzen, K. (1994). Effects of 1,25-dihydroxyvitamin D3 and the analogues MC903 and KH1060 on interleukin-1 beta-induced inhibition of rat pancreatic islet beta-cell function in vitro. *Immunology Letters 41*, 73-77.

[141] Riachy, R., Vandewalle, B., Belaich, S., Kerr-Conte, J., Gmyr, V., Zerimech, F., d'Herbomez, M., Lefebvre, J. & Pattou, F. (2001). Beneficial effect of 1,25 dihydroxyvitamin D3 on cytokine-treated human pancreatic islets. *Journal of Endocrinology, 169*, 161-168

[142] Riachy, R., Vandewalle, B., Kerr C.J., Moerman, E., Sacchetti, P., Lukowiak, B., Gmyr, V., Bouckenooghe, T., Dubois, M. & Pattou, F. (2002). 1,25-dihydroxy-vitamin D3 protects RINm5F and human islet cells against cytokine-induced apoptosis: implication of the antiapoptotic protein A20. *Endocrinology, 143*, 4809-4819.

[143] Hahn H.J., Kuttler B., Mathieu C. & Bouillon R (1997). 1,25-Dihydroxyvitamin D3 reduces MHC antigen expression on pancreatic beta-cells in vitro. *Transplantation Proceedings, 29*, 2156-2157.

[144] Virtanen, S.M., Jaakkola, L., Rasanen, L., Ylonen, K., Aro, A., Lounamaa, R., Akerblom, H.K. & Tuomilehto, J. (1994). Nitrate and nitrite intake and the risk for type 1 diabetes in Finnish children. Childhood Diabetes in Finland Study Group. *Diabetic Medicine, 11*, 656-662.

[145] Dahlquist, G.G., Blom, L., Persson, L.A., Sandstrom, A.I.M. & Wall, S.G.I. (1990). Dietary factors and the risk of developing of insulin-dependent diabetes in childhood. *British Medical Journal, 300*, 1302-1306.

[146] Kostraba, J.N., Gay, E.C., Rewers, M. & Hamman, R.F. (1992). Nitrate levels in community drinking waters and risk of IDDM. *Diabetes Care, 15*, 1505–1508.

[147] Parslow, R.C., McKinney, P.A., Law, G.R., Staines, A., Williams, R. & Bodansky H.J. (1997). Incidence of childhood diabetes mellitus in Yorkshire, northern England, is associated with nitrate in drinking water: an ecological analysis. *Diabetologia, 40*, 550–556.

[148] Zeisel, S.H., DaCosta, K.A. & Fox, J.G. (1985). Endogenous formation of dimethylamine. *Biochemical Journal, 232*, 402-408.

[149] Eizirik, D.L., Pipeleers, D.G., Ling, Z., Welsh, N., Hellestrom, C. & Andersson, A. (1994). Major species differences between humans and rodents in the susceptibility to pancreatic beta-cell injury. *Proceedings of the National Academy of Sciences of the USA, 9*1, 9253-9256.

[150] Szkudelski, T., Kandulska, K. & Okulicz, M. (1998). Alloxan in vivo does not only exert deleterious effects on pancreatic B cells. *Physiological Research, 47*, 343-346.

[151] Kliber, A., Szkudelski, T., Chichlowska, J. (1996). Alloxan stimulation and subsequent inhibition of insulin release from in situ perfused rat pancreas. *Journal of Physiology and Pharmacology, 47*, 321-328.

[152] Boquist, L., Nelson, L. & Lorentzon, R. (1983). Uptake of labeled alloxan in mouse organs and mitochondria in vivo and in vitro. *Endocrinology, 113*, 943-948.

[153] Lenzen, S. & Munday, R. (1991). Thiol-group reactivity, hydrophylicity and stability of alloxan, its reduction products and N-methyl derivatives and a comparison with ninhydrin. *Biochemical Pharmacology, 42*, 1385-1391.

[154] Heikkila, R.E. & Cohen, G. (1975). Cytotoxic aspects of the interaction of ascorbic acid with alloxan and 6-hydroxydopamine. *Annals of new York Academy of Sciences, 258*, 221-230.

[155] Munday, R. (1988). Dialuric acid autooxidation. Effects of transition metals on the reaction and on the generation of “active oxygen” species. *Biochemical Pharmacology, 37*, 409-413.

[156] Sakurai, K. & Ogiso, T. (1995). Effect of ferritin on λDNA breaks in the reaction system of alloxan plus NADPH-cytochrome P450 reductase: ferritin’s role in diabetogenic action of alloxan. *Biological and Pharmaceutical Bulletin, 18*, 262-266.

[157] Lenzen, S., Freytag, S. & Panten, U. (1988). Inhibition of glucokinase by alloxan through interaction with sugar-binding site of the enzyme. *Molecular Pharmacology, 34*, 395-400.

[158] Jorns, A., Munday, R., Tiedge, M. & Lenzen, S. (1997). Comparative toxicity of alloxan, N-alkylalloxans and ninhydrin to isolated pancreatic islets in vitro. *Journal of Endocrinology, 155*, 283-293.

[159] Pipeleers, D.G. & van de Winkel, M. (1986). Pancreatic B-cells possess defence mechanism against cell-specific toxicity. *Proceedings of the National Academy of USA, 83*, 5267-5271.

[160] Sakurai, K. & Ogiso, T. (1991). Inhibitory effect of glutathione on the generation of hydroxyl radicals in the reaction system of glutathione-alloxan. *Chemical and Pharmaceutical Bulletin, 39*, 737-742.

[161] Grankvist, K., Marklund, S., Sehlin, J., Taljedal, I.B. (1979). Superoxide dismutase, catalase and scavengers of hydroxyl radical protect against the toxic action of alloxan om pancreatic islet cells in vitro. *Biochemical Journal, 182*, 17-25.

[162] Jorns, A., Tiedge, M. & Lenzen, S. (1999). Effect of superoxide dismutase, catalase, chelating agents, and free radical scavengers on the toxicity of alloxan to isolated pancreatic islets in vitro. *Free Radical Biology and Medicine, 26*, 1300-1304.

[163] Kim, H.R., Rho, H.W., Park, J.W., Kim, J.S., Kim, U.H. & Chung, M.I. (1994). Role of Ca^{2+} in alloxan-induced pancreatic beta-cell damage. *Biochimica and Biophysica Acta, 1227,* 87-91.

[164] Dean, P.M. & Matthews, E.K. (1972). The bioelectrical properties of pancreatic islet cells: effect of diabetogenic agents. *Diabetologia, 8*, 173-178.

[165] Katsumata, K., Katsumata, K., Jr. & Katsumata Y. (1992). Protective effect of diltiazem hydrochloride on the occurence of alloxan- and streptozotocin-induced diabetes in rats. *Hormone and Metabolism Research, 24*, 508-510.

[166] West, E., Simon, O.R. & Morrison, E.Y. (1996). Streptozotocin alters pancreatic beta-cell responsiveness to glucose within six hours of injection into rats. *West Indian Medical Journal, 45*, 60-62.

[167] Nukatsuka, A., Yoshimura, Y., Nishida, M., Kawada, J. (1990). Importance of the concentration of ATP in rat pancreatic beta cells in the mechanism of the streptozotocin-induced cytotoxicity. *Journal of Endocrinology, 127*, 161-165.

[168] Bedoya, F.J., Solano, F. & Lucas, M. (1996). N-monomethyl-arginine and nicotinamide prevent streptozotocin-induced double strand DNA break formation in pancreatic rat islets. *Experientia, 52*, 344-347.

[169] Wang, Z. & Gleichmann, H. (1998). GLUT2 in pancreatic islets: crucial target molecule in diabetes induced with multiple low doses of streptozotocin in mice. *Diabetes, 47*, 50-56.

[170] Delaney, C.A., Dunger, A., Di Matteo, M., Cunnungham, J.M., Green, M.H. & Green, J.C. (1995). Comparison of inhibition of glucose-stimulated insulin secretion in rat islets of Langerhans by streptozotocin and methyl and ethyl nitrosoureas and methanesulphonates. Lack of correlation with nitric-releasing or O^6-alkylating ability. *Biochemical Pharmacology, 50*, 2015-2020.

[171] Morgan, N.G., Cable, H.C., Newcombe, N.R. & Williams, G.T. (1994). Treatment of cultured pancreatic B-cells with streptozotocin induces cell death by apoptosis. *Bioscience Reports, 14*, 243-250.

[172] Elsner, M., Guldbakke, B., Tiedge, M., Munday, R. & Lenzen, S. (2000). Relative importance of transport and alkylation for pancreatic beta-cell toxicity of streptozotocin. *Diabetologia, 43*, 1528-1533.

[173] Masiello, P., Nvelli, M., Fierabracci, V. & Bergamini, E. (1990). Protection by 3-aminobenzamidine and nicotinamide against streptozotocin-induced beta-cell cytotoxicity in vivo and in vitro. *Research Communications in Chemistry, Pathology and Pharmacology, 69*, 17-32.

[174] Pieper, A.A., Brat, D.J., Krug, D.K., Watkins, S.S., Gupta, A., Blackshaw, S., Verma, A., Wang, Z.Q. & Snyder, S.H. (1999). Poly(ADP-ribose) polymerase-deficient mice are protected from streptozotocin-induced diabetes. *Proceedings of the National Academy of USA, 96*, 3059-3064.

[175] Turk, J., Gorbett, J.A., Ramanadham, S., Bohrer, A. & McDaniel, M.L. (1993). Biochemical evidence for nitric oxide formation fom streptozotocin in isolated pancreatic islets. *Biochemical and Biophysical Research Communications, 197*, 1458-1464.

[176] Kroncke, K.D., Fehsel, K., Sommer, A., Rodriguez, M.L. & Kolb-Bachofen, V. (1995). Nitric oxide generation during cellular metabolization of the diabetogenic N-methyl-N-nitroso-urea streptozotocin contrinutes to islet DNA damage. *Biology and Chemistry Hoppe-Seyler, 376*, 179-185.

[177] Welsh, N. & Sandler, S. (1994). Protective action by hemin against interleukin-1 beta induced inhibition of rat pancreatic islet function. *Molecular and Cellular Endocrinology, 103*, 109-114.

[178] Nukatsuka, M., Yoshimura, Y., Nishida, M. & Kawada, J. (1988). Enchancement by streptozonin of O_2^- radical generation by the xanthine oxydase system of pancreatic beta-cells. *FEBS Letters, 239*, 295-298.

[179] Helgason, T. & Jonasson, M.R. (1981). Evidence for a food additive as a cause of ketosis-prone diabetes. *Lancet, ii*, 716-720.

[180] Siemiatucki, J., Colle, E., Campbell, S., Dewar, R.A.D. & Belmonte, M.M. (1989). Case-control study of IDDM. *Diabetes Care, 12*, 209-216.

[181] Johansson, C., Samuelsson, U. & Ludvigsson, J. (1994). A high weight gain early in life is associated with an increased risk of type 1 (insulin-dependent) diabetes mellitus. *Diabetologia, 37*, 91-94.

[182] Bruining, C.J. (2000). Association between infant growth before onset of juvenile type-1 diabetes and autoantibodies to IA-2. Netherlands Kolibrie Study Group of Childhood Diabetes. *Lancet, 356*, 655-656.

[183] Sabbah, E., Savola, K., Kulmala, P., Veijola, R., Vahasalo, P., Karjalainen, T., Akerblom, H.K. & Knip, M.; the Childhood Diabetes in Finland Study Group. (1999). Diabetes-associated autoantibodies in relation to clinical characteristics and natural course of children with newly diagnosed type 1 diabetes. *Journal of Clinical Endocrinology and Metabolism, 84*, 1534-1539.

[184] Hypponen, E., Kenward, M.G., Virtanen, S.M., Piitulainen, A., Virta-Autio, P., Tuomilehto, J., Knip, M. & Akerblom, H.K.; the Childhood Diabetes in Finland (DiMe) Study Group (1999). Infant feeding, early weight gain, and risk of type 1 diabetes. *Diabetes Care, 22*, 1961-1965.

[185] Hypponen, E., Virtanen, S.M., Kenward, M.G., Knip, M. & Akerblom, H.K.; Childhood Diabetes in Finland Study Group (2000). Obesity, increased linear growth, and risk of type 1 diabetes in children. *Diabetes Care, 23*, 1755-1760.

[186] Wilkin, T.J. (2001). The accelerator hypothesis: weight gain as the missing link between Type I and type II diabetes. *Diabetologia, 44*, 914-922.

[187] Hagglof, B., Blom, L., Dahlquist, G., Lonnberg, G. & Sahlin, B. (1991). The Swedish childhood diabetes study: indication of severe psychological stress as a risk factor for type 1 (insulin-dependent) diabetes mellitus in childhood. *Diabetologia, 34*, 757-762.

[188] Franzeze, A., Valerio, G., Arganzizano, A., De Filippo, G., Ianucci, M.P., Buono, P., Alfonsi, L. & Pisacane, A. (1997). Social deprivation influences illness onset of diabetic children. *Diabetologia, 40*, 988-989.

[189] Thernlund, G.M., Dahlquist, G., Hansson, K., Ivarsson, S.A., Ludvigsson, J., Sjoblad, S. & Hagglof, B. (1995). Psychological stress and the onset of IDDM in children: a case-control study. *Diabetes Care, 18*, 1323-1329.

[190] Dahlquist, G. & Kallen, B. (1992). Maternal-child blood group incomaptibility and other perinatal events increase the risk for early onset type 1 (insulin-dependent) diabetes mellitus. *Diabetologia, 35*, 671-675.

[191] McKinney, P.A., Parslow, R., Gurney, K., Law, G., Bodansky, H.J. & Williams, D.R.R. (1997). Antenatal factors for childhood diabetes mellitus; a case-control study of medical record data in Yorkshire, UK. *Diabetologia, 40*, 933-939.

[192] Dahlquist, G.G., Ivarsson, E., Lindberg, B. & Forsgren, B. (1995). Maternal enteroviral infection during pregnancy. *Diabetes, 44*, 408-413.

[193] Hyoty, H., Hiltunen, M., Knip, M., Laakkonen, M., Vahasalo, P., Karjalainen, J., Koskela, P., Roivanen, M., Leinikki, P., Hovi, T. & Akerblom, H.K.; Childhood Diabetes in Finland Study Group (1995). A prospective study of the role of Coxsackie B and other enterovirus infections in the pathogenesis of IDDM. *Diabetes, 44*, 652-657.

[194] Blay, R.A., Bigley, N.J. & Giron, D.J. (1985). A murine model of insulin-dependent diabetes mellitus resulted from the cumulative effects of the nondiabetogenic strain of encephalomyocarditis virus and a single low dose of streptozotocin. *Diabetes, 34*, 1288-1292.

[195] Patterson, C.C., Dahlquist, G., Soltesz, G. & Green, A. (2001). Is childhood onset type I diabetes a wealth-related disease? An ecological analysis of European incidence rates. *Diabetologia, 44 (Suppl.3)*, B9-B16.

[196] Tauriainen, S., Salminen, K. & Hyoty, H. (2003). Can enteroviruses cause type 1 diabetes? *Annals of New York Academy of Sciences, 1005*, 13-22.

[197] Bruserud, O., Jervell, J. & Thorsby, E. (1985). HLA-DR3 and -DR4 control T-lymphocyte responses to mumps and Coxsackie B4 virus: studies on patients with type 1 (insulin-dependent) diabetes and healthy subjects. *Diabetologia, 28*, 420-426.

[198] Schernthaner, G., Banatvala, J.E., Scherbaum, W., Bryant, J., Borkenstein, M., Schober, E. & Mayr, W.R. (1985) Coxsackie-B-virus-specific IgM responses, complement-fixing islet-cell antibodies, HLA DR antigens, and C-peptide secretion in insulin-dependent diabetes mellitus. *Lancet, 2*, 630-632.

[199] Sadeharju, K., Knip, M., Hiltunen, M., Akerblom, H.K. & Hyoty, H. (2003). The HLA-DR phenotype modulates the humoral immune response to enterovirus antigens. *Diabetologia, 46*, 1100-1105.

[200] Gupta, M., Nikitina-Zake, L., Landin-Olsson, M., Kockum, I. & Sanjeevi, C.B. (2003). Coxsackie virus B antibodies are increased in HLA DR3-MICA5.1 positive type 1 diabetes patients in the Linkoping region of Sweden. *Human Immunology, 64*, 874-879.

[201] Kostraba, J.N., Cruickshanks, K.J., Lawler-Heavner, J., Jobim, L.F., Rewers, M.J., Gay, E.C., Chase, H.P., Klingensmith, G. & Hamman, R.F. (1993). Early exposure to cow's milk and solid foods in infancy, genetic predisposition and risk of IDDM. *Diabetes, 42*, 288-295.

[202] Saukkonen, T., Virtanen, S.M., Karppinen, M., Reijonen, H., Ilonen, J., Rasanen, L., Akerblom, H.K. & Savilahti, E. (1998). Significance of cow's milk protein antibodies as risk factor for childhood IDDM: interactions with dietary cow's milk intake and HLA-DQB1 genotype. Childhood Diabetes in Finland Study Group. *Diabetologia, 41*, 72-78.

[203] Norris, J.M., Beaty, B., Klingensmith, G., Liping, Y., Hoffman, M., Chase, H.P., Erlich, H.A., Hamman, R.F., Eisenbarth, G.S. & Rewers, M. (1996). Lack of

association between early exposure to cow's milk protein and beta-cell autoimmunity. Diabetes Autoimmunity Study in the Young (DAISY). *Journal of American Medical Association, 276*, 609-614.

[204] Martikainen, A., Saukkonen, T., Kulmala, P.K., Reijonen, H., Ilonen, J., Teramo, K., Koskela, P., Knip, M. & Akerblom, H.K. (1996). Disease-associated antibodies in offspring of mothers with IDDM. *Diabetes, 45*, 1706-1710.

[205] Knip, M. & Akerblom, H. (1999). Environmental factors in the pathogenesis of type 1 diabetes mellitus. *Experimental and Clinical Endocrinology and Diabetes, 107* (Suppl.3), S93-S100.

[206] Hanahan, D. (1998). Peripheral antigen-expressing cells in thymic medulla: factors in self-tolerance and autoimmunity. *Current Opinion in Immunology, 10*, 656-662.

[207] Kurts, C., Sutherland, R.M., Davey, G., Li, M., Lew, A.M., Blanas, E., Carbone, F.R., Miller, J.F. & Heath, W.R. (1999). CD8 T cell ignorance or tolerance to islet antigens depends on antigen dose. *Proceedings of the National Academy of USA, 96*, 12703-12707.

[208] Miller, J.F., Kurts, C., Allison, J., Kosaka, H., Carbone, F., Heath, W.R. (1998). Induction of peripheral CD8+ T-cell tolerance by cross-presentation of self- antigens. *Immunological Reviews, 165*, 267-277.

[209] Asano, M., Toda, M., Sakaguchi, N. & Sakaguchi, S. (1996). Autoimmune disease as a consequence of developmental abnormality of a T cell subpopulation. *Journal of Experimental Medicine, 184*, 387-396.

[210] Seddon, B., Saoudi, A., Nicholson, M. & Mason, D. (1996). CD4+CD8- thymocytes that express L-selectin protect rats from diabetes upon adoptive transfer. *European Journal of Immunology, 26*, 2702-2708.

[211] Boitard, C., Yasunami, R., Dardenne, M. & Bach, J.F. (1989). T cell-mediated inhibition of the transfer of autoimmune diabetes in NOD mice. *Journal of Experimental Medicine, 169*, 1669-1680.

[212] Herbelin, A., Gombert, J.M., Lepault, F., Bach, J.F. & Chatenoud, L. (1998). Mature mainstream TCR alpha beta(+)CD4(+) thymocytes expressing L-selectin mediate “active tolerance” in the nonobese diabetic mouse. *Journal of Immunology, 161*, 2620-2628.

[213] Salomon, B., Lenshow, D.J., Rhee, L., Ashourian, N., Singh, B., Sharpe, A. & Bluestone, J.A. (2000). B7/CD28 costimulation is essential for the homeostasis of the CD4+CD25+ immunoregulatory T cells that control autoimmune diabetes. *Immunity, 12*, 431-440.

[214] Lepault, F. & Gagnerault, M.C. (2000). Characterization of peripheral regulatory CD4(+) T cells that prevent diabetes onset in nonobese diabetic mice. *Journal of Immunology, 164*, 240-247.

[215] Trembleau, S., Penna, G., Bosi, E., Mortara, A., Gately, M.K. & Adorini, L. (1995). Interleukin 12 administration induces T helper type 1 cells and accelerates autoimmune diabetes in NOD mice. *Journal of Experimental Medicine, 181*, 817-821.

[216] Debray-Sachs, M., Carnaud, C., Boitard, C., Cohen, H., Gresser, I., Bedossa, P. & Bach, J.F. (1991). Interferon-gamma impacts at multiple points during the progression

of autoimmune diabetes. *Proceedings of the National Academy of Sciences of USA, 94*, 13844-13849.

[217] Wang, B., Gonzales, A., Benoist, C. & Mathis. D. (1996). The role of CD8+ T cells in the initiation of insulin-dependent diabetes mellitus. *European Journal of Immunology, 26*, 1762-1769.

[218] Hehmke, B., Michaelis, D., Gens, E., Laube, F. & Kohnert, K.D. (1995). Aberrant activation of CD8+ T-cell and CD8+ T-cell subsets in patients with newly diagnosed IDDM. *Diabetes, 44*, 1414-1419.

[219] Hayashi, T., Morimoto, M., Iwata, H. & Onodera, T. (1998). Interferon-gamma plays a role in pancreatic islet-cell destruction of reovirus type 2-induced diabetes-like syndrome in DBA/1 suckling mice. *International Journal of Experimental Pathology, 79*, 313-320.

[220] Toyoda, H. & Formby, B. (1998). Contribution of T cells to the development of autoimmune diabetes in the NOD mouse model. *Bioessays, 20*, 750-757.

[221] Atkinson, M.A., Bowman, M.A., Campbell, L., Darrow, B.L., Kaufman, D.L. & McLaren, N.K. (1994). Cellular immunity to a determinant common to glutamate decarboxylase and Coxsackie virus in insulin-dependent diabetes. *Journal of Clinical Investigations, 94*, 2125-2129.

[222] Albert, L.J. & Inman, R.D. (1999). Molecular mimicry and autoimmunity. *New England Journal of Medicine, 341*, 2068-2074.

[223] Bottazzo, G.F., Dean, B.M., McNally, J.M., MacKay, E.H., Swift, P.G. & Gamble, D.R. (1985). In situ characterization of autoimmune phenomena and expression of HLA molecules in the pancreas in diabetic insulitis. *New England Journal of Medicine, 313*, 353-360.

[224] Foulis, A.K. & Farquharson, M.A. (1986). Aberrant expression of HLA-DR antigens by insulin-containing beta-cells in recent-onset type I diabetes mellitus. *Diabetes, 35*, 1215-1224.

[225] Bach, J.F., Koutouzov, S. & Van Endert, P.M. (1998). Are there unique autoantigens triggering autoimmune disease? *Immunological Reviews, 164*, 139-155.

[226] Posnett, D.N. (1993). Do superantigens play a role in autoimmunity? *Seminars in Immunology, 5*, 65-72.

[227] Conrad, B., Weissmahr, R.N., Boni, J., Arcari, R., Schupbach, J. & Mach, B. (1997). A human endogenous retroviral superantigen as candidate autoimmune gene in type 1 diabetes. *Cell, 90*, 303-313.

[228] Conrad, B., Weldmann, E., Trucco, G., Rudert, W.A., Behboo, R., Ricordi, C., Rodriquez-Rilo, H., Finegold, D. & Trucco, M (1994). Evidence for superantigen involvement in insulin-dependent diabetes mellitus aetiology. *Nature, 371*, 351-355.

[229] Muir, A., Ruan, Q.G., Marron, M.P. & She, J.X. (1999). The IDDMK(1,2)22 retrovirus is not detectable in either mRNA or genomic DNA from patients with type 1 diabetes. *Diabetes, 48*, 219-222.

[230] Badenhoop, K., Donner, H., Neumann, J., Herwig, J., Kurth, R., Usadel, K.H. & Tonjes, R.R. (1999). IDDM patients neither show humoral reactivities against endogenous retroviral envelope protein nor do they differ in retroviral mRNA expression from healthy relatives or normal individuals. *Diabetes, 48*, 215-218.

[231] Sakaguchi, S., Sakaguchi, N., Asano, M., Itoh, M & Toda, M. (1995). Immunologic self-tolerance maintained by activated T cells expressing IL-2 receptor alpha-chains (CD25). Breakdown of a single mechanism of self-tolerance vauses varuous autoimmune diseases. *Journal of Immunology, 155*, 1151-1164.

[232] Suri-Payer, E., Amar, A.Z., Thornton, A.M. & Shevach, E.M. (1998). CD4+CD25+ T cells inhibit both the induction and effector functions of autoreactive T cells and represent a unique lineage of immunomodulatory cells. *Journal of Immunology, 160*, 1212-1218.

[233] Roncarolo, M.G., Bacchetta, R., Bordingon, C., Narula, S. & Levings, M.K. (2001). Type 1 T regulatory cells. *Immunological Reviews, 182*, 68-79.

[234] Kukreja, A., Cost, G., Marker J., Zhang, C., Sun, Z., Lin-Su, K., Ten, S., Sanz, M., Exley, M., Wilson, B., Porcelli, S. & Maclaren, N. (2002). Multiple immuno-regulatory defects in type-1 diabetes. *Journal of Clinical Investigations, 109*, 131-140.

[235] Coon, B., An, L.L., Whitton, J.L. & von Herrath, M.G. (1999). DNA immunization to prevent autoimmune diabetes. *Journal of Clinical Investigation, 104*, 189-194.

[236] Lindley, S., Dayan, C.M., Bishop, A., Roep, B.O., Peakman, M. & Tree, T.I. (2005). Defective suppressor function in CD4(+)CD25(+) T-cells from patients with type 1 diabetes. *Diabetes, 54*, 92-99.

[237] Berzins, S.P., Venanzi, E.S., Benoist, C. & Mathis, D. (2003). T-cell compartments of prediabetic NOD mice. *Diabetes, 52*, 327-334.

[238] Mills, K.H. (2004). Regulatory T cells: friend or foe in immunity to infection? *Nature Reviews Immunology, 4*, 841-855.

[239] Piccirillo, C.A. & Thornton, A.M. (2004). Cornerstone of peripheral tolerance: naturally occurring CD4+CD25+ regulatory T cells. *Trends in Immunology, 25*, 374-380.

[240] Brunkow, M.E., Jeffery, E.W., Hjerrild, K.A., Paeper, B., Clark, L.B., Yasayko, S.A., Wilkinson, J.E., Galas, D., Ziegler, S.F. & Ramsdell, F. (2001). Disruption of a new forkhead/winged-helix protein, scurfin, results in the fatal lymphoproliferative disorder of the scurfy mouse. *Nature Genetics, 27*, 68-73.

[241] Cosmi, L., Liotta, F., Lazzeri, E., Francalanci, M., Angeli, R., Mazzinghi, B., Santarlasci, V., Manetti, R., Vanini, V., Romagnani, P., Maggi, E., Romagnani, S. & Annunziato, F. (2003). Human CD8+CD25+ thymocytes share phenotypic and functional features with CD4+CD25+ regulatory thymocytes. *Blood, 102*, 4107-4114.

[242] Bennett, C.L., Brunkow, M.E., Ramsdell, F., O'Briant, K.C., Zhu, Q., Fuleihan, R.L., Shigeoka, A.O., Ochs, H.D. & Chance, P.F. (2001). A rare polyadenylation signal mutation of the FOXP3 gene (AAUAAA-->AAUGAA) leads to the IPEX syndrome. *Immunogenetics, 53*, 435-439.

[243] Fehervari, Z. & Sakaguchi, S. (2004). (CD4+) Tregs and immune control. *Journal of Clinical Investigations, 114*, 1209-1217.

[244] Grossman, W.J., Verbsky, J.W., Barchet, W., Colonna, M., Atkinson, J.P. & Ley, T.J. (2004). Human T regulatory cells can use the perforin pathway to cause autologous target cell death. *Immunity, 21*, 589-601.

[245] Huang, C.T., Workman, C.J., Flies, D., Pan, X., Marson, A.L., Zhou, G., Hipkiss, E.L., Ravi, S., Kowalski, J., Levitsky, H.I., Powell, J.D., Pardoll, D.M., Drake, C.G. & Vignali, D.A. (2004). Role of LAG-3 in regulatory T cells. *Immunity, 21*, 503-513.

[246] Macon-Lemaitre, L. & Triebel, F. (2005). The negative regulatory function of the lymphocyte-activation gene-3 co-receptor (CD223) on human T cells. *Immunology, 115*,170-178.

[247] Paust, S., Lu, L., McCarty, N. & Cantor, H. (2004). Engagement of B7 on effector T cells by regulatory T cells prevents autoimmune disease. *Proceedings of the National Academy of USA, 101*, 10398-10403.

[248] Szanya, V., Ermann, J., Taylor, C., Holness, C. & Fathman, C.G. (2002). The subpopulation of CD4+CD25+ splenocytes that delays adoptive transfer of diabetes expresses L-selectin and high levels of CCR7. *Journal of Immunology, 169*, 2461-2465.

[249] Maron, R., Melican, N.S. & Weiner, H.L. (1999). Regulatory Th2-type T cell lines against insulin and GAD peptides derived from orally- and nasally-treated NOD mice suppress diabetes. *Journal of Autoimmunity, 12*, 251-258.

[250] Thornton, A.M. & Shevach, E.M. (1998). CD4+CD25+ immunoragulatory T cells suppress polyclonal T cell activation in vitro by inhibiting interleukin 2 production. *Journal of Experimental Medicine, 188*, 287-296.

[251] Tisch R., Liblau, R.S., Yamg, X.D., Liblau, P. & McDevitt, H.O. (1999). Induction of GAD65-specific regulatory T cells inhibits ongoing autoimmune diabetes in nonobese diabetic mice. *Diabetes, 47*, 894-899.

[252] Tisch, R., Wang, B., Weaver, D.J., Liu, B., Bui, T., Arthos, J. & Serreze, D.V. (2001). Antigen-specific mediated suppression of beta cell autoimmunity by plasmid DNA vaccination. *Journal of Immunology, 166*, 2122-2132

[253] Ploix, C., Bergerot, I., Durand, A., Czerkinsky, C., Holmgren, J. & Thivolet, C. (1999). Oral administration of cholera toxin B-insulin conjugates protects NOD mice from autoimmune diabetes by inducing CD4+ regulatory T cells. *Diabetes, 48*, 2150-2156.

[254] Ploix, C., Bergerot, I., Fabien, N., Perche, S., Moulin, V. & Thivolet, C. (1998). Protection against autoimmune diabetes with oral insulin is associated with the presense of IL4-type 2 T cells in the pancreas and pancreatic lymph nodes. *Diabetes, 47*, 39-44.

[255] Mueller, R., Krahl, T. & Sarvetnick, N. (1996). Pancreatic expression of interleukin-4 abrogates insulitis and autoimmune diabetes in nonobese diabetic (NOD) mice. *Journal of Experimental Medicine, 184*, 1093-1099.

[256] Cameron, M.J., Arreaza, G.A., Waldhauser, L., Gauthie, J. & Delovitch, T.L. (2000). Immunotherapy of spontaneous type 1 diabetes in nonobese diabetic mice by systemic interleukin-4 treatment employing adenovirus vector-mediated gene transfer. *Gene Therapy, 7*, 1093-1099.

[257] Ko, K.S., Lee, M., Koh, J.J. & Kim, S.W. (2001). Combined administration of plasmids encoding IL-4 and IL-10 prevents the development of autoimmune diabetes in nonobese diabetic mice. *Molecular Therapy, 4*, 313-316.

[258] Goudy, K, Song, S., Wasserfall, C., Zhang, Y.C., Kapturczak, M., Muir, A., Powers, M., Scott-Jorgensen, M., Campbell-Thompson, M., Crawford, J.M., Ellis, T.M., Flotte, T.R. & Atkinson, M.A. (2001). Adeno-associated virus vector-mediated IL-10 gene delivery prevents type 1 diabetes in NOD mice. *Proceedings of the National Academy of Sciences of USA, 98*, 13913-13918.

[259] Arif, S., Tree, T.I., Astill, T.P., Tremble, J.M., Bishop, A.J., Dayan, C.M., Roep, B.O. & Peakman, M. (2004). Autoreactive T cell responses show proinflammatory polarization in diabetes but a regulatory phenotype in health. *Journal of Clinical Investigations, 113*, 451-463.

[260] Fiorentino, D.F., Zlotnik, A., Vieira, P., Mosmann, T.R., Howard, M., Moore, K.W. & O'Garra, A. (1991). IL-10 acts on the antigen-presenting cell to inhibit cytokine production by Th1 cells. *Journal of Immunology, 146*, 3444-3451.

[261] Moore, K.W., de Waal Malefyt, R., Coffman, R.L. & O'Garra, A. (2001). Interleukin-10 and the interleukin-10 receptor. *Annual Reviews in Immunology, 19*, 683-765.

[262] Piccirillo, C.A., Chang, Y. & Prud'homme, G.J. (1998). TGF-beta1 somatic gene therapy prevents autoimmune disease in nonobese diabetic mice. *Journal of Immunology, 161*, 3950-3956.

[263] King, C., Davies, J., Mueller, R., Lee, M.S., Krahl, T., Yeung, B., O'Connor, E. & Sarvetnick, N. (1998). TGF-beta1 alters APC preference, polarizing islet antigen responses toward a Th2 phenotype. *Immunity, 8*, 601-613.

[264] Lee, M.S., Sawyer, S., Arnush, M., Krahl, T., von Herrath, M., Oldstone, M.A. & Sarvetnick, N. (1996). Transforming growth factor-beta fails to inhibit allograft rejection or virus-induced autoimmune diabetes in transgenic mice. *Transplantation, 61*, 1112-1115.

[265] Sanvito, F., Nichols, A., Herrera, P.L., Huarte, J., Wohlwend, A., Vassalli, J.D., Orci, L. (1995). TGF-beta 1 overexpression in murine pancreas induces chronic pancreatitis and, together with TNF-alpha, triggers insulin-dependent diabetes. *Biochemical and Biophysical Research Communications, 217*, 1279-1286.

[266] Wogensen, L., Lee, M.S. & Sarvetnick, N. (1994). Production of interleukin 10 by islet cells accelerates immune-mediated destruction of beta cells in nonobses diabetic mice. *Journal of Experimental Medicine, 179*, 1379-1384.

[267] Pauza, M.E., Neal, H., Hagenbaugh, A., Cheroutre, H. & Lo, D. (1999). T cell production of an inducible interleukin-10 transgene provides limited protection from autoimmune diabetes. *Diabetes, 48*, 1948-1953.

[268] Choileain, N.N. & Redmond, H.P. (2006). Regulatory T-cells and autoimmunity. *Journal of Surgical Research, 130*, 124-135.

[269] Weiner, H.L. (2001). Induction and mechanism of action of transforming growth factor-beta-secreting Th3 regulatory cells. *Immunological Reviews, 182*, 207-214.

[270] Lan, R.Y., Ansari, A.A., Lian, Z.-X. & Gershwin, E.M. (2005). Regulatory T cells: development, function and role in autoimmunity. *Autoimmunity Reviews, 4*, 351-363.

[271] Gombert, J.M., Herbelin, A., Tancrede-Bohin, E., Dy, M., Carnaud, C. & Bach, J.F. (1996). Early quantitative and functional deficiency of NK1(+)-like thymocytes in the NOD mouse. *European Journal of Immunology, 26*, 2989-2998.

[272] Lehuen, A., Lantz, O., Beaudoin, L., Laloux, V., Carnaud, C., Bendelac, A., Bach, J.F., Monteiro, R.C. (1998). Overexpression of natural killer T cells protects V alpha 14-J alpha 281 transgenic nonobese diabetic mice against diabetes. *Journal of Experimental Medicine, 188*, 1831-1839.

[273] Godfrey, D.I., MacDonald, H.R., Kronenberg, M., Smyth, M.J. & Van Kaer, L. (2004). NKT cells: what's in a name? *Nature Reviews in Immunology, 4*, 231-237.

[274] Shi, F.D., Flodstrom, M., Balasa, B., Kim, S.H., Van Gunst, K., Strominger, J.L., Wilson, S.B. & Sarvetnick, N. (2001). Germ line deletion of the CD1 locus exacerbates diabetes in the NOD mouse. *Proceedings of the National Academy of USA. 98*, 6777-6782.

[275] Wang, B., Cheng, Y.B. & Wang, C.R. (2001). CD1-restricted NK T cells protect nonobese diabetic mice from developing diabetes. *Journal of Experimental Medicine, 194*, 313-320.

[276] Zhou, D., Mattner, J., Cantu, C., III, Schrantz, N., Yin, N., Gao, Y., Sagiv, Y., Hudspeth, K., Wu, Y.P., Yamashita, T., Teneberg, S., Wang, D., Proia, R.L., Levery, S.B., Savage, P.B., Teyton, L. & Bendelac, A. (2004). *Lysosomal glycosphingolipid recognition by NKT cells. Science, 306*, 1687-1689.

[277] Yoshimoto, T., Bendelac, A., Hu-Li, J. & Paul W.E (1995). Defective IgE production by SJL mice is linked to the absence of CD4+, NK1.1+T cells that promptly produce interleukin 4. *Proceedings of the National Academy of USA, 92*, 11931-11934.

[278] Falcone, M., Yeung, B., Tucker, L., Rodriguez, E. & Sarvetnick, N. (1999). A defect in interleukin 12-induced activation and interferon gamma secretion of peripheral natural killer T cells in nonobese diabetic mice suggests new pathogenic mechanisms for insulin-dependent diabetes mellitus. *Journal of Experimental Medicine, 190*, 963-972.

[279] Sobel, D.O., Gan, J., Williams, J., Yoon, J.W., Jun, H.S. & Ahvazi, B (2002). Gamma interferon paradoxically inhibits the development of diabetes in the NOD mouse. *Journal of Autoimmunity, 19*, 129-137.

[280] Chen Y.G., Choisy-Rossi, C.M., Holl, T.M., Chapman, H.D., Besra, G.S., Porcelli, S.A., Shaffer, D.J., Roopenian, D., Wilson, S.B. & Serreze, D.V. (2005). Activated NKT cells inhibit autoimmune diabetes through tolerogenic recruitment of dendritic cells to pancreatic lymph nodes. *Journal of Immunology, 174*, 1196-1204.

[281] Delovitch, T.L. & Singh, B. (1997). The nonobese diabetic mouse as a model of utoimmune diabetes: immune dysregulation gets the NOD. *Immunity, 7*, 1669-1680.

[282] Sharif, F., Arreaza, G.A., Zucker, P., Mi, Q.S., Sondhi, J., Naidenko, O.V., Kronenberg, M., Koezuka, Y., Delovitch, T.L., Gombert, J.M., Leite-De-Moraes, M., Gouarin, C., Zhu, R., Hameg, A., Nakayama, T., Taniguchi, M., Lepault, F., Lehuen, A., Bach, J.F. & Herbelin, A. (2001). Activation of natural killer T cells by alpha-galactosylceramide treatment prevents the onset and recurrence of autoimmune Type 1 diabetes. *Nature Medicine, 7*, 1057-1062.

[283] Beaudoin, L., Laloux, V., Novak, J., Lucas B. & Lehuen, A. (2002). NKT cells inhibit the onset of diabetes by impairing the development of pathogenic T cells specific for pancreatic beta cells. *Immunity, 17*, 1954-1961.

[284] Novak, J., Beaudoin, L., Griseri, T. & Lehuen, A. (2005). Inhibition of T cell differentiation into effectors by NKT requires cell contacts. *Journal of Immunology, 174*, 1954-1961.

[285] Wilson, S.B., Kent, S.C., Horton, H.F., Hill, A.A., Bollyky, P.L., Hafler, D.A., Strominger, J.L. & Byrne, M.C. (2000). Multiple differences in gene expression in regulatory Valpha 24Jalpha Q T cells from identical twins discordant for type I diabetes. *Proceedings of the National Academy of Sciences of USA, 97*, 7411-7416.

[286] Oikawa, Y., Shimada, A., Yamada, S., Motohashi, Y., Nakagawa, Y., Irie, J., Maruyama, T., Saruta, T. (2002). High frequency of valpha24(+) vbeta11(+) T-cells observed in type 1 diabetes. *Diabetes Care, 25*, 1818-1823.

[287] Lee, P.T., Putnam, A., Benlagha, K., Teyton, L., Gottlieb, P.A. & Bendelac, A. (2002). Testing the NKT cell hypothesis of human IDDM pathogenesis. *Journal of Clinical Investigations, 110*, 793-800.

[288] Berzins, S.P., Kuparissoudis, K., Pelicci, D.G., Hammond, K.J., Sidobre, S., Baxter, A., Smyth, M.J., Kronenberg, M. & Godfrey, D.I. (2004). Systemic NKT cell deficiency in NOD mice is not detected in peripheral blood: implications for human studies. *Immunology and Cell Biology, 82*, 247-252.

[289] Baekkeskov, S., Nielsen, J.H., Marner, B., Bilde, T., Ludvigsson, J. & Lernmark, A. (1982). Autoantibodies in newly diagnosed diabetic children immunoprecipitate human pancreatic islet cell proteins. *Nature, 288*, 167-169.

[290] Baekkeskov, S., Aanstoot, H.-J., Christgau, S., Reetz, A., Solimena, M., Cascalho, M., Folli, F., Richter-Olesen, H. & De Camilli, P. (1990). Identification of the 64 K autoantigen in insulin-dependent diabetes as the GABA-synthesizing enzyme glutamic acid decarboxylase. *Nature, 347*, 151-156.

[291] Okada, Y, Taniguchi, H. & Shimada, C. (1976). High concentration of GABA and high glutamate decarboxylase activity in rat pancreatic islets and human insulinoma. *Science, 194*, 620-622.

[292] Gilon, P., Bertrand, G., Loubatieres-Mariani, M.M., Remacle, C. & Henquin, J.C. (1991). The influence of γ-aminobutyric acid on hormone release by the mouse and rat endocrine pancreas. *Endocrinology, 129*, 2521-2529.

[293] Lernmark, A. (1996). Glutamic acid decarboxylase: gene to antigen to disease. *Journal of Internal Medicine, 240*, 259-277.

[294] Falorni, A., Ortqvist, E., Persson, B. & Lernmark, A. (1995). Radioimmunoassays for glutamic acid decarboxylase (GAD65) and GAD65 autoantibodies using ^{35}S and ^{3}H recombinant human ligands. *Journal of Immunological Methods, 186*, 89-99.

[295] Seissler, J., Amann, J., Mauch, L., Haubruck, H., Wolfahrt, S., Bieg, S., Richter, W., Holl, R., Heinze, E., Northemann, W. & Scherbaum, W.A. (1993). Prevalence of autoantibodies to the 65- and 67-kD isoforms of glutamate decarboxylase in insulin-dependent diabetes mellitus. *Journal of Clinical Investigantions*, 1394-1399.

[296] Scmidli, R.S., Colman, P.G. & Bonifacio, E. (1995). Disease sensitivity and specificity of 52 assays for glutamic acid decarboxylase antibodies. The Second International Glutamic Acid Workshop. *Diabetes, 44*, 636-640.

[297] Schranz, D.B. & Lernmark, A. (1998). Immunology in diabetes: an update. *Diabetes and Metabolism Reviews, 14*, 3-29.

[298] Karslen, A.E., Hagopian, W.A., Grubin, C.E., Dube S., Disteche, C.M., Adler, D.A., Barmeier, H., Mathewes, S., Grant, F.J., Foster, D. & Lernmark, A. (1991). Cloning and primary structure of a human islet isoform of glutamic acid decarboxylase from chromosome 10. *Proceedings of the National Academy of Sciences of USA. 88*, 8337-8341.

[299] Grubin, C.E., Daniels, T., Toivola, B., Landin-Olsson, M., Hagopian, W.A., Li, K., Karlsen, A.E., Boel, E., Michelsen, B. & Lernmark, A. (1994). A novel radioligand binding assay to determine diagnostic accuracy of isoform-specific glutamic acid decarboxylase antibodies in childhood IDDM. *Diabetologia, 37*, 344-350.

[300] Luo, D., Rogers, C.N., Hampe, C.S. & Lernmark, A. (2003). Molecular engineering of biotin-glutamic acid decarboxylase 65 fusion protein (Biotin-GAD65) for non-radioactive GAD65 antibody assay. *Journal of Biotechnology, 103*, 249-255.

[301] Luo, D., Rogers, C.N., Steed, J.T., Gilliam, L.K., Hampe, C.S. & Lernmark, A. (2004). Development of glutamic acid decarboxylase 65 (GAD65) autoantibody assay using biotin-GAD65 fusion protein. *Journal of Biotechnology, 111*, 97-104.

[302] Hallengren, B., Falorni, A., Landin-Olsson, M., Lernmark, A., Papadopoulos, K.I. & Sundkvist, G. (1996). Islet cell and glutamic acid decarboxylase antibodies in hyperthyroid patients: at diagnosis and following treatment. *Journal of Internal Medicine, 239*, 63-68.

[303] Tsuruoka, A., Matsuba, I., Toyota, T., Isshiki, G., Nagataki, S. & Ikeda, Y. (1995). Antibodies to GAD in Japanese diabetic patients: a multicenter study. *Diabetes Research and Clinical Practice, 28*, 191-199.

[304] Maugendre, D., Verite, F., Guilhem, I., Genetet, B., Allannic, H. & Delamaire, M. (1997). Anti-pancreatic autoimmunity and Graves' disease: study of a cohort of 600 Caucasian patients. *European Journal of Endocrinology, 137*, 503-510.

[305] Lindholm, E., Hallengren, B. & Agardh, C.D. (2004). Gender differences in GAD antibody-positive diabetes mellitus in relation to age at onset, C-peptide and other endocrine autoimmune diseases. *Diabetes Metabolism Research and Reviews, 20*, 158-164.

[306] Galli-Tsinopoulou, A., Nousia-Arvanitakis, S., Dracoulacos, D., Xefteri, M. & Karamouzis, M. (1999). Autoantibodies predicting diabetes mellitus type I in celiac disease. *Hormone Research, 52*, 119-124.

[307] Toscano, V., Conti, F.G., Anastasi, E., Mariani, P., Tiberti, C., Poggi, M., Montuori, M., Monti, S., Laureti, S., Cipolletta, E., Gemme, G., Caiola, S., Di Mario, U. & Bonamico, M. (2000). Importance of gluten in the induction of endocrine autoantibodies and organ dysfunction in adolescent celiac patients. *American Journal of Gastroenterology, 95*, 1742-1748.

[308] Tuomi. T., Bjorses, P., Falorni, A., Partanen, J., Perheentupa, J., Lernmark, A. & Miettinen, A. (1996). Antibodies to glutamic acid decarboxylase and insulin-dependent diabetes in patients with autoimmune polyendocrine syndrome type 1. *Journal of Clinical Endocrinology and Metabolism, 81*, 1488-1494.

[309] Vandemalle, C.L., Falorni, A., Svanholm, S., Lernmark, A., Pipeleeers, D.G. & Gorus, F.K. (1995). High diagnostic sensitivity of glutamate decarboxylase autoantibodies in insulin-dependent diabetes mellitus with clinical onset between age 20 and 40 years.

The Belgian Diabetes Registry. *Journal of Clinical Endocrinology and Metabolism, 80*, 846-851.

[310] Bonifacio, E., Genovese, S., Braghi, S., Bazzigaluppi, E., Lampasona, V., Bingley, P.J., Rogge, L., Pastore, M.R., Bognetti, E., Botazzo, G.F., Gale, E.A.M & Bosi, E. (1995). Iselt autoantibody markers in IDDM: risk assessment strategies yielding high sensitivity. *Diabetologia, 38*, 816-822.

[311] Yu, L., Chase, H.P., Falorni, A., Rewers, M., Lernmark, A. & Eisenbarth, G.S. (1995). Sexual dimorphism in transmission to offspring of expression of islet autoantibodies. *Diabetologia, 38*, 1353-1357.

[312] Yu, L., Rewers, M, Gianani, R., Kawasaki, E., Zhang, Y., Verge, C., Chase, P., Klingensmith, G., Erlich, H., Norris, J. & Eisenbarth, G.S. (1996). Anti islet autoantibodies usually develop sequentially rather then simultaneously. *Journal of Clinical Endocrinology and Metabolism, 81*, 4264-4267.

[313] Kaufman, D.J., Erlander, M.G., Clare-Salzler, M., Atkinson, M.A., Maclaren & Tobin, A.J. (1992). Autoimmunity to two forms of glutamate decarboxylase in insulin-dependent diabetes mellitus. *Journal of Clinical Investigations, 89*, 283-292.

[314] Richter, W., Northemann, W., Muller, M. & Bohm, B.O. (1996). Mapping of an autoreactive epitope with glutamate decarboxylase using a diabetes-associated monoclonal antibody and an epitope cDNA library. *Hybridoma, 15*, 103-108.

[315] Richter, W., Endl, J., Eirmann, T.H., Brandt, M., Kientsch-Engel, R., Thivolet, C., Jungfer, H. & Scherbaum, W.A. (1992). Human monoclonal islet cell antibodies from a patient with insulin-dependent diabetes mellitus reveal glutamate decarboxylase as the target antigen. *Proceedings of the National Academy of Sciences of USA, 89*, 846-847.

[316] Richter, W., Jury, K.M., Loeffler, D., Manfras, B.J., Eiermann, T.H. & Boehm, B.O. (1995). Immunoglobulin variable gene analysis of human autoantibodies reveals antigen-driven immune response to glutamate decarboxylase in Type 1 diabetes mellitus. *European Journal of Immunology, 25*, 1703-1712.

[317] Madec, A.M., Rousset, F., Ho, S., Robert, F., Thivolet, C., Orgiazzi, J. & Lebesque, S. (1996). Four IgG anti-islet human monoclonal antibodies isolated from a Type 1 diabetes patients recognize distinct epitopes of glutamic acid decarboxylase 65 and are somatically mutated. *Journal of Immunology, 156*, 3541-3549.

[318] Falorni, A., Askefors, M., Carlsberg, C., Daniels, T., Persson, B., Robertson, J. & Lernmark, A. (1996). Diagnostic sensitivity of immunodominant epitopes of glutamic acid decarboxylase (GAD) autoantibodies epitopes in childhood IDDM. *Diabetologia, 39*, 1091-1098.

[319] Daw, K. & Powers, A.C. (1995). Two distinct glutamic acid decarboxylase auto-antibody specificities in IDDM target difference epitopes. *Diabetes, 44*, 216-220.

[320] Quinn, A. & Sercarz, E.E. (1996). T cells with multiple fine specificities are used by non-obese diabetic (NOD) mice in the response to GAD(524-543). *Journal of Autoimmunity, 9*, 365-370.

[321] Quinn, A., McInerney, B., Reich, E.P., Kim, O., Jensen, K.P. & Sercarz, E.E. (2001). Regulatory and effector CD4 T cells in nonobese diabetic mice recognize overlapping

determinants on glutamic acid decarboxylase and use distinct V beta genes. *Journal of Immunology, 166*, 2982-2991.

[322] Masewicz, S.A., Meldrum, N., Gersuk, V., Gaur, L., Hagopian, W., Moriarity, L. & Nepom, G.T. (2001). Complexity of human immune response profiles for CD4+ T cell epitopes from the diabetes autoantigen GAD65. *Autoimmunity, 34*, 231-240.

[323] Gebe, J.A., Falk, B.A., Rock, K.A., Kochik, S.A., Heninger, A.K., Reijonen, H., Kwok, W.W. & Nepom, G.T. (2003). Low-avidity recognition by CD4+ T cells directed to self-antigens. *European Journal of Immunology, 33*, 1409-1417.

[324] Reijonen, H., Mallone, R., Heninger, A.K., Laughlin, E.M., Kochik, S.A., Falk, B., Kwok, W.W., Greenbaum, C. & Nepom, G.T. (2004). GAD65-specific CD4+ T-cells with high antigen avidity are prevalent in peripheral blood of patients with type 1 diabetes. *Diabetes, 53*, 1987-1994.

[325] Uemura, Y., Senju, S., Maenaka, K., Iwai, L.K., Fujii, S., Tabata, H., Tsukamoto, H., Hirata, S., Chen, Y.Z. & Nishimura, Y. (2003). Systematic analysis of the combinatorial nature of epitopes recognized by TCR leads to identification of mimicry epitopes for glutamic acid decarboxylase 65-specific TCRs. *Journal of Immunology, 170*, 947-960.

[326] Lonnrot, M., Hyoty, H., Knip, M., Roivainen, M., Kulmala, P., Leinikki, P. & Akerblom, H.K. (1996). Antibody cross-reactivity induced by the homologous regions in glutamic acid decarboxylase (GAD65) and 2C protein of coxsackievirus B4. Childhood Diabetes in Finland Study Group. *Clinical and Experimental Immunology, 104*, 398-405.

[327] Jones, D.B. & Crosby, I. (1996). Proliferative lymphocyte responses to virus antigens homologous to GAD65 in IDDM. *Diabetologia, 39*, 1318-1324.

[328] Vreugdenhil, G.R., Geluk, A., Ottenhoff, T.H., Melchers, W.J., Roep, B.O. & Galama, J.M. (1998). Molecular mimicry in diabetes mellitus: the homologous domain in coxsackie B virus protein 2C and islet autoantigen GAD65 is highly conserved in the coxsackie B-like enteroviruses and binds to the diabetes associated HLA-DR3 molecule. *Diabetologia, 41*, 40-46.

[329] Sarugeri, E., Dozio, N., Meschi, F., Pastore, M.R. & Bonifacio, E. (2001). T cell responses to type 1 diabetes related peptides sharing homologous regions. *Journal of Molecular Medicine, 79*, 213-220.

[330] Wicker, L.S., Chen, S.L., Nepom, G.T., Elliott, J.F., Freed, D.C., Bansal, A., Zheng, S., Herman, A., Lernmark, A., Zaller, D.M., Peterson, L.B., Rothbard, J.B., Cummings, R. & Whiteley, P.J. (1996). Naturally processed T cell epitopes from human glutamic acid decarboxylase identified using mice transgenic for the type 1 diabetes-associated human MHC class II allele, DRB1*0401. *Journal of Clinical Investigations, 98*, 2597-2603.

[331] Reijonen, H., Elliott, J.F., van Endert, P. & Nepom, G. (1999). Differential presentation of glutamic acid decarboxylase 65 (GAD65) T cell epitopes among HLA-DRB1*0401-positive individuals. *Journal of Immunology, 163*, 1674-1681.

[332] Greening, J.E., Tree, T.I., Kotowicz, K.T., van Halteren, A.G., Roep, B.O., Klein, N.J. & Peakman, M. (2003). Processing and presentation of the islet autoantigen GAD by

vascular endothelial cells promotes transmigration of autoreactive T-cells. *Diabetes, 52*, 717-725.

[333] Reijonen, H., Daniels, T.L., Lernmark, A. & Nepom, G.T. (2000). GAD65-specific autoantibodies enhance the presentation of an immunodominant T-cell epitope from GAD65. *Diabetes, 49*, 1621-1626.

[334] Palmer, J.P., Asplin, C.M., Clemons, P., Lyen, K., Tatpati, O., Raghu, P.K. & Paquette, T.L. (1983). Insulin antibodies in insulin-dependent diabetes before insulin treatment. *Science, 222*, 1337-1339.

[335] Vardi, P., Keller, R., Dib, S., Eisenbarth, G.S & Soeldner, J.S. (1988). Log-linear correlation of CIAA with age of in a new onset type I diabetes. *Diabetes, 37*, 28A.

[336] Srikanta, S., Ricker, A.T., McCulloch, D.K., Soeldner, J.S., Eisenbarth, G.S. & Palmer, J.P. (1986). Autoimmunity to insulin, beta cell dysfunction, and development of insulin-dependent diabetes mellitus. *Diabetes, 35*, 139-142.

[337] Landin-Olsson, M., Palmer, J.P., Lernmark, A., Blom, L., Sundkvist, G., Nystrom, L. & Dahlquist, G. (1992). Predictive value of islet cell and insulin autoantibodies for type 1 (insulin-dependent) diabetes mellitus in a population-based study of newly-diagnosed diabetic and matched control children. *Diabetologia, 35*, 1068-1073.

[338] Graham, J., Hagopian, W.A., Kockum, I., Li, L.S., Sanjeevi, C.B., Lowe, R.M., Schaefer, J.B., Zarghami, M., Day, H.L., Landin-Olsson, M., Palmer, J.P., Janer-Villanueva, M., Hood, L., Sundkvist, G., Lernmark, A., Breslow, N., Dahlquist, G. & Blohme, G.; Diabetes Incidence in Sweden Study Group; Swedish Childhood Diabetes Study Group. (2002). Genetic effects on age-dependent onset and islet cell autoantibody markers in type 1 diabetes. *Diabetes, 51*, 1346-1355.

[339] Palmer, J.P., Wilkin, T.J., Kurtz, A.B. & Bonifacio, E. (1990). The third international workshop on the standardization of insulin autoantibody measurement. *Diabetologia, 33*, 60-61.

[340] Kuglin, B., Kolb, H., Greenbaum, C., Maclaren, N.K., Lernmark, A. & Palmer, J.P. (1990). The fourth international workshop on the standardization of insulin autoantibody measurement. *Diabetologia, 33*, 638-639.

[341] Williams, A.J.K., Bingley, P.J., Bonifacio, E., Palmer, J.P. & Gale, E.A.M. (1997). A novel micro-assay for insulin autoantibodies. *Journal of Autoimmunity, 10*, 473-478.

[342] Oneda, H. & Inouye, K. (2004). Detection of antigen-antibody reaction using a fluorescent probe and its application to homogeneous competitive-type immunoassay for insulin. *Bioscience, Biotechnology and Biochemistry, 68*, 2190-2192.

[343] Bae, Y.M., Oh, B.K., Lee, W., Lee, W.H. & Choi, J.W. (2004). Detection of insulin-antibody binding on a solid surface using imaging ellipsometry. *Biosensors and Bioelectronics, 20*, 895-902.

[344] Campbell, S.C. & Macfarlane, W.M. (2003). Detection of insulin production by immunohistochemistry. *Methods in Molecular Medicine, 83*, 47-49.

[345] Nakayama, M., Abiru, N., Moriyama, H., Babaya, N., Liu, E., Miao, D., Yu, L., Wegmann, D.R., Hutton, J.C., Elliott, J.F. & Eisenbarth, G.S. (2005). Prime role for an insulin epitope in the development of type 1 diabetes in NOD mice. *Nature, 12*, 435, 220-223.

[346] Abiru, N., Wegmann, D., Kawasaki, E., Gottlieb, P., Simone, E. & Eisenbarth, G.S. (2000). Dual overlapping peptides recognized by insulin peptide B: 9-23 T cell receptor AV13S3 T cell clones of the NOD mouse. *Journal of Autoimmunity, 14*, 231-237.

[347] Wong, F.S., Moustakas, A.K., Wen, L., Papadopoulos, G.K. & Janeway, C.A., Jr. (2002). Analysis of structure and function relationships of an autoantigenic peptide of insulin bound to H-2K(d) that stimulates CD8 T cells in insulin-dependent diabetes mellitus. *Proceedings of the National Academy of Sciences of USA, 99*, 5551-5556.

[348] Astill, T.P., Ellis, R.J., Arif, S., Tree, T.I. & Peakman, M. (2003). Promiscuous binding of proinsulin peptides to Type 1 diabetes-permissive and -protective HLA class II molecules. *Diabetologia, 46*, 496-503.

[349] Pugliese, A., Bugawan, R., Moromisato, R., Awdeh, Z.L., Alper, C.A., Jackson, R.A., Erlich, H.A. & Eisenbarth, G.S. (1994). Two subtypes of HLA-DQA1 alleles mark phenotypic variation in levels of insulin autoantibodies in first-degree relatives at risk for insulin-dependent diabetes. *Journal of Clinical Investigations, 93*, 2447-2452.

[350] Kimpimaki, T., Kupila, A., Hamalainen, A.M., Kukko, M., Kulmala, P., Savola, K., Simell, T., Keskinen, P., Ilonen, J., Simell, O. & Knip, M. (2001). The first signs of beta-cell autoimmunity appear in infancy in genetically susceptible children from the general population: the Finnish Type 1 Diabetes Prediction and Prevention Study. *Journal of Clinical Endocrinology and Metabolism, 86*, 4782-4788.

[351] Schenker, M., Hummel, M., Ferber, K., Walter, M., Keller, E., Albert, E.D., Janka, H.U., Kastendiek, C., Sorger, M., Louwen, F. & Ziegler, A.G. (1999). Early expression and high prevalence of islet autoantibodies for DR3/4 heterozygous and DR4/4 homozygous offspring of parents with Type I diabetes: the German BABYDIAB study. *Diabetologia, 42*, 671-677.

[352] Knip, M., Kukko, M., Kulmala, P., Veijola, R., Simell, O., Akerblom, H.K. & Ilonen, J. (2002). Humoral beta-cell autoimmunity in relation to HLA-defined disease susceptibility in preclinical and clinical type 1 diabetes. *American Journal of Medical Genetics, 115*, 48-54.

[353] Kent, S.C., Chen, Y., Bregoli, L., Clemmings, S.M., Kenyon, N.S., Ricordi, C., Hering, B.J. & Hafler, D.A. (2005) Expanded T cells from pancreatic lymph nodes of type 1 diabetic subjects recognize an insulin epitope. *Nature, 435*, 224-228.

[354] Hutton, J.C., Penn, E.J. & Peshavaria, M. (1983). Low-molecular-weight constituents of isolated insulin-secretory granules. Bivalent cations, adenine nucleotides and inorganic phosphate. *Biochemical Journal, 210*, 297-305.

[355] Vardi, P., Ziegler, A.G., Mattews, J.H., Diub, S., Keller, R.J., Ricker, A.T., Wolfsdorf, J., Herskowitz, R.D., Rabizadeh, A. & Eisenbarth, G.S. (1988). Concentration of insulin antibodies at onset of type 1 diabetes: inverse log-linear correlation with age. *Diabetes Care, 9*, 736-739.

[356] Gorus, F.K., Vandewalle, C.L., Dorchy, H., Van Crombrugge, P., Schuit, F.C. & Pipeleers, D.G.; The Belgian Diabetes Registry (1994). Influence of age on the associations among insulin autoantibodies, islet cell antibodies, and HLA DQA1*0301-DQB1*0302 and siblings of patients with type 1 (insulin-dependent) diabetes mellitus. *Journal of Clinical Endocrinology and Metabolism, 78*, 1172-1178.

[357] Strebelow, M., Schlosser, M., Ziegler, B., Rjasanowski, I. & Ziegler, M. (1999). Karlsburg Type I diabetes risk study of a general population: frequencies and interactions of the four major Type I diabetes-associated autoantibodies studied in 9419 schoolchildren. *Diabetologia, 42*, 661-670.

[358] Kukko, M., Kimpimaki, T., Korhonen, S., Kupila, A., Simell, S., Veijola, R., Simell, T., Ilonen, J., Simell, O. & Knip, M. (2005). Dynamics of diabetes-associated autoantibodies in young children with human leukocyte antigen-conferred risk of type 1 diabetes recruited from the general population. *Journal of Clinical Endocrinology and Metabolism, 90*, 2712-2717.

[359] Schmidli, R.S., Colman, P.G. & Harrison, L.C. (1994). Do glutamic acid decarboxylase antibodies improve the prediction of IDDM in first-degree relatives at risk for IDDM? *Journal of Autommunity, 7*, 873-879.

[360] Jaeger, C., Hatziagelaki, E., Stroedter, A., Becker, F., Scherer, S., Petzoldt, R., Federlin, K. & Bretzel, R.G. (1999). The Giessen-Bad Oeynhausen family study: improved prediction of type I diabetes in a low incidence population of relatives using combinations of islet autoantibodies in a dual step model. *Experimental and Clinical Endocrinology and Metaboilsm, 107*, 496-505.

[361] Thivolet, C., Nicolino, M., Monbeig, S., Estour, B., Halimi, S., Robert, M., Orgiazzi, J. & Chatelain, P.; GRADI study. (2002). Combination of autoantibody markers and risk for development of type 1 diabetes: results from a large french cohort of family members. *Diabetes and Metabolism, 28*, 279-285.

[362] Verge, C.F., Gianani, R., Kawasaki, E., Yu, L., Pitropaolo, M., Jackson, R.A., Chase, H.P. & Eisenbarth, G.S. (1996). Prediction of type 1 diabetes in first-degree relatives using a combination of insulin, GAD, and ICA512bdc/IA-2 autoantibodies. *Diabetes, 45*, 926-933.

[363] Colman, P.G., McNair, P., Margetts, H., Schmidli, R.S., Werther, G.A., Alford, F.P., Ward, G.M., Tait, B.D., Honeyman, M.C. & Harrison, L.C. (1998). The Melbourne Pre-Diabetes Study: prediction of type 1 diabetes mellitus using antibody and metabolic testing. *Medical Journal of Australia, 169*, 81-84.

[364] Dittler, J., Seidel, D., Schenker, M. & Ziegler, A.G. (1998). GADIA2-combi determination as first-line screening for improved prediction of type 1 diabetes in relatives. *Diabetes, 47*, 592-597.

[365] Verge, C.F., Gianani, R., Kawasaki, E., Yu, L., Pietropaolo, M., Chase, H.P. & Eisenbarth, G.S. (1996). Number of autoantibodies (against insulin, GAD or ICA512/IA2) rather than particular autoantibody specificities determines risk of type I diabetes. *Journal of Autoimmunity, 9*, 379-383.

[366] Christie, M.R., Vohra, G., Champagne, P., Daneman, D. & Delovitch, T.L. (1990). Distinct antibody specificities to a 64-kD islet cell antigen in Type 1 diabetes as revealed by trypsin treatment. *Journal of Experimental Medicine, 172*, 789-794.

[367] Christie, M.R., Hollands, J.A., Brown, T.J., Michelsen, B.M. & Delovitch, T.L. (1993). Detection of pancreatic islet 64,000 Mr autoantigens in insulin-dependent diabetes distinct from glutamate decarboxylase. *Journal of Clinical Investigations, 92*, 240-248.

[368] Rabin, D.U., Pleasic, S.M., Shapiro, J.A., Yoo-Warreb, H., Oles, J., Hicks, J.M., Goldstein, D.E., Rae, P.M. (1994). Iselt cell antigen 512 is a diabetes-specific ilset autoantigen related to protein tyrosine phosphatases. *Journal of Immunology, 152*, 3183-3188.

[369] Lan, M.S., Lu, J., Goto, Y. & Notkins, A.L. (1994). Molecular cloning and identification of receptor-type protein tyrosine phosphatase, IA-2, from human insulinoma. *DNA Cell Biology*, 505-514.

[370] Krueger, N.X., Streuli, M. & Saito, H. (1990). Structural diversity and evolution of human receptor-like protein tyrosine phosphatases. *EMBO Journal, 9*, 3241-3252.

[371] Passini, N., Larigan, J.D.., Genovese, S., Appella, E., Sinigaglia, F. & Rogge, L. (1995). The 37/40 kilodalton autoantigen in insulin-dependent diabetes mellitus is a putative tyrosine phosphatase IA-2. *Proceedings of the National Academy of Sciences of USA. 92*, 9412-9416.

[372] Solimena, M., Dirkx, R.J., Hermel, J.M., Pleasic-Williams, S., Shapiro, J.A., Caron, L. & Rabin, D.U. (1996). ICA512, an autoantigen of type 1 diabetes, is an intrinsic membrane protein of neurosecretory granules. *EMBO Journal, 15*, 2012-2014.

[373] Xie, H., Notkins, A.L. & Lan, M.S. (1996). IA-2, a transmemmbrane protein tyrosine phosphatase, is expressed in human lung cancer cell lines with neuroendocrine phenotype. *Cancer Research, 56*, 2742-2744.

[374] Hermel, J.M., Dirkx, R., Jr. & Solimena, M. (1999). Post-translational modifications of ICA512, a receptor tyrosine phospatase-loke protein of secretory granules. *European Journal of Neuroscience, 11*, 2609-2620.

[375] Ort, T., Maksimova, E., Dirkx, R., Kachinsky, A.M., Berghs, S., Froehner, S.C. & Solimena, M. (2000). The receptor tyrosine phosphatase-like protein ICA512 binds the PDZ domains of beta2-syntrophin and nNOS in pancreatic beta-cells. *European Journal of Cell Biology, 79*, 621-630.

[376] Trajkovski, M., Mziaut, H., Altkruger, A., Ouwendijk, J., Knoch, K.P., Muller, S. & Solimena, M. (2004). Nuclear translocation of an ICA512 cytosolic fragment couples granule exocytosis and insulin expression in β-cells. *Journal of Cell Biology, 167*, 1063-1074.

[377] Harashima, S., Clark, A., Christie, M.R. & Notkins, A.L. (2005). The dense core transmembrane vesicle protein IA-2 is a regulator of vesicle number and insulin secretion. *Proceedings of the National Academy of Sciences of USA, 102*, 8704-8709.

[378] Hu, Y.F., Zhang, H.L., Cai, T., Harashima, S. & Notkins, A.L. (2005). The IA-2 interactome. *Diabetologia, 48*, 2576-2581.

[379] Sejssler, J., Morgenthaler, N.G., Achenbach, P., Lampeter, E.F., Glawe, D., Payton, M., Christie, M., Scherbaum, W.A. & the DENIS Study Group (1996). Combined screening for autoantibodies for IA-2 and antibodies to glutamic acid decarboxylase in first degree relatives of patients with IDDM. *Diabetologia, 39*, 1351-1356.

[380] Gorus, F.K., Goubert, P., Semakula, C., Vandewalle, C.L., Schepper, J.D., Scheen, A., Christie, M.R. & Pipeleers, D.G. (1997). IA-2 autoantibodies complement GAD65 autoantibodies in new-onset IDDM patients and help predict impending diabetes in their siblings. *Diabetologia, 40*, 95-99.

[381] Hawa, M., Rowe, R., Lan, M.S., Notkins, A.L., Pozzilli, P., Christie, M.R. & Leslie, R.D.G. (1997). Value of antibodies to islet protein tyrosine phosphatase-like molecule in predicting Type 1 diabetes. *Diabetes, 46*, 1270-1275.

[382] Schlosser, M., Strebelow, M., Wassmuth, R., Arnold, M.L., Breunig, I., Rjasanowski, I., Ziegler, B. & Ziegler, M. (2002). The Karlsburg type 1 diabetes risk study of a normal schoolchild population: association of beta-cell autoantibodies and human leukocyte antigen-DQB1 alleles in antibody-positive individuals. *Journal of Clinical Endocrinology and Metabolism, 87*, 2254-2261.

[383] Payton, M.A., Hawkes, C.J. & Christie, M.R. (1995). Relationship of the 37,000 and 40,000-M(r) tryptic fragments of islet antigens in insulin-dependent diabetes to the protein tyrosine phosphatase-like molecule IA-2 (ICA512). *Journal of Clinical Investigations, 96*, 1506-1511.

[384] Lamprasona, V., Bearzatto, M., Genovese, S., Bosi, E., Ferrari, M. & Bonifacio, E. (1996). Autoantibodies in insulin-dependent diabetes recognize distinct cytoplasmic domains of the protein tyrosine phosphatase-like IA-2 autoantigen. *Journal of Immunology, 157*, 2707-2711.

[385] Bearzatto, M., Naserke, H., Piquer, S., Koczwara, K., Lampasona, V., Williams, A., Christie, M.R., Bingley, P.J., Ziegler, A.G. & Bonifacio, E. (2002). Two distinctly HLA-associated contiguous linear epitopes uniquely expressed within the islet antigen 2 molecule are major autoantibody epitopes of the diabetes-specific tyrosine phosphatase-like protein autoantigens. *Journal of Immunology, 168*, 4202-4208.

[386] Kawasaki, E., Sera, Y., Fujita, N., Yamauchi, M., Ozaki, M., Abe, T., Yamakawa, K., Uotani, S., Takino, H., Yamasaki, H., Yamaguchi, Y., Uchigata, Y., Matsuura, N. & Eguchi, K. (2001). Association between IA-2 autoantibody epitope specificities and age of onset in Japanese patients with autoimmune diabetes. *Journal of Autoimmunity, 17*, 323-331.

[387] Naserke, H.E., Ziegler, A.G., Lampasona, V. & Bonifacio, E. (1998). Early development and spreading of autoantibodies to epitopes of IA-2 and their association with progression to type 1 diabetes, *The Journal of Immunology, 161*, 6963-6969.

[388] Hoppu, S., Harkonen, T., Ronkainen, M.S., Akerblom, H.K. & Knip, M.; Childhood Diabetes in Finland Study Group. (2004). IA-2 antibody epitopes and isotypes during the prediabetic process in siblings of children with type 1 diabetes. *Journal of Autoimmunity, 23*, 361-370.

[389] Park, Y.S., Kawasaki, E., Kelemen, K., Yu, L., Schiller, M.R., Rewers, M., Mizuta, M., Eisenbarth, G.S. & Hutton, J.C. (2000). Humoral autoreactivity to an alternatively spliced variant of ICA512/IA-2 in Type I diabetes. *Diabetologia, 43*, 1293-1301.

[390] Diez, J., Park, Y., Zeller, M., Brown, D., Garza, D., Ricordi, C., Hutton, J., Eisenbarth, G.S. & Pugliese, A. (2001). Differential splicing of the IA-2 mRNA in pancreas and lymphoid organs as a permissive genetic mechanism for autoimmunity against the IA-2 type 1 diabetes autoantigen. *Diabetes, 50*, 895-900.

[391] Xie, H., Zhang, B.W., Matsumoto, Y., Li. Q., Notkins, A.L. & Lan, M.S. (1997). Autoantibodies to IA-2 and IA-2 beta in insulin-dependent diabetes mellitus recognize conformational epitopes; location of the 37-and 40-kDa fragments determined. *Journal of Immunology, 159*, 3662-3667.

[392] Notkins, A.L., Zhang, B., Matsumoto, Y. & Lan, M.S. (1997). Comparison of IA-2 and IA-2β with six other members of the protein tyrosine phosphatase family: recognition of antigenic determinants by IDDM sera. *Journal of Autoimmunity, 10*, 245-250.

[393] Bonifacio, E., Lampasona, V. & Bingley, P.J. (1998). IA-2 (islet cell antigen 512) is the primary target of humoral autoimmunity against type 1 diabetes-associated tyrosine phosphatase autoantigens. *Journal of Immunology, 161*, 2648-2654.

[394] Kolm-Litty, V., Berlo, S., Bonifacio, E., Bearzatto, M., Engel, A.M., Christie, M., Ziegler, A.G., Wild, T. & Endl, J. (2000). Human monoclonal antibodies isolated from type I diabetes patients define multiple epitopes in the protein tyrosine phosphatase-like IA-2 antigen. *Journal of Immunology, 165*, 4676-4684.

[395] Honeyman, M.C., Stone, N.L. & Harrison, L.C. (1998). T-cell epitopes in type 1 diabetes autoantigen tyrosine phosphatase IA-2: potential for mimicry with rotavirus and other environmental agents. *Molecular Medicine 4*, 231-239.

[396] Harkonen, T., Lankinen, H., Davydova, B., Hovi, T & Roivainen, M. (2002). Enterovirus infection can induce immune responses that cross-react with beta-cell autoantigen tyrosine phosphatase IA-2/IAR. *Journal of Medical Virology, 66*, 340-350.

[397] Davydova, B., Harkonen, T., Kaialainen, S., Hovi, T., Vaarala, O. & Roivainen, M. (2003). Coxsackievirus immunization delays onset of diabetes in non-obese diabetic mice. *Journal of Medical Virology, 69*, 510-520.

[398] Lu, J., Li, Q., Xie, H., Chen, Z.J., Borovitskaya, A.E., Maclaren, N.K., Notkins, A.L. & Lan, M.S. (1996). Identification of a second transmembrane protein tyrosine phosphatase, IA-2β, as an autoantigen in insulin-dependent diabetes mellitus: precursor of the 37 kDa tryptic fragment. *Proceedings of the National Academy of Sciences of USA, 93*, 2307-2311.

[399] Wasmeier, C. & Hutton, J.C. (1996). Molecular cloning of phogrin, a protein tyrosine phospatase homologue localized to insulin secretory granule membranes. *Journal of Biological Chemistry, 271*, 18161-18170.

[400] Li, Q., Borovitskaya, A.E., DeSilva, M.G., Wasserfall, C., Maclaren, N.K., Notkins, A.L. & Lan, M.S. (1997). Autoantigens in insulin-dependent diabetes mellitus: molecular cloning and characterization of human IA-2β. *Proceedings of the Association of American Physicians, 109*, 429-439.

[401] Magistrelli, G., Toma, S. & Isacchi, A. (1996). Substitution of two variant residues in the protein tyrosine phosphatase-like PTP35/IA-2 sequence reconstitutes catalytic activity. *Biochemical and Biophysical Research Communications, 227*, 581-588.

[402] Wasmeier, C. & Hutton, J.C. (1999). Secretagogue-dependent phosphorylation of phogrin, an insulin granule membrane protein tyrosine phosphatase homologue. *Biochemical Journal, 341*, 563-569.

[403] Wasmeier, C. & Hutton, J.C. (2001). Secretagogue-dependent phosphorylation of the insulin granule membrane protein phogrin is mediated by cAMP-dependent protein kinase. *Journal of Biological Chemistry, 276*, 31919-31928.

[404] Lobner, K., Steinbrenner, H., Roberts, G.A., Ling, Z., Huang, G.C., Piquer, S., Pipeleers, D.G., Seissler, J. & Christie, M.R. (2002). Different regulated expression of

the tyrosine phosphatase-like proteins IA-2 and phogrin by glucose and insulin in pancreatic islets: relationship to development of insulin secretory responses in early life. *Diabetes, 51*, 2982-2988.

[405] Doi, A., Shono, T., Nishi, M., Furuta, H., Sasaki, H. & Nanjo, K. (2006). IA-2beta, but not IA-2, is induced by ghrelin and inhibits glucose-stimulated insulin secretion. *Proceedings of the National Academy of Sciences of USA, 103*, 885-890.

[406] Cui, L., Yu, W.-P., DeAizpurua, H.J., Schmidli, R.S. & Pallen, C.J. (1996). Cloning and characterization of ilset antigen-related protein-tyrosine phosphatase (PTP), a novel receptor-like PTP and autoantigen in insulin-dependent diabetes. *Journal of Biological Chemistry, 271*, 24813-24817.

[407] Notkins, A.L., Lan, M.S. & Leslie, R.D.G. (1998). IA-2 and IA-2β: the immune response in IDDM. *Diabetes Metabolism Reviews, 14*, 85-93.

[408] Genovese, S., Bonfanti, R., Bazzigaluppi, E., Lampasona, V., Benazzi, E., Bosi, E., Chiumello, G. & Bonifacio E. (1996). Association of IA-2 autoantibodies with HLA DR4 phenotypes in IDDM. *Diabetologia, 39*, 1223-1226.

[409] Savola, K., Bonifacio, E., Sabbah, E., Kulmala, P., Vahasalo, P., Karjalainen, J., Tuomilehto-Wolf, E., Merilainen, J., Akerblom, H.K. & Knip, M. (1998). IA-2 antibodies - a sensitive marker of IDDM with clinical onset in childhood and adolescence. Childhood Diabetes in Finland Study Group. *Diabetologia, 41*, 424-429.

[410] Kelemen, K., Crawford, M.L., Gill, R.G., Hutton, J.C. & Wegmann, D. (1999). Cellular immune response to phogrin in the NOD mouse: cloned T-cells cause destruction of islet transplants. *Diabetes, 48*, 1529-1534.

[411] Kelemen, K., Wegmann, D.R. & Hutton, J.C. (2001). T-cell epitope analysis on the autoantigen phogrin (IA-2β) in the nonobese diabetic mouse. *Diabetes, 50*, 1729-1734.

[412] Kelemen, K., Gottlieb, P.A., Putnam, A.L., Davidson, H.W., Wegmann, D.R. & Hutton, J.C. (2004). HLA-DQ8-associated T cell responces to the diabetes autoantigen phogrin (IA-2β) in human prediabetes. *Journal of Immunology, 172*, 3955-3962.

[413] Pupilli, C., Giannini, S., Marchetti, P., Lupi, R., Antonelli, A., Malavasi, F., Takasawa, S., Okamoto, H. & Ferrannini, E. (1999). Autoantibodies to CD38 (ADP-ribosyl cyclase/cyclic ADP-ribose hydrolase) in Caucasian patients with diabetes: effects on insulin release from human islets. *Diabetes, 48*, 2309-2315.

[414] Mallone, R., Ortolan, E., Pinach, S., Volante, M., Zanone, M.M., Bruno, G., Baj, G., Lohmann, T., Cavallo-Perin, P. & Malavasi, F. (2002). Anti-CD38 autoantibodies: characterisation in new-onset type I diabetes and latent autoimmune diabetes of the adult (LADA) and comparison with other islet autoantibodies. *Diabetologia, 45*, 1667-1677.

[415] Mallone, R., Ortolan, E., Baj, G., Funaro, A., Giunti, S., Lillaz, E., Saccucci, F., Cassader, M., Cavallo-Perin, P. & Malavasi, F. (2001). Autoantibody response to CD38 in Caucasian patients with type 1 and type 2 diabetes: immunological and genetic characterization. *Diabetes, 50*, 752-762.

[416] Antonelli, A., Tuomi, T., Nannipieri, M., Fallahi, P., Nesti, C., Okamoto, H., Groop, L. & Ferrannini, E. (2002). Autoimmunity to CD38 and GAD in Type I and Type II diabetes: CD38 and HLA genotypes and clinical phenotypes. *Diabetologia, 45*, 1298-1306.

[417] Antonelli, A., Baj, G., Marchetti, P., Fallahi, P., Surico, N., Pupilli, C., Malavasi, F. & Ferrannini, E. (2001). Human anti-CD38 autoantibodies raise intracellular calcium and stimulate insulin release in human pancreatic islets. *Diabetes, 50*, 985-991.

[418] Marchetti, P., Antonelli, A., Lupi, R., Marselli, L., Fallahi, P., Nesti, C., Baj, G. & Ferrannini, E. (2002). Prolonged in vitro exposure to autoantibodies against CD38 impairs the function and survival of human pancreatic islets. *Diabetes, 51 (Suppl. 3)*, S474-S477.

[419] Pietropaolo, M., Castano, L., Babu, S., Buelow, R., Kuo, Y.L., Martin, S., Martin, A., Powers, A.C., Prochazka, M, & Naggert, J. (1993). Islet cell autoantigen 69 kD (ICA69). Molecular cloning and characterization of a novel diabetes-associated autoantigen. *Journal of Clinical Investigation, 92*, 359-371.

[420] Ronningen, K.S., Atrazhev, A., Luo, L., Luo, C., Smith, D.K., Korbutt, G., Rajotte, R.V. & Elliott, J.F. (1998). Anti-BSA antibodies do not cross-react with the 69-kDa islet cell autoantigen ICA69. *Journal of Autoimmunity, 11*, 223-231.

[421] Stassi, G., Schloot, N. & Pietropaolo, M. (1997). Islet cell autoantigen 69 kDa (ICA69) is preferentially expressed in the human islets of Langerhans than exocrine pancreas. *Diabetologia, 40*, 120-122.

[422] Pilon, M., Peng, X.R., Spence, A.M., Plasterk, R.H. & Dosch, H.M. (2000). The diabetes autoantigen ICA69 and its Caenorhabditis elegans homologue, ric-19, are conserved regulators of neuroendocrine secretion. *Molecular Biology of the Cell, 11*, 3277-3288.

[423] Spitzenberger, F., Pietropaolo, S., Verkade, P., Habermann, B., Lacas-Gervais, S., Mziaut, H., Pietropaolo, M. & Solimena M. (2003). Islet cell autoantigen of 69 kDa is an arfaptin-related protein associated with the Golgi complex of insulinoma INS-1 cells. *Journal of Biological Chemistry, 278*, 26166-26173.

[424] Friday, R.P., Pietropaolo, S.L., Profozich, J., Trucco, M. & Pietropaolo, M. (2003). Alternative core promoters regulate tissue-specific transcription from the autoimmune diabetes-related ICA1 (ICA69) gene locus. *Journal of Biological Chemistry, 278*, 853-863.

[425] Mathews, C.E., Pietropaolo, S.L. & Pietropaolo, M. (2003). Reduced thymic expression of islet antigen contributes to loss of self-tolerance. *Annals of the New York Academy of Sciences, 1005*, 412-417.

[426] Lampasona, V., Ferrari, M., Bosi, E., Pastore, M.R., Bingley, P.J. & Bonifacio, E. (1994). Sera from patients with IDDM and healthy individuals have antibodies to ICA69 on western blots but do not immunoprecipitate liquid phase antigen. *Journal of Autoimmunity, 7*, 665-674.

[427] Martin, S., Kardorf, J., Schulte, B., Lampeter, E.F., Gries, F.A., Melchers, I., Wagner, R., Bertrams, J., Roep, B.O. & Pfutzner, A. (1995). Autoantibodies to the islet antigen ICA69 occur in IDDM and in rheumatoid arthritis. *Diabetologia, 38*, 351-355.

[428] Gordon, T.P., Cavill, D., Neufing, P., Zhang, Y.J. & Pietropaolo, M. (2004). ICA69 autoantibodies in primary Sjogren's syndrome. *Lupus, 13*, 483-484.

[429] Karges, W., Gaedigk, R., Hui, M.F., Cheung, R. & Dosch, H.M. (1997). Molecular cloning of murine ICA69: diabetes-prone mice recognize the human autoimmune-

epitope, Tep69, conserved in splice variants from both species. *Biochimica et Biophysica Data, 1360*, 97-101.

[430] Karges, W., Hammond-McKibben, D., Gaedigk, R., Shibuya, N., Cheung, R. & Dosch, H.M. (1997). Loss of self-tolerance to ICA69 in nonobese diabetic mice. *Diabetes, 46*, 1548-1556.

[431] Winer, S., Astsaturov, I., Gaedigk, R., Hammond-McKibben, D., Pilon, M., Song, A., Kubiak, V., Karges, W., Arpaia, E., McKerlie, C., Zucker, P., Singh, B. & Dosch, H.M. (2002). ICA69(null) nonobese diabetic mice develop diabetes, but resist disease acceleration by cyclophosphamide. *Journal of Immunology, 168*, 475-482.

[432] Roep, B.O., Duinkerken, G., Schreuder, G.M., Kolb, H., de Vries, R.R. & Martin S. (1996). HLA-associated inverse correlation between T cell and antibody responsiveness to islet autoantigen in recent-onset insulin-dependent diabetes mellitus. *European Journal of Immunology, 10*, 589-598.

[433] Geluk, A., van Meijgaarden, K.E., Schloot, N.C., Drijfhout, J.W., Ottenhoff, T.H.M. & Roep, B.O. (1998). HLA-DR binding analysis of peptides from islet antigens in IDDM. *Diabetes, 47*, 1594-1601.

[434] Miyazaki, I., Cheung, R.K., Gaedidk, R., Hui, M.F., Vandermeulen, J., Rajotte, R.V. & Dosch, H.M. (1995). T cell activation and anergy to islet cell antigen in type 1 diabetes. *Journal of Immunology*, 1995.

[435] Arden, S.D., Roep, B.O., Neophytou, P.I., Usac, E.F., Duinkerken, G., de Vries, R.R. & Hutton, J.C. (1996). Imogen 38: a novel 38-kD islet mitochondrial autoantigen recognized by T cells from a newly diagnosed type 1 diabetic patient. *Journal of Clinical Investigations, 97*, 551-561.

[436] Geluk, A., van Meijgaarden, K.E., Roep, B.O. & Ottenhoff, T.H. (1998). Altered peptide ligands of islet autoantigen Imogen 38 inhibit antigen specific T cell reactivity in human type-1 diabetes. *Journal of Autoimmunity, 11*, 353-361.

[437] Castano, L., Russo, E., Zhou, L., Lipes, M.A. & Eisenbarth, G.S. (1991). Identification and cloning of a granule autoantigen (carboxypeptidase-H) associated with type I diabetes. *Journal of Clinical Endocrinology and Metabolism, 73*, 1197-1201.

[438] Fiedorek, F.T., Jr & Parkinson, D. (1992). Carboxypeptidase H processing and secretion in rat clonal beta-cell lines. *Endocrinology, 131*, 1054-1062.

[439] Alcalde, L., Tonacchera, M., Costagliola, S., Jaraquemada, D., Pujol-Borrell, R. & Ludgate, M. (1996). Cloning of candidate autoantigen carboxypeptidase H from a human islet library: sequence identity with human brain CPH. *Journal of Autoimmunity, 9*, 525-528.

[440] Aguilar-Diosdado, M., Parkinson, D., Corbett, J.A., Kwon, G., Marshall, C.A., Gingerich, R.L., Santiago, J.V. & McDaniel, M.L. (1994). Potential autoantigens in IDDM. Expression of carboxypeptidase-H and insulin but not glutamate decarboxylase on the beta-cell surface. *Diabetes, 43*, 418-425.

[441] Zhou, Z.G., Yang, L. & Huang, G. (2003). Diagnostic value of carboxypeptidase-H autoantibodies in detecting latent autoimmune diabetes in adults. *Hunan Yi Ke Da Xue Xue Bao, 28*, 549-552.

[442] Res, P., Thole, J. & de Vries, R. (1991). Heat-shock proteins and autoimmunity in humans. *Springer Seminars in Immunopathology, 13*, 81-98.

[443] Takei, I., Kasatani, T., Watanabe, K., Kasuga, A., Shimada, A., Maruyama, T., Saruta, T. & Nomaguchi, H. (1993). Detection of heat shock protein in patients with insulin-dependent diabetes mellitus. *Diabetes Research and Clinical Practice, 21*, 25-29.

[444] Child, D.F., Williams, C.P., Jones, R.P., Hudson, P.R., Jones, M. & Smith, C.J. (1995). Heat shock protein studies in type 1 and type 2 diabetes and human islet cell culture. *Diabetic Medicine, 12*, 595-599.

[445] Scheinin, T., Tran Minh, N.N., Tuomi, T., Miettinen, A. & Kontiainen, S. (1996). Islet cell and glutamic acid decarboxylase antibodies and heat-shock protein 65 responses in children with newly diagnosed insulin-dependent diabetes mellitus. *Immunology Letters, 49*, 123-126.

[446] Horvath, L., Cervenak, L., Oroszlan, M., Prohaszka, Z., Uray, K., Hudecz, F., Baranyi, E., Madacsy, L., Singh, M., Romics, L., Fust, G. & Panczel, P. (2002). Antibodies against different epitopes of heat-shock protein 60 in children with type 1 diabetes mellitus. *Immunology Letters, 80*, 155-162.

[447] Weitgasser, R., Lechleitner, M., Koch, T., Galvan, G., Muhlmann, J., Steiner, K. & Hoppichler, F. (2003). Antibodies to heat-shock protein 65 and neopterin levels in patients with type 1 diabetes mellitus. *Experimental and Clinical Endocrinology and Diabetes, 111*, 127-131.

[448] Qin, H.Y., Mahon, J.L., Atkinson, M.A., Chaturvedi, P., Lee-Chan, E. & Singh, B. (2003). Type 1 diabetes alters anti-hsp90 autoantibody isotype. *Journal of Autoimmunity, 20*, 237-245.

[449] Ozawa, Y., Kasuga, A., Nomaguchi, H., Maruyama, T., Kasatani, T., Shimada, A., Takei, I., Miyazaki, J. & Saruta, T. (1996). Detection of autoantibodies to the pancreatic islet heat shock protein 60 in insulin-dependent diabetes mellitus. *Journal of Autoimmunity, 9*, 517-524.

[450] Birnbaum, G. & Kotilinek, L. (1999). Immunity to heat shock proteins and neurological disorders of women. *Infectious Diseases in Obstetrics and Gynecology, 7*, 39-48.

[451] Harkonen, T., Puolakkainen, M., Sarvas, M., Airaksinen, U., Hovi, T. & Roivainen, M. (2000). Picornavirus proteins share antigenic determinants with heat shock proteins 60/65. *Journal of Medical Virology, 62*, 383-391.

[452] Tracy, S., Drescher, K.M., Chapman, N.M., Kim, K.S., Carson, S.D., Pirruccello, S., Lane, P.H., Romero, J.R. & Leser, J.S. (2002). Toward testing the hypothesis that group B coxsackieviruses (CVB) trigger insulin-dependent diabetes: inoculating nonobese diabetic mice with CVB markedly lowers diabetes incidence. *Journal of Virology, 76*, 12097-12111.

[453] Aanstoot, H.J., Kang, S.M., Kim, J., Lindsay, L.A., Roll, U., Knip, M., Atkinson, M., Mose-Larsen, P., Fey, S., Ludvigsson, J., Landin, L., Bruining, J., Maclaren, N., Akerblom, H.K. & Baekkeskov, S. (1996). Identification and characterization of glima 38, a glycosylated islet cell membrane antigen, which together with GAD65 and IA2 marks the early phases of autoimmune response in type 1 diabetes. *Journal of Clinical Investigations, 97*, 2722-2783.

[454] Roll, U., Turck, C.W., Gitelman, S.E., Rosenthal, S.M., Nolte, M.S., Masharani, U., Ziegler, A.G. & Baekkeskov, S. (2000). Peptide mapping and characterisation of

glycation patterns of the glima 38 antigen recognised by autoantibodies in Type I diabetic patients. *Diabetologia, 43*, 598-608.

[455] Winnock, F., Christie, M.R., Batstra, M.R., Aanstoot, H.J., Weets, I., Decochez, K., Jopart, P., Nicolaij, D. & Gorus, F.K.; Belgian Diabetes Registry. (2001). Autoantibodies to a 38-kDa glycosylated islet cell membrane-associated antigen in (pre)type 1 diabetes: association with IA-2 and islet cell autoantibodies. *Diabetes Care, 24*, 1181-1186.

[456] Honeyman, M.C., Cram, D.S. & Harrison, L.C. (1993). Transcription factor jun-B is target of autoreactive T-cells in IDDM. *Diabetes, 42*, 626-630.

[457] Chang, Y.H., Hwang, J., Shang, H.F. & Tsai, S.T. (1996). Characterization of human DNA topoisomerase II as an autoantigen recognized by patients with IDDM. *Diabetes, 45*, 408-414.

[458] Shiau, M.Y., Tsai, S.T., Hwang, J., Wu, C.Y. & Chang, Y.H. (2000). Relationship between autoantibodies against glutamic acid decarboxylase, thyroglobulin/thyroid microsome and DNA topoisomerase II in the clinical manifestation of patients with type 1 diabetes mellitus in Taiwan. *European Journal of Endocrinology, 142*, 577-585.

[459] Chang, Y.H., Shiau, M.Y., Tsai, S.T. & Lan, M.S. (2004). Autoantibodies against IA-2, GAD, and topoisomerase II in type 1 diabetic patients. *Biochemical and Biophysical Research Communications, 320*, 802-809.

[460] Bingley, P.J., Christie, M.R., Bonifacio, E., Bonfanti, R., Shattock, M., Fonte, M.T., Bottazzo, G.F. & Gale, E.A. (1994). Combined analysis of autoantibodies improves prediction of IDDM in islet cell antibody-positive relatives. *Diabetes, 43*, 1304-1310.

[461] Ziegler, A.G., Standl, E., Albert. E. & Menhert, H. (1999). HLA-associated insulin autoantibody formation in newly diagnosed type I diabetic patients. *Diabetes, 40*, 1146-1149.

[462] Dahlquist, G., Blom, L., Holmgren, G., Hagglof, B., Larsson, Y., Sterky, G. & Wall, S. (1985). The epidemiology of diabetes in Swedish children 0-14 years - a six-year prospective study. *Diabetologia, 28*, 802-808.

[463] Franke, B., Galloway, T.S. & Wilkin, T.J. (2005). Developments in the prediction of type 1 diabetes mellitus, with special reference to insulin autoantibodies. *Diabetes Metabolism Research and Reviews, 21*, 395-415.

[464] Christie, M.R., Roll, U., Payton, M.A., Hatfield, E.C.I. & Ziegler, A.G. (1997). Validity of screening for individuals at risk for type 1 diabetes by combined analysis of antibodies to recombinant proteins. *Diabetes Care, 20*, 965-970.

[465] Jaeger, C., Hatziagelaki, E., Stroedter, A., Becker, F., Scherer, S., Petzoldt, R., Federlin, K. & Bretzel, R.G. (1999). The Giessen-Bad Oeynhausen family study: improved prediction of type I diabetes in a low incidence population of relatives using combinations of islet autoantibodies in a dual step model. *Experimental and Clinical Endocrinology and Diabetes, 107*, 496-505.

[466] Kulmala, P., Savola, K., Petersen, J.S., Vahasalo, P., Karjalainen, J., Lopponen, T., Dyrberg, T., Akerblom, H.K. & Knip, M. (1998). Prediction of insulin-dependent diabetes mellitus in siblings of children with diabetes. A population-based study. The

Childhood Diabetes in Finland Study Group. *Journal of Clinical Investigations, 101*, 327-336.

[467] Kasuga, A., Maruyama, T., Nakamoto, S., Ozawa, Y., Suzuki, Y. & Saruta, T. (1999). High-titer autoantibodies against glutamic acid decarboxylase plus autoantibodies against insulin and IA-2 predicts insulin requirement in adult diabetic patients. *Journal of Autoimmunity, 12*, 131-135.

[468] Greenbaum, C.J., Schatz, D.A., Cuthbertson, D., Zeidler, A., Eisenbarth, C.S. & Krischer, J.P. (2000). Islet cell antibody-positive relatives with human leukocyte antigen DQA1*0102, DQB1*0602: identification by the Diabetes Prevention Trial-type 1. *Journal of Clinical Endocrinology and Metabolism, 85*, 1255-1260.

[469] Greenbaum, C.J., Cuthbertson, D. & Krischer, J.; DPT-1 Study Group. (1999). Undiagnosed hyperglycemia in relatives of type 1 diabetes mellitus. *Diabetes, 47 (Suppl.1)*, A238.

[470] Greenbaum, C.J., Cuthbertson, D. & Krischer, J.; DPT-1 Study Group. (1999). Silent type 1 diabetes. *Diabetes, 47 (Suppl.1)*, A81.

[471] Prigeon, R.L., D'Alessio, D.A. & Greenbaum, C.J. (2000). No difference in insulin sensitivity between 'silent' type 1 diabetes, diabetes prevention trial-type 1, and control subjects. *Diabetes, 49 (Suppl.1)*, A301.

[472] Chase, H.P., Cuthbertson, D. & Dolan, L.M. (1999). First phase insulin release (FRIP) during the initial intravenous glucose tolerance test (IV-GTT) in the Diabetes Prevention Trial (DPT-1). *Diabetes, 48 (Suppl.1)*, A238.

[473] Ziegler, A.G., Hummel, M., Schenker, M. & Bonifacio, E. (1999). Autoantibody appearance and risk for development of childhood diabetes in offspring of parents with type 1 diabetes: the 2-year analysis of the German BABYDIAB Study. *Diabetes, 48*, 460-468.

[474] Yoon, J.W., Jun, H.S. & Santamaria, P.S. (1998). Cellular and molecular mechanisms for the initiation and progression of β-cell destruction resulting from the collaboration between macrophages and T cells. *Autoimmunity, 27*, 109-122.

[475] Yun, H.S., Yoon, C.S., Zbytnuik, L., van Rooijen, N. & Yoon, J.W. (1999). The role of macrophages in T cell-mediated autoimmune diabetes in nonobese diabetic mice. *Journal of Experimental Medicine, 189*, 347-358.

[476] Jun, H.S., Santamaria, P., Lim, H.W., Zhang, M.L. & Yoon, J.W. (1999). Absolute requirement of macrophages for the development and activation of beta-cell cytotoxic CD8+ T-cells in T-cell receptor transgenic NOD mice. *Diabetes, 48*, 34-42.

[477] Mandrup-Poulsen, T., Bendtzen, K., Dinarello, C. & Nerup, J. (1987). Human tumor necrosis factor potentiates human interleukin 1-mediated rat pancreatic beta cell-cytotoxicity. *Journal of Immunology, 139*, 4077-4082.

[478] Brenner, H.H., Burkart, V., Rothe, H. & Kolb, H. (1993). Oxygen radical production is increased in macrophages from diabetes prone BB rats. *Autoimmunity, 15*, 93-98.

[479] Wong, F.S., Wen, L., Tang, M., Ramanathan, M., Visintin, I., Daugherty, J., Hannum, L.G., Janeway, C.A., Jr. & Shlomchik, M.J. (2004). Investigation of the role of B-cells in type 1 diabetes in the NOD mouse. *Diabetes, 53*, 2581-2587.

[480] Noorchashm, H., Greeley, S.A. & Naji, A. (2003). The role of T/B lymphocyte collaboration in the regulation of autoimmune and alloimmune responses. *Immunologic Research, 27*, 443-450.

[481] Noorchashm, H., Lieu, Y.K., Noorchashm, N., Rostami, S.Y., Greeley, S.A., Schlachterman, A., Song, H.K., Noto, L.E., Jevnikar, A.M., Barker, C.F. & Naji, A. (1999) I-Ag7-mediated antigen presentation by B lymphocytes is critical in overcoming a checkpoint in T cell tolerance to islet beta cells of nonobese diabetic mice. *Journal of Immunology, 163*, 743-750.

[482] Like, A.A., Biron, C.A., Weringer, E.J., Byman, K., Sroczynski, E. & Guberski, D.L. (1986). Prevention of diabetes in BioBreeding/Worcester rats with monoclonal antibodies that recognize T lymphocytes or natural killer cells. *Journal of Experimental Medicine, 164*, 1145-1159.

[483] Like, A.A., Kislauskis, E., Williams, R.M. & Rossini, A.A. (1982). Neonatal thymectomy prevents spontaneous diabetes in the BB/W rats. *Science, 216*, 644-646.

[484] Makino, S., Harada, M., Kishimoto, Y. & Hayashi, Y. (1986). Absence of insulitis and overt diabetes in athymic nude mice with NOD genetic background. *Experimental Animals, 35*, 495-499.

[485] Christianson, S.W., Shultz, L.D. & Leiter, E.H. (1993). Adoptive transfer of diabetes into immunidificient NOD-scid/scid mice. Relative contibutions of CD4+ and CD8+ T cells from diabetic versus prediabetic NOD.NON-Thy-1a donors. *Diabetes, 42*, 44-45.

[486] Haskins, K. & McDuffie, M. (1990). Accelaration of diabetes in young NOD mice with CD4+ ilset-specific T cell clone. *Science, 249*, 1433-1436.

[487] Nagata, M. & Yoon, J.W. (1992). Studies on autoimmunity for T-cell-mediated β cell destruction. Distinct difference of β cell destruction between CD4+ and CD8+ T cell clones derived from lymphocytes infiltrating the islets of NOD mice. *Diabetes, 41*, 998-1008.

[488] Wong, S., Visintin, I. & Wen, L. (1996). CD8 T cell clones fom young nonobese diabetic (NOD) islets can transfer rapid onset of diabetes in NOD mice in the absence of CD4 T cells. *Journal of Experimental Medicine, 183*, 67-76.

[489] Su, X., Hu, O. & Kristan, J.M. (2000). Significant role for Fas in the pathogenesis of autoimmune diabetes. *Journal of Immunology, 164*, 2523-2532.

[490] Verdaguer, J., Yoon, J.W. & Averill, N. (1996). Accelaration of diabetes in TCR-β-transgenic nonobese diabetic mise by beta-cytotoxic T cells expressing endogenous TCR-α chains. *Journal of Immunology, 157*, 4726-4735.

[491] Verdaguer, J., Schmidt, D. & Amrani, A. (1997). Spontaneous autoimmune diabetes in monoclonal T cell nonobese diabetic mice. *Journal of Experimental Medicine, 186*, 989-997.

[492] Rabinovitch, A. (1998). An update of cytokines in the pathogenesis of insulin-dependent diabetes mellitus. *Diabetes Metabolism Reviews, 14*, 129-151.

[493] Von Herrath, M. (2005). Insulin trigger for diabetes. *Nature, 435*, 151-152.

[494] Wilson, D.B. (2005). Insulin auto-antigenisity in type 1 diabetes. *Nature, 438*, E5.

[495] Koskenvuo, M., Karpio, J. & Romanov, K. (1992). Twin studies in metabolic diseses. *Annals of Medicine, 24*, 379-381.

[496] Hawkes, C.H. (1997). Twin studies in medicine – what do they tell us? *Queen Journal of Medicine, 90*, 311-321.

[497] Lykken, D.T., McGue, M. & Tellegen, A. (1987). Recruitment bias in twin research: the rule of two-third reconsidered. *Behaviorial Genetics, 17*, 343-362.

[498] Gottlieb, M.S. & Root, H.F. (1968). Diabetes mellitus in twins. *Diabetes, 17*, 693-704.

[499] Pyke, D.A. (1988) Development of diabetes in identical twins.In: Camerini-Davalos, R.A., Cole, H., eds. *Early diabetes: pre-diabetes*. Plenum Press, New York, p. 255-258.

[500] Japanese Diabetes Society. Committee on diabetic twins (1988). Diabetes mellitus in twins: a cooperative study in Japan. *Diabetes Research and Clinical Practice, 5*, 271-280.

[501] Matsuda, A. & Kuzuya, T. (1994). Diabetic twins in Japan. *Diabetes Research and Clinical Practice, 24 (Suppl.)*, S63-S67.

[502] Harvald, B. & Hauge, M. (1963). Selection in diabetes in modern society. *Acta Medica Scandinavica, 173*, 459-465.

[503] Kaprio, J., Tuomilehto, J. & Koskenvuo, M. (1992). Concordance for type 1 (insilin dependent) and type 2 (non insulin dependent) diabetes in a popuation-based cohort of twins in Finland. *Diabetologia, 35*, 1060-1067.

[504] Kyvik, K.O., Green, A., Beck-Nielsen, H. (1995). Concordance rates of insulin dependent diabetes mellitus: a population based study of young Danish twins. *British Medical Journal, 311*, 913-917.

[505] Redondo, M.J., Rewers, M., Yu, L., Garg, S., Pilcher, C.C., Elliott, R.B., Eisenbarth, G.S. (1999). Genetic determination of islet cell autoimmunity in monozygotic twin, dizygotic twin, and non-twin siblings of patients with type 1 diabetes: prospective twin study. *British Medical Journal, 318*, 698-702.

[506] Fava, D., Gardner, S., Pyke, D. & Leslie, R.D. (1998). Evidence that the age at diagnosis of IDDM is genetically determined. *Diabetes Care, 21*, 925-929.

[507] Hyttinen, V., Kaprio, J., Kinnunen, L., Koskenvuo, M. & Tuomilehto, J. (2003). Genetic liability of type 1 diabetes and the onset age among 22,650 young Finnish twin pairs: a nationwide follow-up study. *Diabetes, 52*, 1052-1055.

[508] Petersen, J.S., Kyvik, K.O., Bingley, P.J., Gale, E.A., Green, A., Dyrberg, T. & Beck-Nielsen, H. (1997). Population based study of prevalence of islet cell autoantibodies in monozygotic and dizygotic Danish twin pairs with insulin dependent diabetes mellitus. *British Medical Journal, 31*, 314, 1575-1579.

[509] Gale, E.A.M., Bingley, P.J., Eisenbarth, G.S., Redondo, M.J., Kyvik, K.O. & Petersen, J.S. (2001). Reanalysis of twin studies suggests that diabetes is mainly genetic. *British Medical Journal, 323*, 997.

[510] Redondo, M.J., Fain, P.R., Krischer, J.P., Yu, L., Cuthbertson, D., Winter, W.E. & Eisenbarth, G.S.; DPT-1 Study Group. (2004). Expression of beta-cell autoimmunity does not differ between potential dizygotic twins and siblings of patients with type 1 diabetes. *Journal of Autoimmunity, 23*, 275-279.

[511] Redondo, M.J., Yu, L., Hawa, M. Mackenzie, T., Pyke, D.A., Eisenbarth, G.S. & Leslie, R.D. (2001). Heterogeneity of type I diabetes: analysis of monozygotic twins in Great Britain and the United States. *Diabetologia, 44*, 354-362.

[512] Metcalfe, K.A., Hitman, G.A., Rowe, R.E., Hawa, M., Huang, X., Stewart, T. & Leslie, R.D. (2001). Concordance for type 1 diabetes in identical twins is affected by insulin genotype. *Diabetes Care, 24*, 838-842.

[513] Hawa, M.I., Bonfanti, R., Valeri, C., Delli Castelli, M., Beyan, H. & Leslie, R.D. (2005). No evidence for genetically determined alteration in insulin secretion or sensitivity predisposing to type 1 diabetes: a study of identical twins. *Diabetes Care, 28*, 1415-1418.

[514] Elston, R.C. (1995). The genetic dissection of multifactorial traits. *Clinical and Experimental Allergy, 25 (Suppl. 2)*, 103–106.

[515] Lander, E.S. & Schork, N.J. (1994). Genetic dissection of complex traits, *Science, 265*, 2037–2048.

[516] Hirschhorn, J.N. & Daly, M.J. (2005). Genome-wide association studies for common diseases and complex traits, *Nature Reviews Genetics 6*, 95–108.

[517] Kruglyak, L., Daly, M.J., Reeve-Daly, M.P. & Lander, E.S. (1996). Parametric and nonparametric linkage analysis: a unified multipoint approach. *American Journal of Human Genetics, 58*, 1347–1363.

[518] Morton, N.E. (1955). Sequential tests for the detection of linkage. *American Journal of Human Genetics, 7*, 277–318.

[519] Penrose, L.S. (1953). The general purpose sibpair linkage test. *Annals of Eugenenics, 18*, 120–124.

[520] Suarez, B.K. (1978). The affected sib pair IBD distribution for HLA-linked disease susceptibility genes. *Tissue Antigens, 12*, 87–93.

[521] Hyer, R.N., Julier, C., Buckley, J.D., Trucco, M., Rotter, J. & Spielman, R. (1991). High-resolution linkage mapping for susceptibility genes in human polygenic disease: insulin-dependent diabetes mellitus and chromosome 11q, *American Journal of Human Genetics, 48*, 243–257.

[522] Slager, S.L. & Schaid, D.J. (2001). Case-control studies of genetic markers: power and sample size approximations for Armitage's test for trend. *Human Heredity, 52*, 149–153.

[523] Falk, C.T. & Rubinstein, P. (1987). Haplotype relative risks: an easy reliable way to construct a proper control sample for risk calculations. *Annals of Human Genetics, 51,* 227-233.

[524] Ahsan, H., Hodge, S.E., Heiman, G.A., Begg, M.D. & Susser, E.S. (2002). Relative risk for genetic associations: the case-parent triad as a variant of case-cohort design. *International Journal of Epidemiology, 31*, 669-678.

[525] Ott, J. (1989). Statistical properties of the haplotype relative risk. *Genetic Epidemiology, 6*, 127-130.

[526] Spielman, R.S., McGinnis, R.E. & Ewens, W.J. (1993). Transmission test for linkage disequilibrium: the insulin gene region and insulin-dependent diabetes mellitus (IDDM). *American Journal of Human Genetics, 52*, 506–516.

[527] Sun, F., Flanders, W.D., Yang Q. & Khoury, M.J. (1999). Transmission disequilibrium test (TDT) when only one parent is available: the 1-TDT. *American Journal of Epidemiology, 150*, 97–104.

[528] Sham, P.C. & Curtis, D. (1995). An extended transmission/disequilibrium test (TDT) for multi-allele marker loci. *Annals of Human Genetics, 59*, 323–336.

[529] Cordell, H.J. & Clayton, D.G. (2002) A unified stepwise regression procedure for evaluating the relative effects of polymorphisms within a gene using case/control or family data: application to HLA in type 1 diabetes. *American Journal of Human Genetics, 70*, 124–141.

[530] Morris, R.W. & Kaplan, N.L. (2002). On the advantage of haplotype analysis in the presence of multiple disease susceptibility alleles *Genetic Epidemiology, 23*, 221–233.

[531] Martin, E.R., Lai, E.H., Gilbert, J.R., Rogala, A.R., Afshari, A.J. & Riley, J. (2000) SNPing away at complex diseases: analysis of single-nucleotide polymorphisms around APOE in Alzheimer disease. *American Journal of Human Genetics, 67*, 383–394.

[532] Lie, B.A., Todd, J.A., Pociot, F., Nerup, J., Akselsen, H.E. & Joner, G. (1999). The predisposition to type 1 diabetes linked to the human leukocyte antigen complex includes at least one non-class II gene. *American Journal of Human Genetics, 64*, 793–800.

[533] Thomson, G., Robinson, W.P., Kuhner, M.K., Joe, S., MacDonald, M.J. & Gottschall, J.L. (1988). Genetic heterogeneity, modes of inheritance, and risk estimates for a joint study of Caucasians with insulin-dependent diabetes mellitus. *American Journal of Human Genetics, 43*, 799–816.

[534] Svejgaard, A. & Ryder, L.P. (1994) HLA and disease associations: detecting the strongest association, *Tissue Antigens, 43*, 18–27.

[535] Serreze, D.V. & Letter, E.H. (1995). Insulin dependent diabetes mellitus (IDDM) in NOD mice and BB rats: origins in hematopoietic dtem cell defects and implications for therapy. In: Shafrir, E., ed. *Lessons from Animal Diabetes*. V. London: Smith-Gordon, p.59-73.

[536] Makino, S., Kunimoto, K., Muraoka, Y., Mizushima, Y., Katagiri, K. & Tochino, Y. (1980). Breeding of a non-obese, diabetic strain of mice. *Experimental Animals, 29*, 1–8.

[537] Pomerleau, D.P., Bagley, R.J., Serreze, D.V., Mathews, C.E. & Leiter, E.H. (2005). Major histocompatibility complex-linked diabetes susceptibility in NOD/Lt mice: subcongenic analysis localizes a component of Idd16 at the H2-D end of the diabetogenic H2^{g7} complex. *Diabetes, 54*, 1603–1606.

[538] Yoshida, K. & Kikutani, H. (2000). Genetic and immunological basis of autoimmune diabetes in the NOD mouse. *Reviews in Immunogenetics, 2*, 140-146.

[539] Baxter, AG., Adams, M.A. & Mandel, T.E. (1989). Comparison of high- and low-diabetes incidence NOD mouse strains. *Diabetes, 38*, 96–1300.

[540] Miyazaki, A., Hanafusa, T., Yamada, K., Miyagawa, J., Fujino-Kurihara, H., Nakajima, H., Nonaka, K. & Tarui, S. (1985). Predominance of T lymphocytes in pancreatic islets and spleen of pre-diabetic non-obese diabetic (NOD) mice: a longitudinal study. *Clinical and Experimental Immunology, 60*, 622-630.

[541] Faveeuw, C., Gagnerault, M.C. & Lepault, F. (1995). Isolation of leukocytes infiltrating the islets of Langerhans of diabetes-prone mice for flow cytometric analysis. *Journal of Immunological Methods, 187*, 163–169.

[542] Gaskins, H.R., Prochazka, M., Hamaguchi, K., Serreze, D.V. & Leiter, E.H. (1992). Beta cell expression of endogenous xenotropic retrovirus distinguishes diabetes susceptible NOD/Lt from resistant NON/Lt mice. *Journal of Clinical Investigations, 90*, 2220–2227.

[543] Lafferty, K.J. (1997). Immunobiology of autoimmune diabetes. *Research in Immunology, 148*, 313–319.

[544] Kikutani, H. & Makino, S. (1992). The murine autoimmune diabetes model: NOD and related strains. *Advances in Immunology, 51*, 285–322.

[545] Mathews, C.E., Leiter, E.H., Spirina, O., Bykhovskaya, Y., Gusdon, A.M., Ringquist, S. & Fischel-Ghodsian, N. (2005). Mt-Nd2 Allele of the ALR/Lt mouse confers resistance against both chemically induced and autoimmune diabetes. *Diabetologia, 48*, 261-267.

[546] Lang, J. & Bellgrau, D. (2004). Animal models of type 1 diabetes: genetics and immunological function. *Advances in Experimental Medicine and Biology, 552*, 91-116.

[547] Leiter, E.H. (2005). Nonobese diabetic mice and the genetics of diabetes susceptibility. *Current Diabetes Reports, 5*, 141-148.

[548] Wicker, L.S., Chamberlain, G., Hunter, K., Rainbow, D., Howlett, S., Tiffen, P., Clark, J., Gonzalez-Munoz, A., Cumiskey, A.M., Rosa, R.L., Howson, J.M., Smink, L.J., Kingsnorth, A., Lyons, P.A., Gregory, S., Rogers, J., Todd, J.A. & Peterson, L.B. (2004). Fine mapping, gene content, comparative sequencing, and expression analyses support Ctla4 and Nramp1 as candidates for Idd5.1 and Idd5.2 in the nonobese diabetic mouse. *Journal of Immunology, 173*,164–173.

[549] Hamilton-Williams, E.E., Serreze, D.V., Charlton, B., Johnson, E.A., Marron, M.P., Mullbacher, A. & Slattery, R.M. (2001). Transgenic rescue implicates beta2-microglobulin as a diabetes susceptibility gene in nonobese diabetic (NOD) mice. *Proceedings of the National Academy of Sciences of USA, 98*, 11533–11538.

[550] Lyons, P.A., Armitage, N., Argentina, F., Denny, P., Hill, N.J., Lord, C.J., Wilusz, M.B., Peterson, L.B., Wicker, L.S. & Todd, J.A. (2000). Congenic mapping of the type 1 diabetes locus, ldd3, to a 780-kb region of mouse chromosome 3: identification of a candidate segment of ancestral DNA by haplotype mapping. *Genome Research, 10*, 446–453.

[551] King, C., Ilic, A., Koelsch, K. & Sarvetnick, N. (2004) Homeostatic expansion of T cells during immune insufficiency generates autoimmunity. *Cell, 117*, 265–277.

[552] Podolin, P.L., Denny, P., Lord, C.J., Hill, N.J., Todd, J.A., Peterson, L.B., Wicker L.S. & Lyons, P.A. (1997). Congenic mapping of the insulin-dependent diabetes (Idd) gene, Idd10, localizes two genes mediating the Idd10 effect and eliminates the candidate Fcgr1. *Journal of Immunology, 159*, 1835–1843.

[553] Wang, J.,Yoshida, T., Nakaki, F., Hiai, H., Okazaki, T. & Honjo, T. (2005). Establishment of NOD-Pdcd1-/- mice as an efficient animal model of type I diabetes. *Proceedings of the National Academy of USA, 102*, 11823-11828.

[554] Penha-Goncalves, C., Moule, C., Smink, L.J., Howson, J., Gregory, S., Rogers, J., Lyons, P.A., Suttie, J.J., Lord, C.J., Peterson, L.B., Todd, J.A. & Wicker, L.S. (2003). Identification of a structurally distinct CD101 molecule encoded in the 950-kb Idd10 region of NOD mice. *Diabetes, 52*, 1551–1556.

[555] Maier, L.M., Smyth, D.J., Vella, A., Payne, F., Cooper, J.D., Pask, R., Lowe, C., Hulme, J., Smink, L.J., Fraser, H., Moule, C., Hunter, K.M., Chamberlain, G., Walker, N., Nutland, S., Undlien, D.E., Ronningen, K.S., Guja, C., Ionescu-Tirgoviste, C., Savage, D.A., Strachan, D.P., Peterson, L.B., Todd, J.A., Wicker, L.S. & Twells, R.C. (2005). Construction and analysis of tag single nucleotide polymorphism maps for six human-mouse orthologous candidate genes in type 1 diabetes. *BMC Genetics,* 6:9.

[556] Carnaud, C., Gombert, J., Donnars, O., Garchon, H. & Herbelin, A. (2001). Protection against diabetes and improved NK/NKT cell performance in NOD.NK1.1 mice congenic at the NK complex, *Journal of Immunology, 166*, 2404–2411.

[557] Grimm, C.H., Rogner, U.C. & Avner, P. (2003). Lamp and Bcat1 are candidates for the type I diabetes susceptibility locus Idd6. *Autoimmunity, 36*, 241–246.

[558] Lyons, P.A., Hancock, W.W., Denny, P., Lord, C.J., Hill, N.J., Armitage, N., Siegmund, T., Todd, J.A., Phillips, M.S., Hess, J.F., Chen, S.L., Fischer, P.A., Peterson, L.B. & Wicker, L.S. (2000). The NOD Idd9 genetic interval influences the pathogenicity of insulitis and contains molecular variants of Cd30, Tnfr2, and Cd137. *Immunity, 13*, 107–115.

[559] Brodnicki, T.C., McClive, P., Couper, S. & Morahan, G. (2000). Localization of Idd11 using NOD congenic mouse strains: elimination of Slc9a1 as a candidate gene. *Immunogenetics, 51*, 37–41.

[560] Cannons, J.L., Chamberlain, G., Howson, J., Smink, L.J., Todd, J.A., Peterson, L.B., Wicker, L.S., & Watts, T.H. (2005). Genetic and functional association of the immune signaling molecule 4-1BB (CD137/TNFRSF9) with type 1 diabetes. *Journal of Autoimmunity, 25*, 13-20.

[561] Grattan, M., Mi, Q.S., Meagher, C. & Delovitch, T.L. (2002). Congenic mapping of the diabetogenic locus Idd4 to a 5.2-cM region of chromosome 11 in NOD mice: identification of two potential candidate subloci, *Diabetes, 51*, 215–223.

[562] Brodnicki, T.C., Quirk, F. & Morahan, G. (2003). A susceptibility allele from a non-diabetes-prone mouse strain accelerates diabetes in NOD congenic mice, *Diabetes, 52*, 218–222.

[563] Deruytter, N., Boulard, O. & Garchon, H.J. (2004). Mapping non-class II H2-linked loci for type 1 diabetes in nonobese diabetic mice, *Diabetes, 53*, 3323–3327.

[564] Inoue, K., Ikegami, H., Fujisawa, T., Noso, S., Nojima, K., Babaya, N., Itoi-Babaya, M., Makimo, S. & Ogihara, T. (2004). Allelic variation in class I K gene as candidate for a second component of MHC-linked susceptibility to type 1 diabetes in non-obese diabetic mice, *Diabetologia, 47*, 739–747.

[565] Hattori, M.., Buse, J.B., Jackson, R.A., Glimcher, L., Dorf, M.E., Minami, M., Makino, S., Moriwaki, K., Kuzuya, H. & Imura, H. (1986). The NOD mouse: recessive diabetogenic gene in the major histocompatibility complex. *Science, 231*, 733-735.

[566] Wicker, L.S., Miller, B.J., Coker, L.Z., McNally, S.E., Scott, S., Mullen, Y. & Appel, M.C. (1987). Genetic control of diabetes and insulitis in the nonobese diabetic (NOD) mouse. *Journal of Experimental Medicine, 165*, 1639–1654.

[567] Markees, T.G., Serreze, D.V., Phillips, N.E., Sorli, C.H., Gordon, E.J., Shultz, L.D., Noelle, R.J., Woda, B.A., Greiner, D.L., Mordes, J.P./ & Rossini, A.A. (1999). NOD mice have a generalized defect in their response to transplantation tolerance induction. *Diabetes, 48*, 967-974.

[568] Serreze, D.V. (1998). The identity and ontogenic origins of autoreactive T lymphocytes in NOD mice. In: Leiter, E.H. & Atkinson, M.A., eds. *NOD Mice and Related Strains: Research Applications in Diabetes, AIDS, Cancer, and Other Diseases*. Austin: R.G. Landes, p. 71–99.

[569] Shimada, A., Charlton, B., Rohane, P., Taylor-Edwards, C. & Fathman, C.G. (1996). Immune regulation in type 1 diabetes. *Journal of Autoimmunity, 9*, 263–269.

[570] Carrasco-Marin, E., Shimizu, J., Kanagawa, O. & Unanue, E.R. (1996). The class II MHC class I-A^{g7} molecules from non-obese diabetic mice are poor peptide binders. *Journal of Immunology, 156*, 450–458.

[571] Lie, B.A., Sollid, L.M., Ascher, H., Ek, J., Akselsen, H.E., Ronningen, K.S., Thorsby, E. & Undlien, D.E. (1999). Gene telomeric of the HLA class I region is involved in predisposition to both type 1 diabetes and coeliac disease. *Tissue Antigens, 54*, 162–168.

[572] Hattori, M., Yamato, E., Itoh, N., Senpuku, H., Fujisawa, T., Yoshino, M., Fukuda, M., Matsumoto, E., Toyonaga, T., Nakagawa, I., Petruzzelli, M., McMurray, A., Weiner, H., Sagai, T., Moriwaki, K., Shiroishi, T., Maron, R. & Lund, T. (1999). Cutting edge: homologous recombination of the MHC class I K region defines new MHC-linked diabetogenic susceptibility gene(s) in nonobese diabetic mice. *Journal of Immunology, 163*, 1721-1724.

[573] Melanitou, E., Joly, F., Lanthrop, M., Boitard, C. & Avner, P. (1998). Evidence for the presence of insulin-dependent diabetes-associated alleles on the distal part of mouse chromosome 6. *Genome Research, 8*, 608–620.

[574] Wicker, L.S., Todd, J.A. & Peterson, L.B. (1995). Genetic control of autoimmune diabetes in the NOD mouse. *Annual Reviews in Immunology, 13*,179–200.

[575] Friday, R.P., Trucco, M. & Pietropaolo, M. (1999). Genetics of Type 1 diabetes mellitus. *Diabetes Nutrition and Metabolism, 12*, 3–26.

[576] Graser, R.T., Mathews, C.E., Leiter, E.H. & Serreze, D.V. (1999). MHC characterization of ALR and ALS mice: respective similarities to the NOD and NON strains. *Immunogenetics, 49*, 722–726.

[577] Mathews, C.E., Graser, R.T., Serreze, D.V. & Leiter, E.H. (2000). Reevaluation of the major histocompatibility complex genes of the NOD-progenitor CTS/Shi strain. *Diabetes, 49,*131–134.

[578] Hattori, M., Yamato, E. & Matsumoto, E. (1996). Occurrence of pretype I diabetes (pre-IDDM) and type II diabetes (NIDDM) in BC1 [(NOD X mus spretus) F1 X NOD] mice. In: Shafrir, E., ed. *Lessons from Animal Diabetes*, Vol. VI. Boston: Birkhaüser, p.83–95.

[579] Kennedy, G.C., German, M.S. & Rutter, W.J. (1995). The minisatellite in the diabetes susceptibility locus IDDM2 regulates insulin transcription. *Nature Genetics, 9*, 293-298.

[580] Bennett, S.T., Lucassen, A.M., Gough, S.C., Powell, E.E., Undlien, D.E., Pritchard, L.E., Merriman, M.E., Kawaguchi, Y., Dronsfield, M.J. & Pociot, F. (1995). Susceptibility to human type 1 diabetes at IDDM2 is determined by tandem repeat variation at the insulin gene minisatellite locus. *Nature Genetics, 9*, 284-292.

[581] French, M.B., Allison, J., Cram, D.S., Thomas, H.E., Dempsey-Collier, M., Silva, A., Georgiou, H.M., Kay, T.W., Harrison, L.C. & Lew, A.M. (1997). Transgenic expression of mouse proinsulin II prevents diabetes in non-obese diabetic mice. *Diabetes, 46*, 34–39.

[582] Wong, F.S., Karttunen, J., Dumont, C., Wen, L., Visintin, I., Pilip, I.M., Shastri, N., Pamer, E.G. & Janeway, C.A., Jr. (1999). Identification of an MHC class I-restricted autoantigen in type 1 diabetes by screening an organ-specific cDNA library. *Nature Medicine, 5*, 1026–1031.

[583] Hill, N.J., Lyons, P.A., Armitage, N., Todd, J.A., Wicker, L.S. & Peterson, L.B. (2000). The NOD Idd5 locus controls insulitis and diabetes and overlaps the orthologous CTLA4/IDDM12 and NRAMP1 loci in humans. *Diabetes, 49*, 1744-1747.

[584] Marron, M.P., Raffel, L.J., Garchon, H.J., Jacob, C.O., Serrano-Rios, M., Martinez Larrad, M.T., Teng, W.P., Park, Y., Zhang, Z.X., Goldstein, D.R., Tao, Y.W., Beaurain, G., Bach, J.F., Huang, H.S., Luo, D.F., Zeidler, A., Rotter, J.I., Yang, M.C., Modilevsky, T., Maclaren, N.K. & She, J.X. (1997). Insulin-dependent diabetes-mellitus (IDDM) is associated with CTLA4 polymorphisms in multiple ethnic groups. *Human Molecular Genetics, 6*, 1275–1282.

[585] Uchigata, Y., Okada, T., Gong, J.S., Yamada, Y., Iwamoto, Y. & Tanaka, M. (2002). A mitochondrial genotype associated with the development of autoimmune-related type 1 diabetes. *Diabetes Care, 25*, 2106.

[586] Yao, Y.G., Kong, Q.P. & Zhang, Y.P. (2002). Mitochondrial DNA 5178A polymorphism and longevity. *Human Genetics, 111*, 462–463.

[587] Matsunaga, H., Tanaka, Y., Tanaka, M., Gong, J.S., Zhang, J., Nomiyama, T., Ogawa, O., Ogihara, T., Yamada, Y., Yagi, K. & Kawamori, R. (2001). Antiatherogenic mitochondrial genotype in patients with type 2 diabetes. *Diabetes Care, 24*, 500–503.

[588] Kokaze, A., Ishikawa, M., Matsunaga, N., Yoshida, M., Sekine, Y., Sekiguchi, K., Harada, M., Satoh, M., Teruya, K., Takeda, N., Fukazawa, S., Uchida, Y. & Takashima, Y. (2004). Longevity-associated mitochondrial DNA 5178 A/C polymorphism and blood pressure in the Japanese population. *Journal of Human Hypertension, 18*, 41–45.

[589] Takagi, K., Yamada, K., Gong, J.S., Sone, T., Yokota, M. & Tanaka, M. (2004). Association of a 5178C→A (Leu237Met) polymorphism in the mitochondrial DNA with a low prevalence of myocardial infarction in Japanese individuals. *Atherosclerosis, 175*, 281–286.

[590] Aoki, C.A., Borchers, A.T., Ridgway, W.M., Keen, C.L., Ansari, A.A. & Gershwin, M.E. (2005). NOD mice and autoimmunity. *Autoimmunity Reviews, 4*, 373-379.

[591] Cardell, S.L. (2006). The natural killer T lymphocyte: a player in the complex regulation of autoimmune diabetes in non-obese diabetic mice. *Clinical and Experimental Immunology, 143*, 194-202.

[592] Hammond, K.J., Poulton, L.D., Palmisano, L.J., Silveira, P.A., Godfrey, D.I & Baxter, A.G. (1998). Alpha/beta-T cell receptor $(TCR)^{+}CD4CD8$ (NKT) thymocytes prevent insulin-dependent diabetes mellitus in nonobese diabetic (NOD)/Lt mice by the influence of interleukin (IL)-4 and/or IL-10. Journal *of Experimental Medicine, 187*, 1047–1056.

[593] Biron, C.A., Nguyen, K.B., Pien, G.C., Cousens, L.P. & Salazar-Mather, T.P. (1999). Natural killer cells in antiviral defence: function and regulation by innate cytokines. *Amnnual Reviews in Immunology, 17*, 189-220.

[594] Fox, A. & Harrison, L.C. (2000). Innate immunity and graft rejection. *Immunology Reviews, 173*, 141-147.

[595] Banuelos, S.J., Shultz, L.D., Greiner, D.L., Burzenski, L.M., Gott, B., Lyons, B.L., Rossini, A.A. & Appel, M.C. (2004). Rejection of human islets and human HLA-A2.1 transgenic mouse islets by alloreactive human lymphocytes in immunodeficient NOD-scid and NOD-$Rag1^{null}Prf1^{null}$ mice. *Clinical Immunology, 112*, 273-283.

[596] Nakhooda, A.F., Like, A.A., Chappel, C.I., Murray, F.T. & Marliss, E.B. (1976). The spontaneously diabetic Wistar rat metabolic and morphologic studies. *Diabetes, 26*, 100-112.

[597] Crisa, L., Mordes, J.P. & Rossini, A.A. (1992). Autoimmune diabetes in the BB rat. *Diabetes Metabolism Reviews, 8*, 9-37.

[598] Mordes, J.P., Desemone, J. & Rossini, A.A. (1987). The BB rat. *Diabetes Metabolism Reviews*, 1987, 3, 725-750.

[599] Ellerman, K., Wrobleski, M., Rabinovitch, A. & Like, A. (1993). Natural killer cell depletion and diabetes mellitus in BB/Wor rat (revisited). *Diabetologia, 36*, 596-601.

[600] Greiner, D.L., Mordes, J.P., Handler, E.S., Angelillo, M., Nakamura, N. & Rossini, A.A. (1987). Depletion of RT6.1+ T lymphocytes induces diabetes in resistant Biobreeding/Worcester (BB/W) rats. *Journal of Experimental Medicine, 166*, 461-475.

[601] Sterntal, E., Like, A.A., Sarantis, K., Braverman, L.E. (1981). Lympholytic thyroiditis and diabetes in the BB/W rats. A new model of autoimmune endorinopathy. *Diabetes, 30*, 1058-1061.

[602] Rajatanavin, R., Appel, M.C., Reinhardt, W., Alex, S., Yang, Y.-N. & Braverman, L.E. (1991). Variable prevalence of lympholytic thyriditis among diabetes-prone sublines of BB/Wor rats. *Endocrinology, 128*, 153-157.

[603] Awata, T. & Kanazawa, Y (1994). *Genetic markers for insulin-dependent diabetes mellitus in Japanese, 24 (Suppl.)*, S83-S87.

[604] McKeever, U., Mordes, J.P., Greiner, D.L., Appel, M.C., Rozing, J., Handler, E.S. & Rossini, A.A. (1990). Adoptive transfer of autoimmune diabetes and thyroiditis to athymic rats. *Proceedings of the National Academy of USA, 87*, 7618-7622.

[605] Jacob, H.J., Pettersson, A., Wilson, D., Mao, Y., Lernmark, A. & Lander, E.S. (1992). Genetic dissection of autoimmune type 1 diabetes in the BB rat. *Nature Genetics, 2*, 56–60.

[606] Colle, E., Guttman, R.D., Fuks, A., Seemayer, T.A., Prud'homme, G.J. (1986). Genetics of the spontaneous diabetic syndrome: interaction of MHC and non-MHC associated factors. *Molecular Biology and Medicine 3*, 13–23.

[607] Ellerman, K.E. & Like, A.A. (1995). A major histocompatibility complex class II restriction for BioBreeding Worcester diabetes-inducing T cells. *Journal of Experimental Medicine, 182*, 923–930.

[608] Awata, T., Guberski, D.L. & Like, A.A. (1995). Genetics of the BB rat: association of autoimmune disorders (diabetes, insulitis, and thyroiditis) with lymphopenia and major histocompatibility complex class II *Endocrinology, 136*, 5731–5735.

[609] Holowachuk, E.W. & Greer, M.K. (1989). Unaltered class II histocompatibility antigens and pathogenesis of IDDM in BB rats. *Diabetes, 38*, 267–271.

[610] Chao, N.J., Timmerman, L., McDevitt, H.O. & Jacob, C.O. (1989). Molecular characterization of MHC class II antigens (beta 1 domain) in the BB diabetes-prone and – resistant rat. *Immunogenetics 29*, 231–234.

[611] Hornum, L., Jackerott, M. & Markholst, H. (1995). The rat T-cell lymphopenia resistance gene (Lyp) maps between D4Mit6 and Npy on RNO4. *Mammalian Genome, 6*, 371–372.

[612] Markholst, H., Eastman, S., Wilson, D., Andreasen, B.E. & Lernmark, A. (1991). Diabetes segregates as a single locus in crosses between inbred BB rats prone or resistant to diabetes. *Journal of Experimental Medicine, 174*, 297–300.

[613] Iwakoshi, N.H., Goldschneider, I., Tausche, F., Mordes, J.P., Rossini, A.A. & Greiner, D.L. (1998). High frequency apoptosis of recent thymic emigrants in the liver of lymphopenic diabetes-prone BioBreeding rats. *Journal of Immunology, 160*, 5838–5850.

[614] Bortell, R., Kanaitsuka, T., Stevens, L A., Moss, J., Mordes, J.P., Rossini, A.A. & Greiner, D.L. (1999). The RT6 (Art2) family of ADP-ribosyltransferases in rat and mouse. *Molecular and Cellular Biochemistry, 193*, 61–68.

[615] Koch-Nolte, F., Duffy, T., Nissen, M., Kahl, S., Killeen, N., Ablamunits, V., Haag, F. & Leiter, E.H. (1999). New monoclonal antibody detects a developmentally regulated mouse ecto ADP ribosyltransferase on T cells: subset distribution, inbred strain variation, and modulation by T cell activation. *Journal of Immunology, 163*, 6014–6022.

[616] Hornum, L., Romer, J. & Markholst, H. (2002). The diabetes-prone BB rat carries a frameshift mutation in Ian4, a positional candidate of Iddm1. *Diabetes, 51*, 1972–1979.

[617] MacMurray, A.J., Moralejo, D.H., Kwitek, A.E., Rutledge, E.A., Van Yserloo, B., Gohlke, P., Speros, S.J., Snyder, B., Schaefer, J., Bieg, S., Jiang, J., Ettinger, R.A., Fuller, J., Daniels, T.L., Pettersson, A., Orlebeke, K. Birren, B., Jacob, H.J., Lander, E.S. & Lernmark, A. (2002). Lymphopenia in the BB rat model of type 1 diabetes is due to a mutation in a novel immune-associated nucleotide (Ian)-related gene. *Genome Research, 12*, 1029–1039.

[618] Michalkiewicz, M., Michalkiewicz T., Ettinger, R.A., Rutledge, E.A., Fuller, J.M., Moralejo, D.H., Van Yserloo, B., MacMurray, A.J., Kwitek, A.E., Jacob, H.J., Lander,

E.S. & Lernmark, A. (2004) Transgenic rescue demonstrates involvement of the Ian5 gene in T cell development in the rat. *Physiological Genomics, 19*, 228–232.

[619] Sandal, T., Aumo, L., Hedin, L. Gjertsen, B.T. & Doskeland, S.O. (2003). Irod/Ian5: an inhibitor of gamma-radiation- and okadaic acid-induced apoptosis. *Molecular Biology of the Cell, 14*, 3292–3304.

[620] Daheron, L., Zenz, T. Sirakuza, L.D., Brenner, C. & Calabretta, B. (2001). Molecular cloning of Ian4: a BCR/ABL-induced gene that encodes an outer membrane mitochondrial protein with GTP-binding activity. *Nucleic Acids Research, 29*, 1308–1316.

[621] Andersen, U.N., Markholst, H. & Hornum, L. (2004). The antiapoptotic gene Ian4l1 in the rat: genomic organization and promoter characterization. *Gene, 341*, 141–148.

[622] Poussier, P., Ning, T., Murhy, T., Dabrowski, D. & Ramanathan, S. (2005). Impaired post-thymic development of regulatory $CD4^{+}25^{+}$ T cells contributes to diabetes pathogenesis in BB rats. *Journal of Immunology, 174*, 4081–4089.

[623] Like, A.A., Gubesrki, D.L. & Butler, L. (1986). Diabetic BioBreeding/Worcester (BB/Wor) rats need not be lymphopenic. *Journal of Immunology, 136*, 3254–3258.

[624] Martin, A.M., Blankenhorn, E.P., Maxson, M.N., Zhao, M., Leif, J., Mordes, J.P. & Greiner, D.L. (1999). Non-major histocompatibility complex-linked diabetes susceptibility loci on chromosomes 4 and 13 in a backcross of the DP-BB/Wor rat to the WF rat. *Diabetes, 48*, 50–58.

[625] Kloting, I. & Kovacs, P. (1998). Genes of the immune system cosgregate with the age at onset of diabetes in tge BB/OK rat. *Biochemical and Biophysical Research Communications, 242*, 461–463.

[626] Kloting, I. Van den Brande, J. & Kovacs, P. (1998). Quantitative trait loci for blood glucose confirm diabetes predisposing and protecive genes, IDDM4 and IDDM5, in the spontaneously diabetic BB/OK rat. *International Journal of Molecular Medicine, 2*, 597–601.

[627] Kloting, I., Schmidt, S. & Kovacs, P. (1998). Mapping of novel genes predisposing or protecting diabetes development in the BB/OK rat. *Biochemical and Biophysical Research Communications, 245*, 483–486.

[628] Kloting, I., Vogt, L. & Serikawa, T. (1995). Locus on chromosome 18 cosegregates with diabetes in the BB/OK rat subline. *Diabetes and Metabolism, 21*, 338–344.

[629] Prochazka, M., Leiter, E.H., Serreze, D.V. & Coleman, D.L. (1987). Three recessive loci required for insulin-dependent diabetes in NOD mice. *Science, 237*, 286–289.

[630] Payne, F., Smyth, D.J., Pask, R., Barratt, B.J., Cooper, J.D., Twells, R.C., Walker, N.M., Lam, A.C., Smink, L.J., Nutland, S., Rance, H.E. & Todd, J.A. (2004). Haplotype tag single nucleotide polymorphism analysis of the human orthologues of the rat type 1 diabetes genes Ian4 (Lyp/Iddm1) and Cblb. *Diabetes, 53*, 505–509.

[631] Yoon, J.W. & Jun, H.S. (1999). Cellular and molecular roles of beta cell autoantigens, macrophages and T cells in the pathogenesis of autoimmune diabetes. *Archives of Pharmacal Research, 22*, 437-447.

[632] Takaki, T., Marron, M.P., Mathews, C.E., Guttmann, S.T., Bottino, R., Trucco, M., DiLorenzo, T.P. & Serreze, D.V. (2006). HLA-A*0201-restricted T cells from

humanized NOD mice recognize autoantigens of potential clinical relevance to type 1 diabetes. *Journal of Immunology, 176*, 3257-3265.

[633] Davies, J.L., Kawaguchi, Y., Bennett, S.T., Copeman, J.B., Cordell, H.J., Pritchard, L.E., Reed, P.W., Gough, S.C., Jenkins, S.C. & Palmer, S.M. (1994) A genome-wide search for human type 1 diabetes susceptibility genes. *Nature, 371*, 130–136.

[634] Risch, N. (1987). Assessing the role of HLA-linked and unlinked determinants of disease, *American Journal of Human Genetics, 40*, 1–14.

[635] Cox, N.J., Wapelhorst, B., Morrison, V.A., Johnson, L., Pinchuk, L., Spielman, R.S., Todd, J.A. & Concannon, P. (2001). Seven regions of the genome show evidence of linkage to type 1 diabetes in a consensus analysis of 767 multiplex families, *American Journal of Human Genetics, 69*, 820–830.

[636] Concannon, P., Erlich, H.A., Julier, C., Morahan, G., Nerup, J., Pociot, F., Todd, J.A.& Rich, S.S.; Type 1 Diabetes Genetics Consortium. (2005). Type 1 diabetes: evidence for susceptibility loci from four genome-wide linkage scans in 1,435 multiplex families. *Diabetes, 54,* 2995-3001.

[637] Shiina, T., Inoko, H. & Kulski, J.K. (2004). An update of the HLA genomic region, locus information and disease associations: 2004. *Tissue Antigens, 64*, 631-639.

[638] Herr, M., Dudbridge, F., Zavattari, P., Cucca, F., Guja, C., March, R., Campbell, R.D., Barnett, A.H., Bain, S.C., Todd, J.A. & Koeleman, B.P. (2000). Evaluation of fine mapping strategies for a multifactorial disease locus: systematic linkage and association analysis of IDDM1 in the HLA region of chromosome 6p21. *Human Molecular Genetics 9*, 1291–1301.

[639] Koeleman, B.P., Herr, M.H., Zavattari, P., Dudbridge, F., March, R., Campbell, D., Barnett, A.H., Bain, S.C., Mulargia, A.P., Loddo, M., Amos, W., Cucca, F. & Todd, J.A. (2000). Conditional ETDT analysis of the human leukocyte antigen region in type 1 diabetes. *Annals of Human Genetics, 64*, 215-221.

[640] Ronningen, K.S., Keiding. N. & Green, A.; EURODIAB ACE Study Group. Europe and Diabetes. (2001). Correlations between the incidence of childhood-onset type I diabetes in Europe and HLA genotypes. *Diabetologia, 44 (Suppl.3)*, B51-B59.

[641] Thomson, G., Robinson, W.P., Kuhner, M.K., Joe, S., MacDonald, M.J., Gottschall, J.L., Barbosa, J., Rich S.S., Bertrams, J. & Baur, M.P. (1988). Genetic heterogeneity, modes of inheritance, and risk estimates for a joint study of Caucasians with insulin-dependent diabetes mellitus. *American Journal of Human Genetics, 43*, 799-816.

[642] Pugliese, A., Gianani, R., Moromisato, R., Awdeh Z.L., Alper, C.A., Erlich, H.A., Jackson, R.A. & Eisenbarth, G.S. (1995). HLA-DQB1*0602 is associated with dominant protection from diabetes even among islet cell antibody-positive first-degree relatives of patients with IDDM. *Diabetes, 44*, 608-613.

[643] Baisch, J.M., Weeks, T., Giles, R , Hoover, M., Stastny, P. & Capra, J.D. (1990). Analysis of HLA-DQ genotypes and susceptibility in insulin-dependent diabetes mellitus. *New England Journal of Medicine, 322*, 1836-1841.

[644] Nepom, G.T. (1990). A unified hypothesis for the complex genetics of HLA associations with IDDM. *Diabetes, 39*, 1153-1157.

[645] She, J.-X. (1996). Susceptibility to type 1 diabetes: HLA-DQ and DR revisited. *Immunology Today, 17*: 323-329.

[646] Sheehy, M.J., Scharf, S.J., Rowe, J.R., Neme de Gimenez, M.H., Meske, L.M., Erlich, H.A. & Nepom, B.S. (1989). A diabetes-susceptible HLA haplotype is best defined by a combination of HLA-DR and DQ alleles. *Journal of Clinical Investigations, 83*, 830-835.

[647] Caillat-Zucman, S., Garchon, H.J., Timsit, J., Assan, R., Boitard, C., Djilali-Saiah, I., Bougneres, P. & Bach, J.F. (1992). Age-dependent HLA genetic heterogeneity of type 1 insulin-dependent diabetes mellitus. *Journal Clinical Investigations, 90*, 2242-2250.

[648] Cucca, F., Lampis, R., Frau, F., Macis, D., Angius, E., Masile, P., Chessa, M., Frongia, P., Silvetti, M. & Cao, A. (1995). The distribution of DR4 haplotypes in Sardinia suggests a primary association of type 1 diabetes with DRB1 and DQB1 loci. *Human Immunology, 43*, 301-308.

[649] Undlien, D.E., Friede, T., Rammensee, H.G., Joner, G., Dahl-Jorgensen, K., Sovik, O., Akselsen, H.E., Knutsen, I., Ronningen, K.S. & Thorsby, E. (1997). HLA-encoded genetic predisposition in IDDM: DR4 subtypes may be associated with different degrees of protection. *Diabetes, 46*, 143-149.

[650] Cucca, F., Lampis, R., Congia, M., Angius, E., Nutland, S., Bain, S.C., Barnett, A.H. & Todd, J.A. (2001). A correlation between the relative predisposition of MHC class II alleles to type 1 diabetes and the structure of their proteins. *Human Molecular Genetics, 10*, 2025-2037.

[651] Chao, C.C., Sytwu, H.K., Chen, E.L., Toma, J. & McDevitt, H.O. (1999). The role of MHC class II molecules in susceptibility to type 1 diabetes: identification of peptide epitopes and characterization of the T cell repertoire. *Proceedings of the National Academy of Sciences of USA, 96*, 9299-9304.

[652] Latek, R.R., Suri, A,, Petzold, S.J., Nelson, C.A., Kanagawa, O., Unanue, E.R. & Fremont, D.H. (2000). Structural basis of peptide binding and presentation by the type I diabetes-associated MHC class II molecule of NOD mice. *Immunity, 12*, 699-710.

[653] Stratmann, T., Apostolopoulos, V., Mallet-Designe, V., Corper, A.L., Scott, C.A., Wilson, I.A., Kang, A.S. & Teyton, L. (2000). The I-A^{g7} MHC class II molecule linked to murine diabetes is a promiscuous peptide binder. *Journal of Immunology, 165*, 3214-3225.

[654] Lee, K.H., Wucherpfennig, K.W. & Wiley, D.C. (2001). Structure of a human insulin peptide-HLA-DQ8 complex and susceptibility to type 1 diabetes. *Nature Immunology, 2*, 501-507.

[655] McDevitt, H.O. (2001). Closing in on type 1 diabetes. *New England Journal of Medicine, 345*, 1060-1061.

[656] Kwok, W.W., Domeier, M.E., Johnson, M.L., Nepom, G.T. & Koelle, D.M. (1996). HLA-DQB1 codon 57 is critical for peptide binding and recognition. *Journal of Experimental Medicine, 183*, 1253-1258.

[657] Corper, A.L., Stratmann, T., Apostolopoulos, V., Scott, C.A., Garcia, K.C., Kang, A.S., Wilson, I.A., Teyton, L. (2000). A structural framework for deciphering the link between I-A^{g7} and autoimmune diabetes. *Science, 288*, 505-511.

[658] Awata, T., Kuzuya, T., Matsuda, A., Iwamoto, Y., Kanazawa, Y., Okuyama, M., Juji, T. (1990). High frequency of aspartic acid at position 57 of HLA-DQ beta-chain in Japanese IDDM patients and nondiabetic subjects. *Diabetes, 39*, 266-269.

[659] Yamagata, K., Hanafusa, T., Nakajima, H., Sada, M., Amemiya, H., Noguchi, T., Tanaka, T., Kono, N., Tarui, S. (1991). HLA-DQA1*1 contributes to resistance and A1*3 confers susceptibility to type 1 (insulin-dependent) diabetes mellitus in Japanese subjects. *Diabetologia, 34*, 133-136.

[660] Noble, J.A., Valdes, A.M., Thomson, G. & Erlich, H.A. (2000). The HLA class II locus DPB1 can influence susceptibility to type 1 diabetes. *Diabetes, 49*, 121–125.

[661] Erlich, H.A., Rotter, J.I., Chang, J.D., Shaw, S.J., Raffel, L.J., Klitz, W., Bugawan, T.L. & Zeidler, A. (1996). Association of HLA-DPB1*0301 with IDDM in Mexican-Americans. *Diabetes* 1996; 45, 610-614.

[662] Valdes, A.M., Noble, J.A., Genin, E., Clerget-Darpoux, F., Erlich, H.A. & Thomson, G. (2001) Modeling of HLA class II susceptibility to type I diabetes reveals an effect associated with DPB1. *Genetic Epidemiology, 21*, 212-223.

[663] Johansson, S., Lie, B.A., Pociot, F., Nerup, J., Cambon-Thomsen, A., Kockum, I., Thorsby, E. & Undlien, D.E. (2003). HLA associations in type 1 diabetes: DPB1 alleles may act as markers of other HLA-complex susceptibility genes. *Tissue Antigens, 61*, 344-351.

[664] Cucca, F., Dudbridge, F., Loddo, M., Mulargia, A.P., Lampis, R., Angius, E., De Virgiliis, S., Koeleman, B.P., Bain, S.C., Barnett, A.H., Gilchrist, F., Cordell, H., Welsh, K. & Todd, J.A. (2001). The HLA-DPB1-associated component of the IDDM1 and its relationship to the major loci HLA-DQB1, -DQA1, and -DRB1. *Diabetes, 50*, 1200-1205.

[665] Van Endert, P.M., Liblau, R., Patel, S.D., Fugger, L. Lopez, T., Pociot, F., Nerup, J., McDevitt, H.O. (1994). Major histocompatibility complex-encoded antigen processing gene polymorphism in IDDM. *Diabetes, 43*, 110-117.

[666] Caillat-Zucman, S., Daniel, S., Djilali-Saiah, I., Timsit, J., Garchon, H.J., Boitard, C. & Bach, JF. (1995). Family study of linkage disequilibrium between TAP2 transporter and HLA class II genes. Absence of TAP2 contribution to association with insulin-dependent diabetes mellitus. *Human Immunology, 44*, 80-87.

[667] Undlien, D.E., Akselsen, H.E., Joner, G., Dahl-Jorgensen, K., Sovik, O., Ronningen, K.S. & Thorsby, E. (1997). No independent associations of LMP2 and LMP7 polymorphisms with susceptibility to develop IDDM. *Diabetes* 1997; 46, 307-312.

[668] Thomsen, M., Molvig, J., Zerbib, A., de Preval, C., Abbal, M., Dugoujon, J.M., Ohayon, E., Svejgaard, A., Cambon-Thomsen, A. & Nerup, J. (1988). The susceptibility to insulin-dependent diabetes mellitus is associated with C4 allotypes independently of the association with HLA-DQ alleles in HLA-DR3, 4 heterozygotes. *Immunogenetics, 28*, 320-327.

[669] Pociot, F., Molvig, J., Wogensen, L., de Preval, C., Abbal, M., Dugoujon, J.M., Ohayon, E., Svejgaard, A., Cambon-Thomsen, A. & Nerup, J. (1991). A tumour necrosis factor beta gene polymorphism in relation to monokine secretion and insulin-dependent diabetes mellitus. Journal of Scandinavian *Immunology, 33*, 37-49.

[670] Robinson, W.P., Barbosa, J., Rich, S.S. & Thomson G. (1993) Homozygous parent affected sib pair method for detecting disease predisposing variants-application to insulin-dependent diabetes-mellitus. *Genetic Epidemiology, 10*, 273-288.

[671] Pociot, F., Briant, L., Jongeneel, C.V., Molvig, J., Worsaae, H., Abbal, M., Thomsen, M., Nerup, J. & Cambon-Thomsen, A. (1993). Association of tumor necrosis factor (TNF) and class II MHC alleles with the secretion of TNFa and TNFb by human mononuclear cells: a possible link to insulin-dependent diabetes mellitus. *European Journal of Immunology, 23*, 224-231.

[672] Bidwell, J., Keen, L., Gallagher, G., Kimberly, R., Huizinga, T., McDermott, M.F., Oksenberg, J., McNicholl, J., Pociot, F., Hardt, C. & D'Alfonso, S. (1999) Cytokine gene polymorphism in human disease: on-line databases. *Genes and Immunity, 1*, 3-19.

[673] Bidwell, J., Keen, L., Gallagher, G., Kimberly, R., Huizinga, T., McDermott, M.F., Oksenberg, J., McNicholl, J., Pociot, F., Hardt, C. & D'Alfonso, S. (2001) Cytokine gene polymorphism in human disease: on-line databases, supplement 1. *Genes and Immunity, 2*, 61-70.

[674] Nejentsev, S., Reijonen, H., Adojaan, B., Kovalchuk, L., Sochnevs, A., Schwartz, E.I., Akerblom, H.K. & Ilonen, J. (1997). The effects of HLA-B allele on the IDDM risk defined by DRB1*04 subtypes and DQB1*0302. *Diabetes, 46*, 1888–1892.

[675] Moghaddam, P.H., Zwinderman, A.H., de Knijff, P., Roep, B.O., Schipper, R.F., Van der Auwera, B., Naipal, A., Gorus, F., Schuit, F., Giphart, M.J. (1997). TNFa microsatellite polymorphism modulates the risk of IDDM in Caucasians with the high-risk genotype HLA DQA1*0501- DQB1*0201 DQA1*0301- DQB1*0302. Belgian Diabetes Registry. *Diabetes, 46*, 1514-1515.

[676] Lie, B.A., Todd, J.A., Pociot, F., Nerup, J., Akselsen, H.E., Joner, G., Dahl-Jorgensen, K., Ronningen, K.S., Thorsby, E. & Undlien, D.E. (1999). The predisposition to type 1 diabetes linked to the human leukocyte antigen complex includes at least one non-class II gene. *American Journal of Human Genetics, 64*, 793-800.

[677] Nejentsev, S., Gombos, Z., Laine, A.P., Veijola, R., Knip, M., Simell, O., Vaarala, O., Akerblom, H.K. & Ilonen, J. (2000) Non-class II HLA gene associated with type 1 diabetes maps to the 240-kb region near HLA-B. *Diabetes, 49*, 2217-2221.

[678] Herr, M., Dudbridge, F., Zavattari, P., Cucca, F., Guja, C., March, R., Campbell, R.D., Barnett, A.H., Bain, S.C., Todd, J.A. & Koeleman, B.P. (2000). Evaluation of fine mapping strategies for a multifactorial disease locus: systematic linkage and association analysis of IDDM1 in the HLA region on chromosome 6p21. *Human Molecular Genetics, 9*, 1291-1301.

[679] Cordell, H.J. & Clayton, D.G. (2002). A unified stepwise regression procedure for evaluating the relative effects of polymorphisms within a gene using casecontrol or family data: application to HLA in type 1 diabetes. *American Journal of Human Genetics, 70*, 124-141.

[680] Zavattari, P., Lampis, R., Motzo, C., Loddo, M., Mulargia, A., Whalen, M., Maioli, M., Angius, E., Todd, J.A. & Cucca, F. (2001). Conditional linkage disequilibrium analysis of a complex disease superlocus, IDDM1 in the HLA region, reveals the presence of independent modifying gene effects influencing the type 1 diabetes risk encoded by the major HLA-DQB1, -DRB1 disease loci. *Human Molecular Genetics* 2001; 10, 881-889.

[681] Wong, F.S. & Wen, L. (2003). The study of HLA class II and autoimmune diabetes. *Current Molecular Biology, 3*, 1-15.

[682] Cosgrove, D., Gray, D., Dierich, A., Kaufman, J., Lemeur, M., Benoist, C. & Mathis, D. (1991). Mice lacking MHC class II molecules. *Cell, 66*, 1051-1066.

[683] Wen, L., Wong, F.S., Burkly, L., Altieri, M., Mamalaki, C., Kioussis, D., Flavell, R.A. & Sherwin, R.S. (1998). Induction of insulitis by glutamic acid decarboxylase peptide-specific and HLA-DQ8-restricted CD4(+) T cells from human DQ transgenic mice. *Journal of Clinical Investigations, 102*, 947-957.

[684] Abraham, R.S., Kudva, Y.C., Wilson, S.B., Strominger, J.L & David, C.S. (2000). Co-expression of HLA DR3 and DQ8 results in the development of spontaneous insulitis and loss of tolerance to GAD65 in transgenic mice. *Diabetes, 49*, 548-554.

[685] Liu, J., Purdy, L.E., Rabinovitch, S., Jevnikar, A.M. & Elliott, J.F. (1999). Major DQ8-restricted T-cell epitopes for human GAD65 mapped using human CD4, DQA1*0301, DQB1*0302 transgenic IA(null) NOD mice. *Diabetes, 48*, 469-477.

[686] Patel, S.D., Cope, A.P., Congia, M., Chen, T.T., Kim, E., Fugger, L., Wherrett, D., Sonderstrup-McDevitt, G. (1997). Identification of immunodominant T cell epitopes of human glutamic acid decarboxylase 65 by using HLA-DR (alpha1*0101, beta1*0401) transgenic mice. *Proceedings of the National Academy of Sciences of USA, 94*, 8082-8087.

[687] Boyton, R.J., Lohmann, T., Londei, M., Kalbacher H, Halder T, Frater AJ, Douek DC, Leslie DG, Flavell RA, Altmann DM. (1998). Glutamic acid decarboxylase T lymphocyte responses associated with susceptibility or resistance to type I diabetes: analysis in disease discordant human twins, non-obese diabetic mice and HLA-DQ transgenic mice. *International Immunology, 10*, 1765-1776.

[688] Herman, A.E., Tisch, R.M., Patel, S.D., Parry, S.L., Olson, J., Noble, J.A., Cope, A.P., Cox, B., Congia, M., McDevitt, H,O. (1999). Determination of glutamic acid decarboxylase 65 peptides presented by the type I diabetes-associated HLA-DQ8 class II molecule identifies an immunogenic peptide motif. *Journal of Immunology, 163*, 6275-6282.

[689] Geluk, A., van Meijgaarden, K.E., Schloot, N.C., Drijfhout, J.W., Ottenhoff, T.H. & Roep, B.O. (1998). HLA-DR binding analysis of peptides from islet antigens in IDDM. *Diabetes, 47*, 1594-1601.

[690] Abraham, R.S., Wen, L., Marietta, E.V. & David S.S. (2001). Type 1 diabetes-predisposing MHC alleles influence the selection of glutamic acid decarboxylase (GAD) 65-specific T cells in a transgenic model. *Journal of Immunology, 166*, 1370-1379.

[691] Raju, R., Munn, S.R. & David, C.S. (1997). T cell recognition of human pre-proinsulin peptides depends on the polymorphism at HLA DQ locus: a study using HLA DQ8 and DQ6 transgenic mice. *Human Immunology, 58*, 21-29.

[692] Congia, M., patel, S., Cope, A.P., De Virgiliis, S., Sonderstup, G. (1998). T cell epitopes of insulin defined in HLA-DR4 transgenic mice are derived from preproinsulin and proinsulin. *Proceedings of the National Academy of Sciences of USA, 95*, 3833-3838.

[693] Kudva, Y.C., Deng, Y.J., Govindarajan, R., Abraham, R.S., Marietta, E.V., Notkins, A.L., David, C.S. (2001). HLA-DQ8 transgenic and NOD mice recognize different epitopes within the cytoplasmic region of the tyrosine phosphatase-like molecule, IA-2. *Human Immunology, 62*, 1099-1105.

[694] Hugues, S., Mougneau, E., Ferlin, W., Jeske, D., Hofman, P., Homann, D., Beaudoin, L., Schrike, C., Von Herrath, M., Lehuen, A. & Glaichenhaus, N. (2002). Tolerance to islet antigens and prevention from diabetes induced by limited apoptosis of pancreatic beta cells. *Immunity, 16*, 169-181.

[695] Guarder, S., Picarella, D.E., Linsley, P.S. & Flavell, R.A. (1994). Costimulator B7-1 confers antigen-presenting-cell function to parenchymal tissue and in conjuction with tumor necrosis alpha leads to autoimmunity in transgenic mice. *Proccedings of the National Academy of USA. 91*, 5138-5142.

[696] Wen, L., Wong, F.S., Tang, J., Chen, N.Y., Altieri, M., David, C., Flavell, R. & Sherwin, R. (2000). In vivo evidence for the contribution of human histocompatibility leukocyte antigen (HLA)-DQ molecules to the development of diabetes. *Journal of Experimental Medicine, 191*, 97-104.

[697] Wen, L., Chen, N.Y., Tnag, J., Sherwin, R., Wong, F.S. (2001). The regulatory role of DR4 in a spontaneous diabetes DQ8 transgenic mice. *Journal of Clinical Investigations, 107*, 871-880.

[698] Lipes, M. (2002). Differential progression to diabetes in human DQ8 transgenic mice. *Diabetes Metabolism Research and Reviews, 18*, S2.

[699] Stewart, T.A., Hultgern, B., Huang, X., Pitts-Meek, S., Hully, J. & MacLachlan, N.J. (1993). Induction of type 1 diabetes by interferon-alpha in transgenic mice. *Science, 260*, 1942-1946.

[700] Nepom, B.S., Schwarz, D., Palmer, J.P. & Nepom, G.T. (1987). Transcomplementation of HLA genes in IDDM. HLA-DQ alpha- and beta-chains produce hybrid molecules in DR3/4 heterozygotes. *Diabetes, 36*, 114-117.

[701] Kudva, Y.C., Rajagopalan, G., Raju, R., Abraham, R.S., Smart, M., Hanson, J. & David, C.S. (2002). Modulation of insulitis and type 1 diabetes by transgenic HLA-DR3 and DQ8 in NOD mice lacking endogenous MHC class II. *Human Immunology, 63,* 987-999.

[702] Sheehy, M.J. (1992). HLA and insulin-dependent diabetes. A protective perspective. *Diabetes, 41*, 123-129.

[703] Undlien, D.E., Friede, T., Rammensee, H.G., Joner, G., Dahl-Jorgensen, K., Sovik, O., Akselsen, H.E., Knutsen, I., Ronningen, K.S. & Thorsby, E. (1997). HLA-encoded genetic predisposition in IDDM: DR4 subtypes may be associated with different degrees of protection. *Diabetes, 46*, 143-149.

[704] Fennessy, M., Metcalfe, K., Hitman, G.A., Niven, M., Biro, P.A., Tuomilehto, J. & Tuomilehto-Wolf E. (1994). A gene in the HLA class I region contributes to susceptibility to IDDM in the Finnish population. Childhood Diabetes in Finland (DiMe) Study Group. *Diabetologia, 37*, 937-944.

[705] Noble, J.A., Valdes, A.M., Bugawan, T.L., Apple, R.J., Thomson, G. & Erlich, H.A. (2002). The HLA class I A locus affects susceptibility to type 1 diabetes. *Human Immunology, 63*, 657-664.

[706] Breban, M., Hacquard-Bouder, C. & Falgarone, G (2004). Animal models of HLA-B27-associated diseases. *Current Molecular Medicine, 4*, 31-40.

[707] Marron, M.P., Graser, R.T., Chapman, H.D. & Serreze, D.V. (2002). Functional evidence for the mediation of diabetogenic T cell responces by HLA-A2.1 MHC class I molecules through transgenic expression in NOD mice. *Proceedings of the National Academy of Sciences of USA, 99*, 13753-13758.

[708] Hassainya, Y., Garcia-Pons, F., Kratzer, R., Lindo, V., Greer, F., Lemonnier, F.A., Niedermann, G. & van Endert, P.M. (2005). Identification of naturally processed HLA-A2--restricted proinsulin epitopes by reverse immunology. *Diabetes, 54*, 2053-2059.

[709] Brown, J.H., Jardetzky, T., Saper, M.A., Samraoui, B., Bjorkman, P.J. & Wiley, D.C. (1988). A hypothetical model of the foreign antigen binding site of class II histocompatibility molecules. *Nature, 332*, 845–850.

[710] Ettinger, R.A. & Kwok, W.W. (1998). A peptide binding motif for HLA-DQA1*0102/DQB1*0602, the class II MHC molecule associated with dominant protection in insulin-dependent diabetes mellitus. *Journal of Immunology, 160*, 2365–2373.

[711] Kwok, W.W., Domeier, M.E., Raymond, F.C., Byers, P. & Nepom, G.T. (1996). Allele-specific motifs characterize HLA-DQ interactions with a diabetes-associated peptide derived from glutamic acid decarboxylase. *Journal of Immunology, 156*, 2171–2177.

[712] Vartdal, F., Johansen, B.H., Friede, T., Thorpe, C.J., Stevanovic, S., Eriksen, J.E., Sletten, K., Thorsby, E., Rammensee, H.G. & Sollid, L.M. (1996). The peptide binding motif of the disease associated HLA-DQ (alpha 1*0501, beta 1*0201) molecule. *European Journal of Immunology, 26*, 2764–2772.

[713] Dessen, A., Lawrence, C.M., Cupo, S., Zaller, D.M. & Wiley, D.C. (1997). X-ray crystal structure of HLA-DR4 (DRA*0101, DRB1*0401) complexed with a peptide from human collagen II. *Immunity, 7*, 473-481.

[714] Todd, J.A., Bell, J.I. & McDevitt, H.O. (1987). HLA-DQ beta gene contributes to susceptibility and resistance to insulin-dependent diabetes mellitus. *Nature, 329*, 599-604.

[715] Nepom, G.T. & Erlich, H. (1991). MHC class-II molecules and autoimmunity. *Annual Reviews in Immunology*, *9*, 493-525.

[716] Awata, T., Kuzuya, T., Matsuda A., Iwamoto, Y., Kanazawa, Y., Okuyama, M. & Juji, T. (1990). High frequency of aspartic acid at position 57 of HLA-DQ beta-chain in Japanese IDDM patients and nondiabetic subjects. *Diabetes, 39*, 266-269.

[717] Brown, J.H., Jardetzky, T.S., Gorga, J.C., Stern, L.J., Urban, R.G., Strominger, J.L. & Wiley, D.C. (1993). Three-dimensional structure of the human class II histocompatibility antigen HLA-DR1. *Nature, 364*, 33-39.

[718] Stern, L.J., Brown, J.H., Jardetzky, T.S., Gorga, J.C., Urban, R.G., Strominger, J.L. & Wiley, D.C. (1994). Crystal structure of the human class II MHC protein HLA-DR1 complexed with an influenza virus peptide. *Nature, 368*, 215-221.

[719] Reizis, B., Eisenstein, M., Bockova, J., Konen-Waisman, S., Mor, F., Elias, D. & Cohen, I.R. (1997). Molecular characterization of the diabetes-associated mouse MHC class II protein, I-Ag7. *International Immunology, 9*, 43-51.

[720] Kwok, W.W., Domeier, M.E., Johnson, M.L., Nepom, G.T. & Koelle, D.M. (1996). HLA-DQB1 codon 57 is critical for peptide binding and recognition. *Journal of Experimental Medicine, 183*, 1253-1258.

[721] Kinouchi, R., Kobayasi, H., Sato, K., Kimura, S. & Katagiri, M. (1994). Peptide motifs of HLA-DR4/DR53 (DRB1*0405/DRB4*0101) molecules. *Immunogenetics, 40*, 376-378.

[722] Quarsten, H., Paulsen, G., Johansen, B.H., Thorpe, C.J., Holm, A., Buus, S. & Sollid, L.M. (1998). The P9 pocket of HLA-DQ2 (non-Aspbeta57) has no particular preference for negatively charged anchor residues found in other type 1 diabetes-predisposing non-Aspbeta57 MHC class II molecules. *International Immunology, 10*, 1229-1236.

[723] Nepom, B.S., Nepom, G.T., Coleman, M. & Kwok, W.W. (1996). Critical contribution of beta chain residue 57 in peptide binding ability of both HLA-DR and -DQ molecules. *Proceedings of the National Academy of Sciences of USA, 93*, 7202-7206.

[724] Sato, A.K., Sturniolo, T., Sinigaglia, F. & Stern, L.J. (1999). Substitution of aspartic acid at beta57 with alanine alters MHC class II peptide binding activity but not protein stability: HLA-DQ (alpha1*0201, beta1*0302) and (alpha1*0201, beta1*0303). *Human Immunology, 60*, 1227-1236.

[725] Garboczi, D.N., Ghosh, P., Utz, U., Fan, Q.R., Biddison, W.E. & Wiley, D.C. (1996). Structure of the complex between human T-cell receptor, viral peptide and HLA-A2. *Nature, 384*, 34-41.

[726] Hennecke, J., Carfi, A. & Wiley, D.C. (2000). Structure of a covalently stabilized complex of human alphabeta T-cell receptor, influenza HA peptide and MHC class II molecule, HLA-DR1. *EMBO Journal, 19*, 5611-5624.

[727] Signorelli, K.L., Watts, L.M. & Lambert, L.E. (1995). The importance of DR4Dw4 beta chain residues 70, 71 and 86 in peptide binding and T cell recognition. *Cellular Immunology, 162*, 217-224.

[728] Coppin, H.L., Carmichael, P., Lombardi, G., L'Faqihi, F.E., Salter, R., Parham, P., Lechler, R.I. & de Preval, C. (1993). Position 71 in the alpha helix of the DR beta domain is predicted to influence peptide binding and plays a central role in allorecognition. *European Journal of Immunology, 23*, 343-349.

[729] Reichstetter, S., Papadopoulos, G.K., Moustakas, A.K., Swanson, E., Liu, A.W., Beheray, S., Ettinger, R.A., Nepom, G.T. & Kwok, W.W. (2002). Mutational analysis of critical residues determining antigen presentation and activation of HLA-DQ0602 restricted T-cell clones. *Human Immunology, 63*, 185-193.

[730] De Oliveira, D.B., Harfouch-Hammoud, E., Otto, H., Papandreou, N.A., Stern, L.J., Cohen, H., Boehm, B.O., Bach, J., Caillat-Zucman, S., Walk ,T., Jung, G., Eliopoulos, E., Papadopoulos, G.K. & van Endert, P.M. (2001). Structural analysis of two HLA-DR-presented autoantigenic epitopes: crucial role of peripheral but not central peptide residues for T-cell receptor recognition. *Molecular Immunology, 37*, 813-825.

[731] Nepom, G.T., Lippolis, J.D., White, F.M., Masewicz, S., Marto, J.A., Herman, A., Luckey, C.J., Falk, B., Shabanowitz, J., Hunt, D.F., Engelhard, V.H. & Nepom, B.S. (2001). Identification and modulation of a naturally processed T cell epitope from the diabetes-associated autoantigen human glutamic acid decarboxylase 65 (hGAD65). *Proccedings of the National Academy of Sciences of USA, 98*, 1763-1768.

[732] Ettinger, R.A., Liu, A.W., Nepom, G.T. & Kwok, W.W. (1998). Exceptional stability of the HLA-DQA1*0102/DQB1*0602 alpha beta protein dimer, the class II MHC molecule associated with protection from insulin-dependent diabetes mellitus. *Journal of Immunology, 161*, 439-445.

[733] Rayner, M.L., Mijovic, C.H. & Barnett, G.T. (2002). Aspartate at residue β57 is important for the stability and antigen-binding ability of the DQ6.2 molecule. *Diabetic Medicine, 19*, P154.

[734] Ettinger, R.A., Liu, A.W., Nepom, G.T. & Kwok, W.W. (2000). Beta 57-Asp plays an essential role in the unique SDS stability of HLA-DQA1*0102/DQB1*0602 alpha beta protein dimer, the class II MHC allele associated with protection from insulin-dependent diabetes mellitus. *Journal of Immunology 165*, 3232-3238.

[735] Nepom, G.T. & Kwok, W.W. (1998). Molecular basis for HLA-DQ associations with IDDM. *Diabetes, 47*, 1177-1184.

[736] Schmidt, D., Verdaguer, J., Averill, N. & Santamaria, P. (1997). A mechanism for the major histocompatibility complex-linked resistance to autoimmunity. *Journal of Experimental Medicine, 186*, 1059-1075.

[737] Luhder, F., Katz, J., Benoist, C. & Mathis, D. (1998). Major histocompatibility complex class II molecules can protect from diabetes by positively selecting T cells with additional specificities. *Journal of Experimental Medicine, 187*, 379-387.

[738] Lucassen, A.M., Julier, C., Beressi, J.-P., Boitard, C., Froguel, P., Lathrop, M. & Bell, J.I. (1993). Susceptibility to insulin dependent diabetes mellitus maps to a 4.1 kb segment of DNA spanning the insulin gene and associated VNTR. *Nature Genetics, 4*, 305-310.

[739] Bell, G.I., Selby, M.I. & Rutter, M.J. (1982). The highly polymorphic region near the human insulin gene is composed of simple tandemly repeated sequences. *Nature, 295*, 31-35.

[740] Rotwein, P., Yokoyama, S., Didier, D.K. & Chrigwin, J.M. (1986). Genetic analysis of the hypervariable region flanking of the insulin gene in diabetes mellitus. *Diabetes, 31*, 275-277.

[741] Bell, G.I., Horita, S. & Karam, J.H. (1984). A polymprhic locus near the human insulin gene is associated with insulin-dependent diabetes mellitus. *Diabetes, 33*, 1504-1509.

[742] Julier, C., Hyer, R.N., Davies, J., Merlin, F., Soularue, P., Briant, L., Cathelineau, G., Deschamps, I., Rotter, J.I. & Froguel, P. (1991). Insulin-IGF2 region on chromosome 11p encodes a gene implicated in HLA-DR4-dependent diabetes susceptibility. *Nature, 354*, 144-159.

[743] Owerbach, D. & Gabbay, K.H. (1993). Localization of type I diabetes susceptibility locus to the variable tndem repeat region flanking the insulin gene. *Diabetes, 42*, 1708-1714.

[744] Julier, C., Lucassen, A., Velledieu, P., Delepine, M., Levy-Marchal, C., Danze, P.M., Bianchi, F., Boitard, C., Froguel, P. & Bell, J. (1994). Multiple DNA variant association analysis: application to the insulin gene region in type 1 diabetes. *American Journal of Human Genetics, 55*, 1247-1254.

[745] Undlien, D.E., Bennett, S.T., Todd, J.A., Akselsen, H.E., Ikaheimo, I., Rejionen, H. , Knip, M., Thorsby, E., & Ronningen, K.S. (1995). Insulin gene region-encoded susceptibility to IDDM maps upstream of the insulin gene. *Diabetes, 44*, 620-625.

[746] Bennett, S.T., Wilson, A.J., Cucca, F., Nerup, J., Pociot, F., McKinney, P.A., Barnett, A.H., Bain, S.C. & Todd, J.A. (1996). IDDM2-VNTR-encoded susceptibility to type 1 diabetes: dominant protection and parental transmission of alleles of the insulin gene-linked minisatellite locus. *Journal of Autoimmunity, 9*, 415-421.

[747] Bennett, S.T., Wilson, A.J., Esposito, L., Bouzekri, N., Undlien, D.E., Cucca, F., Nistico, L., Buzzetti, R., Bosi, E., Pociot, F., Nerup, J., Cambon-Thomsen, A., Pugliese, A., Shield. J.P., McKinney, P.A., Bain, S.C., Polychronakos, C. & Todd, J.A. (1997). Insulin VNTR allele-specific effect in type 1 diabetes depends on identity of untransmitted paternal allele. The IMDIAB Group. *Nature Genetics, 17*, 350-352.

[748] Stead, J.D., Buard, J., Todd, J.A & Jeffreys, A.J. (2000). Influence of allele lineage on the role of the insulin minisatellite in susceptibility to type 1 diabetes. *Human Molecular Genetics, 9*, 2929-2935.

[749] Vafiadis, P., Ounissi-Benkalha, H., Palumbo, M., Grabs, R., Rousseau, M., Goodyer, C.G. & Polychronakos, C. (2001). Class III alleles of the variable number of tandem repeat insulin polymorphism associated with silencing of thymic insulin predispose to type 1 diabetes. *Journal of Clinical Endocrinology and Metabolism, 86*, 3705-3710.

[750] Stead, D.H., Hurles, M.E. & Jeffreys, A.J. (2003). Global haplotype diversity in the human insulin gene region. *Genome Research, 13*, 2101-2111.

[751] Aly, T.A., Ide, A., Humphrey, K., Barker, J.M., Steck, A., Erlich, H.A., Yu, L., Miao, D., Redondo, M.J., McFann, K., Roberts, C.M., Babu, S.R., Norris, J.M., Eisenbarth, G.S. & Rewers, M.J. (2005). Genetic prediction of autoimmunity: initial oligogenic prediction of anti-islet autoimmunity amongst DR3/DR4-DQ8 relatives of patients with type 1A diabetes. *Journal of Autoimmunity, 25*, 40-45.

[752] Hearne, C.M., Ghosh, S. & Todd, J.A. (1992). Microsatellites for linkage analysis of genetic traits. *Trends in Genetics, 8*, 288-294.

[753] Bennett, S.T., Lucassen, A.M., Gough, S.C., Powell, E.E., Undlien, D.E., Pritchard, L.E., Merriman, M.E., Kawaguchi, Y., Dronsfield, M.J. & Pociot, F. (1995). Susceptibility to human type 1 diabetes at IDDM2 is determined by tandem repeat variation at the insulin gene minisatellite locus. *Nature Genetics, 9*, 284-292.

[754] Awata, T., Kurihara, S., Kikuchi, C., Takei, S., Inoue, I., Ishii, C., Takanashi, K., Negishi, K., Yoshida, Y., Hagura, R., Kanazawa, Y. & Katayama, S. (1997). Evidence for association between the class I subset of the insulin gene minisatellite (IDDM2 locus) and IDDM in the Japanese population. *Diabetes, 46*, 1637-1642.

[755] Berka, N., Nunlee-Bland, G., Erabhaoui, E., Belmamoun, M. & Dunston, G.M. (2004). IDDM2 and the polymorphism of the human tyrosine hydroxylase gene (hTH) gene in African Americans with type-1 diabetes. *Journal of the National Medical Association, 96*, 1042-1046.

[756] Vafiadis, P., Bennett, S.T., Colle, E., Grabs, R., Goodyer, C.G. & Polychronakos, C. (1996). Imprinted- and genotype-specific expression of genes in the IDDM2 locus in pancreas and leucocytes. *Journal of Autoimmunity, 9*, 937-403.

[757] Owerbach, D., Poulsen, S., Billesbolle, P. & Nerup, J. (1982). DNA insertion sequences near the imnsulin gene affect glucose regulation. *Lancet, i*, 880-883.

[758] Permutt, M.A., Rotwein, P., Andreone, T., Ward, W.K. & Porte, D., Jr. (1985). Islet beta-cell function and polymorphism in the 5'-flanking region of the human insulin gene. *Diabetes, 34*,311-314.

[759] Cocozza, S., Riccardi, G., Monticelli, A., Capaldo, B., Genovese, S., Krogh, V., Celentano, E., Farinaro, E., Varrone, S. & Avvedimento, V.E. (1988). Polymorphism at the 5'end flanking region of the insulin gene is associated with reduced insulin secretion in healthy individuals. *European Journal of Clinical Investigations, 18*, 582-586.

[760] Weaver, J.U., Kopelman, P.G & Hitman, G.A. (1992). Central obesity and hyperinsulinaemia in women is associated with polymorphism in the 5'flanking region of the human insulin gene. *European Journal of Clinical Investigations, 22*, 265-270.

[761] Lucassen, A.M., Screaton, G.R., Julier, C., Elliott T.J., Lathrop, M. & Bell, J.I. (1995). Regulation of insulin gene expression by the IDDM-associated insulin locus haplotype. *Human Molecular Genetics, 4*, 501-506.

[762] Lew, A., Rutter, W.J. & Kennedy, G.C. (2000). Unusual DNA structure of the diabetes susceptibility locus IDDM2 and its effect on transcription levels correlated with allelic variation at the INS VNTR-IDDM2 susceptibility locus for type 1 diabetes. *Nature Genetics, 15*, 293-297.

[763] Vafiadis, P., Bennett, S.T., Todd, J.A., Nadeau J., Grabs, R., Goodyer, C.G., Wickramasinghe, S., Colle, E. & Polychronakos, C. (1997). Insulin expression in human thymus is modulated by INS VNTR alleles at the IDDM2 locus. *Nature Genetics, 15*, 289-292.

[764] Pugliese, A., Zeller, M., Fernandez, A., Jr, Zalcberg, L.J., Bartlett, R.J., Ricordi, C., Pietropaolo, M., Eisenbarth, G.S., Bennett, S.T. & Patel, D.D. (1997). The insulin gene is transcribed in the human thymus and transcription levels correlated with allelic variation at the INS VNTR-IDDM2 susceptibility locus for type 1 diabetes. *Nature Genetics, 15*, 293-297.

[765] Chentoufi, A.A. & Polychronakos, C. (2002). Insulin expression levels in the thymus modulate insulin-specific autoreactive T-cell tolerance. The mechanism by which the IDDM2 locus may predispose to diabetes. *Diabetes, 51*, 1383-1390.

[766] Durinovic-Bello I, Jelinek E, Schlosser M, Eiermann T, Boehm BO, Karges W, Marchand L, Polychronakos C. (2005). Class III alleles at the insulin VNTR polymorphism are associated with regulatory T-cell responses to proinsulin epitopes in HLA-DR4, DQ8 individuals. *Diabetes, 54 (Suppl.2)*, S18-S24.

[767] Vafiadis, P., Grabs, Goodyer, C.G., Colle, E. & Polychronakos, C. (1998). A functional analysis of the role of IGF2 in IDDM2-encoded susceptibility in type 1 diabetes. *Diabetes, 47*, 831-836.

[768] Vafiadis, P., Bennett, S.T., Todd, J.A., Grabs, R. & Polychronakos, C. (1998). Divergence between genetic determinants of IGF2 transcription levels in leukocytes

and of IDDM2-encoded susceptibility to type 1 diabetes. *Journal of Clinical Endocrinology and metabolism, 83*, 2933-2939.

[769] Paquette, J., Giannoukakis, N., Polychronakos, C., Vafiadis, P. & Deal, C. (1998). The INS 5'variable number of tandem repeats is associated with IGF2 expression in humans. *Journal of Biological Chemistry, 273*, 14158-14164.

[770] Dahlquist, G., Bennich, S.S. & Kallen, B. (1996). Intrauterine growth pattern and risk of childhood onset insulin dependent (type 1) diabetes: population based case-control study. *British Medical Journal, 313*, 1174-1177.

[771] Nistico, L., Buzzetti, R.,Pritchard, L.E., Van der Auwera, B., Giovannini, C., Bosi, E., Larrad, M.T., Rios, M.S., Chow, C.C., Cockram, C.S., Jacobs, K., Mijovic, C., Bain, S.C., Barnett, A.H., Vandewalle, C.L., Schuit, F., Gorus, F.K., Tosi, R., Pozzilli, P. & Todd, J.A. (1996). The CTLA-4 gene region of chromosome 2q33 is linked to, and associated with, type 1 diabetes. *Human Molecular Genetics, 5*, 1075-1080.

[772] Ling, V., Wu, P.W., Finnerty, H.F., Agostino, M.J., Graham, J.R., Chen, S., Jussiff, J.M., Fisk, G.J., Miller, C.P. & Collins, M. (2001). Assembly and annotation of human chromosome 2q33 sequence containing the CD28, CTLA4, and ICOS gene cluster: analysis by computational, comparative, and microarray approaches. *Genomics, 78*, 155-168.

[773] Marron, M.P., Raffel, L.J., Garchon, H.J., Jacob, C.O., Serrano-Rios, M., Martinez Larrad, M.T., Teng, W.P., Park, Y., Zhang, Z.X., Goldstein, D.R., Tao, Y.W., Beaurain, G., Bach, J.F., Huang, H.S., Luo, D.F., Zeidler, A., Rotter, J.I., Yang, M.C., Modilevsky, T., Maclaren, N.K. & She, J.X. (1997). Insulin-dependent diabetes mellitus (IDDM) is associated with CTLA4 polymorphisms in multiple ethnic groups. *Human Molecular Genetics, 6*, 1275-1282.

[774] Pociot, F. & McDermott, M.F. (2002). Genetics of type 1 diabetes mellitus. *Genes and Immunity, 3*, 235-249.

[775] Kavvoura, F.K. & Ioannidis, J.P. (2005). CTLA-4 gene polymorphisms and susceptibility to type 1 diabetes mellitus: a HuGE Review and meta-analysis. *American Journal of Epidemiology, 162*, 3-16.

[776] Ihara, K., Ahmed, S., Nakao, F., Kinukawa, N., Kuromaru, R., Matsuura, N., Iwata, I., Nagafuchi, S., Kohno, H., Miyako, K. & Hara, T. (2001). Association studies of CTLA-4, CD28, and ICOS gene polymorphisms with type 1 diabetes in the Japanese population. *Immunogenetics, 53*, 447-454.

[777] Wood, J.P., Pani, M.A., Bieda, K., Meyer, G., Usadel, K.H. & Badenhoop, K. (2002). A recently described polymorphism in the CD28 gene on chromosome 2q33 is not associated with susceptibility to type 1 diabetes. *European Journal of Immunogenetics, 29*, 347-349.

[778] Bouqbis, L., Izaabel, H., Akhayat. O., Perez-Lezaun, A., Calafell, F., Bertranpetit, J. & Comas, D. (2003). Association of the CTLA4 promoter region (-1661G allele) with type 1 diabetes in the South Moroccan population. *Genes and Immunity, 4*, 132-137.

[779] Baniasadi, V., Narain, N., Goswami, R., Das, S.N. (2006). Promoter region -318 C/ T and -1661 A/G CTLA-4 single nucleotide polymorphisms and type 1 diabetes in North Indians. *Tissue Antigens, 67*, 383-389.

[780] Anjos, S.M., Tessier, M.C. & Polychronakos, C. (2004). Association of the cytotoxic T lymphocyte-associated antigen 4 gene with type 1 diabetes: evidence for independent effects of two polymorphisms on the same haplotype block. *Journal of Clinical Endocrinology and Metabolism. 89*, 6257-6265.

[781] Steck, A.K., Bugawan, T.L., Valdes, A.M., Emery, L.M., Blair, A., Norris, J.M., Redondo, M.J., Babu, S.R., Erlich, H.A., Eisenbarth, G.S. & Rewers, M.J. (2005). Association of non-HLA genes with type 1 diabetes autoimmunity. *Diabetes, 54*, 2482-2486.

[782] Ligers, A., Teleshova, N. , Masterman, T., Huang, W.X. & Hillert J. (2001). CTLA-4 gene expression is influenced by promoter and exon 1 polymorphisms. *Genes and Immunity, 2*, 145-152.

[783] Wang, X.B., Zhao, X., Giscombe, R. & Lefvert, A.K. (2002). A CTLA-4 gene polymorphism at position -318 in the promoter region affects the expression of protein. *Genes and Immunity, 3*, 233-234.

[784] Chistiakov, D.A., Savost'anov, K.V., Turakulov, R.I., Efremov, I.A. & Demurov, L.M. (2006). Genetic analysis and functional evaluation of the C/T(-318) and A/G(-1661) polymorphisms of the CTLA-4 gene in patients affected with Graves' disease. *Clinical Immunology, 118*, 233-242.

[785] Perkins, D., Wang, Z., Donovan, C., He, H., Mark, D., Guan, G., Wang, Y., Walunas, T., Bluestone, J., Listman, J. & Finn, P.W. (1996). Regulation of CTLA-4 expression during T cell activation. *Journal of Immunology, 156*, 4154-4159.

[786] Ling, V., Wu, P.W., Finnerty, H.F., Sharpe, A.H., Gray, G.S. & Collins, M. (1999). Complete sequence determination of the mouse and human CTLA4 gene loci: cross-species DNA sequence similarity beyond exon borders. *Genomics, 60*, 341–355.

[787] Lindsten, T., Lee, K.P., Harris, E.S., Petryniak, B., Craighead, N., Reynolds, P.J., Lombard, D.B., Freeman, G.J., Nadler, L.M. & Gray, G.S. (1993). Characterization of CTLA-4 structure and expression on human T cells. *Journal of Immunology, 151*, 3489–3499

[788] Kristiansen, O.P., Larsen, Z.M. & Pociot, F. (2000). CTLA-4 in autoimmune diseases – a general susceptibility gene to autoimmunity? *Genes and Immunity, 1*, 170-184.

[789] Anjos, S., Nguyen, A., Ounissi-Benhalha, H., Tessier, M.H. & Polychronakos, C. (2002). A common autoimmunity predisposing signal peptide variant of the cytotoxic T-lymphocyte antigen 4 results in inefficient glycosylation of the susceptibility allele. *Journal of Biological Chemistry, 277*, 46478-46486.

[790] Anjos, S. & Polychronakos, C. (2004). Mechanisms of genetic susceptibility to type I diabetes: beyond HLA. *Molecular Genetics and Metabolism, 81*, 187-195.

[791] Maurer, M., Loserth, S., Kolb-Maurer, A., Ponath, A., Wiese, S., Kruse, N. & Rieckmann, P. (2002). A polymorphism in the human cytotoxic T-lymphocyte antigen 4 (CTLA4) gene (exon 1 +49) alters T-cell activation. *Immunogenetics, 54*, 1-8.

[792] Ban, Y., Taniyama, M., Tozaki, T., Yanagawa, T., Yamada, S., Maruyama, T., Kasuga, A., Tomita, M. & Ban, Y. (2001). No association of type 1 diabetes with a microsatellite marker for CTLA-4 in a Japanese population. *Autoimmunity, 34*, 39-43.

[793] Chistiakov, D.A., Savost'anov, K.V. & Nosikov, V.V. (2001). CTLA4 gene polymorphisms are associated with, and linked to, insulin-dependent diabetes mellitus in a Russian population. *BMC Genetics*, 2:6.

[794] Turpeinen, H., Lainem A.P., Hermann, R., Simell, O., Veijola, R., Knip, M. & Ilonen, J. (2003). A linkage analysis of the CTLA4 gene region in Finnish patients with type 1 diabetes. *European Journal of Immunogenetics, 30*, 289-293.

[795] Lowe, R.M., Graham, J., Sund, G., Kockum, I., Landin-Olsson, M., Schaefer, J.B., Torn, C., Lernmark, A. & Dahlquist, G. (2000). The length of the CTLA-4 microsatellite (AT)n-repeat affects the risk for type 1 diabetes. *Autoimmunity, 32*, 173-180.

[796] Wang, X.B., Kakoulidou, M., Giscombe, R., Qiu, Q., Huang, D., Pirskanen, R., Lefvert, A.K. (2002). Abnormal expression of CTLA-4 by T cells from patients with myasthenia gravis: effect of an AT-rich gene sequence. *Journal of Neuroimmunology, 130*, 224-232.

[797] Huang, D., Giscombe, R., Zhou, Y., Pirskanen, R., Lefvert, A.K. (2000). Dinucleotide repeat expansion in the CTLA-4 gene leads to T cell hyper-reactivity via the CD28 pathway in myasthenia gravis. *Journal of Neuroimmunology, 105*, 69-77.

[798] Takara, M., Kouki, T. & De Groot, L.J. (2003). CTLA-4 AT-repeat polymorphism reduces the inhibitory function of CTLA-4 in Graves' disease. Thyroid, 13, 1083-1089.

[799] Finn, P.W., He, H., Wang, Y., Wang, Z., Guan, G., Listman, J. & Perkins, D.L. (1997). Synergistic induction of CTLA-4 expression by costimulation with TCR plus CD28 signals mediated by increased transcription and messenger ribonucleic acid stability. *Journal of Immunology, 158*, 4074-4081.

[800] Gingerich, T.J., Feige, J.J. & LaMarre, J. (2003). AU-rich elements and the control of gene expression through regulated mRNA stability. *Animal Health Research and Reviews, 5*, 49-63.

[801] Ueda, H., Howson, J.M., Esposito, L.,Heward, J., Snook, H., Chamberlain, G., Rainbow, D.B., Hunter, K.M., Smith, A.N., Di Genova, G., Herr, M.H., Dahlman, I., Payne, F., Smyth, D., Lowe, C., Twells, R.C., Howlett, S., Healy, B., Nutland, S., Rance, H.E., Everett, V., Smink, L.J., Lam, A.C., Cordell, H.J., Walker, N.M., Bordin, C., Hulme, J., Motzo, C., Cucca, F., Hess, J.F., Metzker, M.L., Rogers, J., Gregory, S., Allahabadia, A., Nithiyananthan, R., Tuomilehto-Wolf, E., Tuomilehto, J., Bingley, P., Gillespie, K.M., Undlien, D.E., Roningen, K.S., Guja, C., Ionescu-Tirgoviste, C., Savage, D.A., Maxwell, A.P., Carson D.J., Patterson, C.C., Franklyn, J.A., Clayton, D.G., Peterson, L.B., Wicker, L.S., Todd, J.A. & Gough, S.C. (2003). Association of the T-cell regulatory gene CTLA4 with susceptibility to autoimmune disease. *Nature, 423*, 506-511.

[802] Magistrelli, G., Jeannin, P., Herbault, N., Benoit De Coignac, A., Bonnefoy, J.Y. & Delneste, Y. (1999). A soluble form of CTLA-4 generated by alternative splicing is expressed by nonstimulated human T cells. *European Journal of Immunology, 29*, 3596-3602.

[803] Oaks, M.K., Hallett, K.M., Penwell, R.T., Stauber, E.C., Warren, S.J. & Tector, A.J. (2000). A native soluble form of CTLA-4. *Cell Immunology, 201*, 144-153.

[804] Pawlak, E., Kochanowska, I.E., Frydecka, I., Kielbinski, M., Potoczek, S. & Bilinska, M. (2005). The soluble CTLA-4 receptor: a new marker in autoimmune diseases. *Archivum Immunologiae and Therapiae Expeimentalis, 53*, 336-341.

[805] Purohit, S., Podolsky, R., Collins, C., Zheng, W., Schatz, D., Muir, A., Hopkins, D., Huang, Y.H. & She, J.X. (2005). Lack of correlation between the levels of soluble cytotoxic T-lymphocyte associated antigen-4 (CTLA-4) and the CT-60 genotypes. *Journal of Autoimmune Diseases*, 2:8.

[806] Anjos, S.M., Shao, W., Marchand, L. & Polychronakos, C. (2005). Allelic effects on gene regulation at the autoimmunity-predisposing CTLA4 locus: a re-evaluation of the 3' +6230G>A polymorphism. *Genes and Immunity, 6*, 305-311.

[807] Vijayakrishnan, L., Slavik, J.M., Illes, Z., Greenwald, R.J., Rainbow, D., Greve, B., Peterson, L.B., Hafler, D.A., Freeman, G.J., Sharpe, A.H., Wicker, L.S. & Kuchroo, V.K. (2004). An autoimmune disease-associated CTLA-4 splice variant lacking the B7 binding domain signals negatively in T cells. *Immunity, 20*, 563-575.

[808] Johnson, G.C., Esposito, L., Barratt, B.J., Heward, J., Di Genova, G., Ueda, H., Cordell, H.J., Eaves, I.A., Dudbridge, F., Twells, R.C., Payne, F., Hughes, W., Nutland, S., Stevens, H., Carr, P., Tuomilehto-Wolf, E., Tuomilehto, J., Gough, S.C., Clayton, D.G. & Todd, J.A. (2001). Haplotype tagging for the identification of common disease genes. *Nature Genetics, 29*, 233-237.

[809] Holopainen, P.M. & Partanen, J.A. (2001). Technical note: linkage disequilibrium and disease-associated CTLA4 polymorphisms. Jounal of Immunology, 167, 2457-2458.

[810] Halldorsson, B.V., Istrail, S., De La Vega, F.M. (2004). Optimal selection of SNP markers for disease association studies. *Human Heredity, 58*, 190-202.

[811] Wang, X.B., Zheng, C.Y., Giscombe, R. & Lefvert, A.K. (2001). Regulation of surface and intracellular expression of CTLA-4 on human peripheral T cells. *Scandinavian Journal of Immunology, 54*, 453-458.

[812] Waterhouse, P., Penninger, J.M., Timms, E., Wakeham, A., Shahinian, A., Lee, K.P., Thompson, C.B., Griesser, H. & Mak, T.W. (1995). Lymphoproliferative disorders with early lethality in mice deficient in Ctla-4. *Science, 270*, 985-988.

[813] Tivol, E.A., Borriello, F., Schweitzer, A.N., Lynch, W.P., Bluestone, J.A. & Sharpe, A.H. (1995). Loss of CTLA-4 leads to massive immunoproliferation and fatal multiorgan tissue destruction, revealing a critical negative regulatory role of CTLA-4. *Immunity, 3*, 541-547.

[814] Chambers, C.A., Cado, D., Truong, T. & Allison, P. (1997). Thymocyte development in normal and CTLA-4-deficient mice. *Proceedings of the National Academy of Sciences of USA, 94*, 9296-9301.

[815] Waterhouse, P., Bachman, M.F., Penninger, J.M., Oshashi, P.S. & Mack, T.W. (1997). Normal thymic selection, normal viability and decreased lymphoproliferation in T cell receptor-transgenic CTLA-4-deficient mice. *European Journal of Immunology, 27*, 1887-1892.

[816] Linsley, P.S., Brady, W., Urnes, M., Grosmaire, L.S., Damle, N.K. & Ledbetter, J.A. (1991). CTLA-4 is a second receptor for the B cell activation antigen B7. *Journal of Experimental Medicine, 174*, 561-569.

[817] Tivol, E.A., Boyd, S.D., McKeon, S., Borriello, F., Nickerson, P., Strom, T.B. & Sharpe AH. (1997). CTLA4Ig prevents lymphoproliferation and fatal multiorgan tissue destruction in CTLA-4-deficient mice. *Journal of Immunology, 158*, 5091-5094.

[818] Balzano, C., Buonavista, N., Rouvier, E. & Golstein, P. (1992). CTLA-4 and CD28: similar proteins, neighboring genes. *International Journal of Cancer Supplement, 7*, 28-32.

[819] Linsley, P.S., Clark, E.A. & Ledbetter, J.A. (1990). T-cell antigen CD28 mediates adhesion with B cells by interacting with activation antigen B7/BB-1. *Proceedings of the National Academy of Sciences of USA, 87*, 5031-5035.

[820] Tivol, E.A., Schweitzer, A.N. & Sharpe, A.H. (1996). Costimulation and autoimmunity. *Current Opinion in Immunology, 8*, 822-830.

[821] Linsley, P.S., Green, J.L., Brady, W., Bajorath, J., Ledbetter, J.A. & Peach, R. (1994). Human B7-1 (CD80) and B7-2 (CD86) bind with similar avidities but distinct kinetics to CD28 and CTLA-4 receptors. *Immunity, 1*, 793-801.

[822] van der Merwe, P.A. & Davis, S.J. (2003). Molecular interactions mediating T cell antigen recognition. *Annual Reviews in Immunology, 21*, 659-684.

[823] Stamper, C.C., Zhang, Y., Tobin, J.F., Erbe, D.V., Ikemizu, S., Davis, S.J., Stahl, M.L., Seehra, J., Somers, W.S. & Mosyak, L. (2003). Crystal structure of the B7-1/CTLA-4 complex that inhibits human immune responses. *Nature, 410*, 608-611.

[824] Zhang, Z., Schwartz, J.C., Almo, S.C. & Nathenson, S.G. (2003). Crystal structure of the receptor-binding domain of human B7-2: insights into organization and signaling. *Proceedings of the National Academy of Sciences of USA, 100*, 2568-2591.

[825] Collins, A.V., Brodie, D.W., Gilbert, R.J., Iaboni, A., Manso-Sancho, R., Walse, B., Stuart, D.I., van der Merwe, P.A. & Davis, S.J. (2002). The interaction properties of costimulatory molecules revisited. *Immunity, 17*, 201-210.

[826] Chikuma, S., Abbas, A.K. & Bluestone, J.A. (2005). B7-independent inhibition of T cells by CTLA-4. *Journal of Immunology, 175*, 177-181.

[827] Shiratori, T., Miyatake, S., Ohno, H., Nakaseko, C., Isono, K., Bonifacino, J.S. & Saito, T. (1997). Tyrosine phosphorylation controls internalization of CTLA-4 by regulating its interaction with clathrin-associated adaptor complex AP-2. *Immunity, 6*, 583-589.

[828] Davis, D.M. & Dustin, M.L. (2004). What is the importance of the immunological synapse: variations in assembly and function? *Current Opinion in Immunology, 16*, 345-352.

[829] Carreno, B.M., Bennett, F., Chau, T.A., Ling, V., Luxenberg, D., Jussif, J., Baroja, M.L. & Madrenas, J. (2000). CTLA-4 (CD152) can inhibit T cell activation by two different mechanisms depending on its level of cell surface expression. *Journal of Immunology, 165*, 1352-1356.

[830] Linsley, P.S., Bradshaw, J., Greene, J., Peach, R., Bennett, K.L. & Mittler, R.S. (1996). Intracellular trafficking of CTLA-4 and focal localization toward sites of TCR engagement. *Immunity, 4*, 535-543.

[831] Cinek, T., Sadra, A. & Imboden, J.B. (2000). Cutting edge: tyrosine-independent transmission of inhibitory signals of CTLA-4 function in vivo. *Journal of Immunology, 164*, 5319-5327.

[832] Darlington, P.J., Baroja, M.L., Chau, T.A., Siu, E., Ling, V., Carreno, B.M. & Madrenas, J. (2002). Surface cytotoxic T-lymphocyte-associated antigen 4 partitions within lipid rafts and relocates to the immunological synapse under conditions of inhibition of T cell activation. *Journal of Experimental Medicine, 195*, 1337-1347.

[833] Fraser, J.H., Rincon, M., McCoy, K.D. & Le Gros, G. (1999). CTLA-4 ligation attenuates AP-1, NFAT and NF-κB activity in activated T cells. *European Journal of Immunology, 29*, 838-844.

[834] Brunner, M.C., Chambers, C.A., Chan, F.K., Hanke, J., Winoto, A. & Allison, J.P. (1999). CTLA-4-mediated inhibition of early events of T cell proliferation. *Journal of Immunology, 162*, 5813-5820.

[835] Li, D., Gal, I., Vermes, C., Alegre, M.L., Chong, A.S., Chen, L., Shao, Q., Adarichev, V., Xu, X., Koreny, T., Mikecz, K., Finnegan, A., Glant, T.T. & Zhang, J. (2004). Cutting edge: Cbl-b: one of the key molecules tuning CD28- and CTLA-4-mediated T cell costimulation. *Journal of Immunology, 173*, 7135-7139.

[836] Bachmaier, K., Krawczyk, C., Kozieradzki, I., Kong, Y.Y., Sasaki, T., Oliveira-dos-Santos, A., Mariathasan, S., Bouchard, D., Wakeham, A., Itie, A., Le, J., Ohashi, P.S., Sarosi, I., Nishina, H., Lipkowitz, S. & Penninger, J.M. (2000). Negative regulation of lymphocyte activation and autoimmunity by the molecular adaptor Cbl-b. *Nature, 403*, 211-216.

[837] Miyatake, S., Nakaseko, C., Umemori, H., Yamamoto, T. & Saito, T. (1998). Src family tyrosine kinases associate with and phosphorylate CTLA-4 (CD152). *Biochemical and Biophysical Research Communications, 249*, 444-448.

[838] Schneider, H., Schwarzberg, P.L. & Rudd, C.E. (1998). Resting lymphocyte kinase (Rlk/Txk) phosphorylates the YVKM motif and regulates PI 3-kinase binding to T-cell antigen CTLA-4. *Biochemical and Biophysical Research Communications, 252*, 14-19.

[839] Chikuma, S., Murakami, M., Tanaka, K. & Uede, T. (2000). Janus kinase 2 is associated with box 1-like motif and phosphorylates a critical tyrosine residue in the cytoplasmic region of cytotoxic T lymphocyte associated molecule-4. *Journal of Cellular Biochemistry, 78*, 241-250.

[840] Baroja, M.L., Luxenberg, D., Chau, T., Ling, V., Strathdee, C.A., Carreno, B.M. & Madrenas, J. (2000). The inhibitory function of CTLA-4 does not require its tyrosine phosphorylation. *Journal of Immunology, 164*, 49-55.

[841] Schneider, H., Mandelbrot, D.A., Greenwald, R.J., Ng, F., Lechler, R., Sharpe, A.H. & Rudd, C.E. (2002). Cutting edge: CTLA-4 (CD152) differentially regulates mitogen-activated protein kinases (extracellular signal-regulated kinase and c-Jun N-terminal kinase) in CD4+ T cells from receptor/ligand-deficient mice. *Journal of Immunology, 169*, 3475-3479.

[842] Baroja, M.L., Vijayakrishnan, L., Bettelli, E., Darlington, P.J., Chau, T.A., Ling, V., Collins, M., Carreno, B.M., Madrenas, J. & Kuchroo, V.K. (2002). Inhibition of CTLA-4 function by the regulatory subunit of serine/threonine phosphatase 2A. *Journal of Immunology, 168*, 5070-5078.

[843] Chuang, E., Fisher, T.S., Morgan, R.W., Robbins, M.D., Duerr, J.M., Vander Heiden, M.G., Gardner, J.P., Hambor, J.E., Neveu, M.J. & Thompson, C.B. (2000). The CD28

and CTLA-4 receptors associate with the serine/threonine phosphatase PP2A. *Immunity, 13*, 313-322.

[844] Janssens, V. & Goris, J. (2001). Protein phosphatase 2A: a highly regulated family of serine/threonine phosphatases implicated in cell growth and signaling. *Biochemical Journal, 353*, 417-439.

[845] Resjo, S., Goransson, O., Harndahl, L., Zolnierowicz, S., Manganiello, V. & Degerman, E. (2002). Protein phosphatase 2A is the main phosphatase involved in the regulation of protein kinase B in rat adipocytes. *Cell Signalling, 14*, 231-238.

[846] Jago, C.B., Yates, J., Camara, N.O., Lechler, R.I. & Lombardi, G. (2004). Differential expression of CTLA-4 among T cell subsets. *Clinical and Experimental Immunology, 136*, 463-471.

[847] Chatfield, K. & Eastman, A. (2004). Inhibitors of protein phosphatases 1 and 2A differentially prevent intrinsic and extrinsic apoptosis pathways. *Biochemical and Biophysical Research Communications, 323*, 1313-1320.

[848] Mandelbrot, D.A., McAdam, A.J. & Sharpe, A.H. (1999). B7-1 or B7-2 is required to produce the lymphoproliferative phenotype in mice lacking cytotoxic T lymphocyte-associated antigen 4 (CTLA-4). *Journal of Experimental Medicine, 189*, 435-440.

[849] Wu, Y., Guo, Y., Huang, A., Zheng, P. & Liu, Y. (1997). CTLA-4-B7 interaction is sufficient to costimulate T cell clonal expansion. *Journal of Experimental Medicine, 185*, 1327-1335.

[850] Madrenas, J., Chau, L.A., Teft, W.A., Wu, P.W., Jussif, J., Kasaian, M., Carreno, B.M. & Ling, V. (2004). Conversion of CTLA-4 from inhibitor to activator of T cells with a bispecific tandem single-chain Fv ligand. *Journal of Immunology, 172*, 5948-5956.

[851] Takanashi, T., Tagami, T., Yamazaki, S. Uede, T., Shimizu, J., Sakaguchi, N., Mak, T.W. & Sakaguchi, S. (2000). Immunologic self-tolerance maintained by CD25+CD4+ regulatory T cells constitutively expressing cytotoxic T lymphocyte-associated antigen 4. *Journal of Experimental Medicine, 192*, 303-310.

[852] Mellor, A.L. & Munn, D.H. (2004). IDO expression by dendritic cells: tolerance and tryptophan catabolism. *Nature Reviews Immunology, 4*, 762-774.

[853] Chen, W., Jin, W. & Wahl, S.M. (1998). Engagement of cytotoxic T lymphocyte-associated antigen 4 (CTLA-4) induces transforming growth factor β (TGF-β) production by murine CD4+ T cells. *Journal of Experimental Medicine, 188*, 1849-1857.

[854] Annunziato, F., Cosmi, L., Liotta, F., Lazzeri, E., Manetti, R., Vanini, V., Romagnani, P., Maggi, E., & Romagnani, S. (2001). Phenotype, localization, and mechanism of suppression of CD4+CD25+ human thymocytes. *Journal of Experimental Medicine, 196*, 379-387.

[855] Chikuma, S., Bluestone, J.A. (2003). CTLA-4 and tolerance: the biochemical point of view. *Immunologic Research, 28*, 241-253.

[856] Eggena, M.P., Walker, L.S.K., Nagabhushaman, V., Barron, L., Chodos, A. & Abbas, A.A. (2004). Cooperative roles of CTLA-4 and regulatory T cells in tolerance to an islet cell antigen. *Journal of Experimental Medicine, 199*, 1725-1730.

[857] Egen, J.G. & Allison, J.P. (2002). Cytotoxic T lymphocyte antigen-4 accumulation in the immunological synapse is regulated by TCR signal strength. *Immunity, 16*, 23-35.

[858] Brand, O., Gough, S. & Heward, J. (2005). HLA, CTLA-4 and PTPN22: the shared genetic master-key to autoimmunity? *Expert Reviews in Molecular Medicine, 7*, 1-15.

[859] Gjorloff-Wingren, A., Saxena, M., Williams, S., Hammi, D. & Mustelin T. (1999). Characterization of TCR-induced receptor-proximal signaling events negatively regulated by the protein tyrosine phosphatase PEP. *European Journal of Immunology, 29*, 3845-3854.

[860] Wicker, L.S., Clark, K., Fraser, H.K., Garner, V.E., Gonzales-Munoz, A., Healy, B., Howlett, S., Hunter, K., Rainbow, D., Rosa, R.L., Smink, L.J., Todd, J.A. & Peterson, L.B. (2005). Type 1 diabetes genes and pathways shared by humans and NOD mice. *Journal of Autoimmunity, 25*, 29-33.

[861] Mustelin T. & Tasken, K. (2003). Positive and negative regulation of T-cell activation through kinases and phosphatases. *Biochemical Journal, 371*, 15-27.

[862] Cloutier , J.-F. & Veillette, A. (1999). Cooperative inhibition of T-cell antigen receptor signaling by a complex between a kinase and a phosphatase. *Journal of Experimental Medicine, 189*, 111-121.

[863] Cloutier, J.-F. & Veillette, A. (1995). Association of inhibitory tyrosine protein kinase p50csk with protein phosphatase PEP in T cells and other hamatopoietic cells. *EMBO Journal, 15*, 4909-4918.

[864] Siminovitch, K.A. (2004). PTPN22 and autoimmune disease. *Nature Genetics, 12*, 1248-1249.

[865] Hasegawa, K., Martin, F., Huang, G., Tumas, D., Diehl, L. & Chan, A.C. (2004). PEST domain-enriched tyrosine phosphatase (PEP) regulation of effector/memory T cells. *Science, 303*, 685-689.

[866] Luzina, I.G., Atamas, S.P., Stotter C.E., daSilva, L.C., Kelsoe, G., Papadimitriou, J.C. & Handwerger, B.S. (2001). Spontaneous formation of germinal centers in autoimmune mice. *Journal of Leukocyte Biology, 70*, 578-584.

[867] Brenner, M., Meng, H.C., Yarlett, N.C., Griffiths, M.M., Remmers, E.F., Wilder, R.L. & Gulko, P.S. (2005). The non-major histocompatibility complex quantitative trait locus Cia10 contains a major arthritis gene and regulates disease severity, pannus formation, and joint damage. *Arthritis and Rheumatism, 52*, 322-332.

[868] Yokoi, N., Komeda, K., Wang, H.Y., Yano, H., Kitada, K., Saitoh, Y., Seino, Y., Yasuda, K., Serikawa, T. & Seino S. (2002). Cblb is a major susceptibility gene for rat type 1 diabetes mellitus. *Nature Genetics, 31*, 391-394.

[869] Yokoi, N., Namae, M., Fuse, M., Wang, H.Y., Hirata, T., Seino, S. & Komeda, K. (2003). Establishment and characterization of the Komeda diabetes-prone rat as a segregating inbred strain. *Experimental Animals, 52*, 295-301.

[870] Sakaguchi, N., Takahashi, T., Hata, H., Nomura T., Tagami, T., Yamazaki, S., Sakihama, T., Matsutani, T., Negishi, I., Nakatsuru, S. & Sakaguchi, S. (2003). Altered thymic T-cell selection due to a mutation of the ZAP-70 gene causes autoimmune arthritis in mice. *Nature, 426*, 454-460.

[871] Cohen, S., Dadi, H., Shaoul, N. & Roifman, C.M. (1999). Cloning and characterization of a lymphoid-specific, inducible human protein tyrosine phosphatase, Lyp. *Blood, 93*, 2013-2024.

[872] Ghose, R., Shekhtman, A., Coger, M.J., Ji., H. & Cowburn, D. (2001). A novel, specific interaction, involving the Csk SH3 domain and its natural ligand. *Nature Structural Biology, 8*, 998-1004.

[873] Hill, R.J., Zozulya, S., Lu, Y.L., Ward, K., Gishizky, M. & Jallal, B. (2002). The lymphoid protein tyrosine phosphatase Lyp interacts with the adaptor molecule Grb2 and functions as a negative regulator of T-cell activation. *Experimental Hematology, 30*, 237-244.

[874] Bottini, N., Musumeci, L., Alonso, A., Rahmouni, S., Nika, K., Rostamkhani, M., MacMurray, J., Meloni, G.F., Lucarelli, P., Pelecchia, M., Eisenbarth, G.S., Comings, D. & Mustelin, T. (2004). A functional variant of lymphoid tyrosine phosphatase is associated with type I diabetes. *Nature Genetics, 36*, 337-338.

[875] Smyth, D., Cooper, J.D., Collins, J.E., Heward, J.M., Franklyn, J.A., Howson, J.M., Vella, A., Nutland, S., Rance, H.E., Maier, L., Barratt, B.J., Guja, C., Ionescu-Tirgoviste, C., Savage, D.A., Dunger, D.B., Widmer, B., Strachan, D.P., Ring, S.M., Walker, N., Clayton, D.G., Twells, R.C., Gough, S.C. & Todd, J.A. (2004). Replication of an association between the lymphoid tyrosine phosphatase locus (LYP/PTPN22) with type 1 diabetes, and evidence for its role as a general autoimmunity locus. *Diabetes, 53*, 3020-3023.

[876] Zheng, W. & She, J.X. (2005). Genetic association between a lymphoid tyrosine phosphatase (PTPN22) and type 1 diabetes. *Diabetes, 54*, 906-908.

[877] Zhernakova, A., Eerligh, P., Wijmenga, C., Barrera, P., Roep, B.O. & Koeleman, B.P. (2005). Differential association of the PTPN22 coding variant with autoimmune diseases in a Dutch population. *Genes and Immunity, 6*, 459-461.

[878] Gomez, L.M., Anaya, J.M., Gonzalez, C.I., Pineda-Tamayo, R., Otero, W., Arango, A. & Martin, J. (2005). PTPN22 C1858T polymorphism in Colombian patients with autoimmune diseases. *Genes and Immunity, 6*, 628-631.

[879] Kahles, H., Ramos-Lopez, E., Lange, B., Zwermann, O., Reincke, M. & Badenhoop K. (2005). Sex-specific association of PTPN22 1858T with type 1 diabetes but not with Hashimoto's thyroiditis or Addison's disease in the German population. *European Journal of Endocrinology, 153*, 895-899.

[880] Hermann, R., Lipponen, K., Kiviniemi, M., Kakko, T., Veijola, R., Simell, O., Knip, M. & Ilonen, J. (2006). Lymphoid tyrosine phosphatase (LYP/PTPN22) Arg620Trp variant regulates insulin autoimmunity and progression to type 1 diabetes. *Diabetologia, 49*, 1198-1208.

[881] Fedetz, M., Matesanz, F., Caro-Maldonado, A., Smirnov, I.I., Chvorostinka, V.N., Moiseenko, T.A. & Alcina, A. (2006). The 1858T PTPN22 gene variant contributes to a genetic risk of type 1 diabetes in a Ukrainian population. *Tissue Antigens, 67*, 430-433.

[882] Onengut-Gumuscu, S., Ewens, K.G., Spielman, R.S. & Concannon, P. (2004). A functional polymorphism (1858C/T) in the PTPN22 gene is linked and associated with type I diabetes in multiplex families. *Genes and Immunity, 5*, 678-680.

[883] Ladner, M.B., Bottini, N., Valdes, A.M. & Noble, J.A. (2005). Association of the single nucleotide polymorphism C1858T of the PTPN22 gene with type 1 diabetes. *Human Immunology, 66*, 60-64.

[884] Criswell, L.A., Pfeiffer, K.A., Lum, R.F., Gonzales B., Novitzke, J., Kern, M., Moser, K.L., Begovich, A.B., Carlton, V.E., Li, W., Lee, A.T., Ortmann, W., Behrens, T.W. & Gregersen, P.K. (2005). Analysis of families in the multiple autoimmune disease genetics consortium (MADGC) collection: the PTPN22 620W allele associates with multiple autoimmune phenotypes. *American Journal of Human Genetics, 76*, 561-571.

[885] Qu, H., Tessier, M.C., Hudson, T.J. & Polychronakos, C. (2005). Confirmation of the association of the R620W polymorphism in the protein tyrosine phosphatase PTPN22 with type 1 diabetes in a family based study. *Journal of Medical Genetics, 42*, 266-270.

[886] Kawasaki, E., Awata, T., Ikegami, H., Kobayashi, T., Maruyama, T., Nakanishi, K., Shimada, A., Uga, M., Kurihara, S., Kawabata, Y., Tanaka, S., Kanazawa, Y., Lee, I. & Eguchi, K. (2006). Systematic search for single nucleotide polymorphisms in a lymphoid tyrosine phosphatase gene (PTPN22): association between a promoter polymorphism and type 1 diabetes in Asian populations. *American Journal of Medical Genetics, 140*, 586-593.

[887] Cucca, F., Goy, J.V., Kawaguchi, Y., Esposito, L., Merriman, M.E., Wilson, A.J., Gordell, H.J., Bain, S.C. & Todd, J.A. (1998). A male-female bias in type 1 diabetes and linkage to chromosome Xp in MHC HLA-DR3-positive patients. *Nature Genetics, 19*, 301-302.

[888] Contu, D., Morelli, L., Zavaratti, P., Lampis, R., Angius, F., Frongia, P. Murru, D., Maioli, M., Francalacci, P., Todd, J.A. & Cucca F. (2002). Sex-related bias and exlusion mapping of the nonrecombinant portion of chromosome Y in human type 1 diabetes in the isolated founder population of Sardinia. *Diabetes, 51*, 3573-3576.

[889] Aly, T.A., Ide, A., Humphrey, K., Barker, J.M., Steck, A., Erlich, H.A., Yu, L., Miao, D., Redondo, M.J., McFann, K., Roberts, C.M., Babu, S.R., Norris, J.M., Eisenbarth, G.S. & Rewers, M.J. (2005). Genetic prediction of autoimmunity: initial oligogenic prediction of anti-islet autoimmunity amongst DR3/DR4-DQ8 relatives of patients with type 1A diabetes. *Journal of Autoimmunity, 25*, 40-45.

[890] Mori, M., Yamada, R., Kobayashi, K., Kawaida, R. & Yamamoto, K. (2005). Ethnic differences in allele frequency of autoimmune-disease-associated SNPs. *Journal of Human Genetics, 50*, 264-266.

[891] Takahashi, T., Tanaka, H., Iguchi, N., Kitamura, K., Chen, Y., Maekawa, M., Nishimura, H., Ohta, H., Miyagawa, Y., Matsumiya, K., Okuyama, A. & Nishimune, Y. (2004). Rosbin: a novel homeobox-like protein gene expressed exclusively in round spermatids. *Biology of Reproduction, 70*, 1485-1492

[892] Carlton, V.E., Hu, X., Chokkalingam, A.P., Schrodi, S.J., Brandon, R., Alexander, H.C., Chang, M., Catanese, J.J., Leong, D.U., Ardlie, K.G., Kastner, D.L., Seldin, M.F., Criswell, L.A., Gregersen, P.K., Beasley, E., Thomson, G., Amos, C.I. & Begovich, A.B. (2005). PTPN22 genetic variation: evidence for multiple variants associated with rheumatoid arthritis. *American Journal of Human Genetics, 77*, 567-581.

[893] Gregorieff, A., Cloutier, J.F. & Veillette, A. (1998). Sequence requirements for association of protein-tyrosine phosphatase PEP with the Src homology 3 domain of

inhibitory tyrosine protein kinase p50(Sck). *Journal of Biological Chemistry, 273*, 13217-13222.

[894] Vang, T., Congia, M., Macis, M.D., Musumeci, L., Orru, V., Zavattari, P., Nika, K., Tautz, L., Tasken, K., Cucca, F., Mustelin, T. & Bottini, N. (2005). Autoimmune-associated lymphoid tyrosine phosphatase is a gain-of-function variant. *Nature Genetics, 37*, 1317-1319.

[895] Bottini, N., Vang, T., Cucca, F. & Mustelin, T. (2006). Role of PTPN22 in type 1 diabetes and other autoimmune diseses. *Seminars in Immunology, 18*, 207-213.

[896] Gregersen, P.K. (2005). Gaining insight into PTPN22 and autoimmunity. *Nature Genetics, 37*, 1300-1301

[897] Rapoport, M.J., Lazarus, A.H., Jaramillo, A., Speck, E. & Delovitch, T.L. (1993). Thymic T cell anergy in autoimmune nonobese diabetic mice is mediated by deficient T cell receptor regulation of the pathway of p21ras activation. *Journal of Experimental Medicine, 177*, 1221-1226.

[898] Salojin, K., Zhang, J., Cameron, M., Gill, B., Arreaza, G., Ochi, A. & Delovitch, T.L. (1997). Impaired plasma membrane targeting of Grb2-murine son of sevenless (mSOS) complex and differential activation of the Fyn-T cell receptor (TCR)-zeta-Cbl pathway mediate T cell hyporesponsiveness in autoimmune nonobese diabetic mice. *Journal of Experimental Medicine, 186*, 887-897.

[899] Haussler, M.R., Haussler, C.A., Jurutka, P.W., Thompson, P.D., Hsieh, J.C., Remus, l.S., Selznick, S.H. & Whitefield, G.K. (1997). The vitamin D hormone and its nuclear receptor: molecular actions and disease states. *Journal of Endocrinology, 154 (Suppl.1)*, S57-S73.

[900] Cantorna, M.T. & Mahon, B.D. (2004). Mounting evidence for vitamin D as an environmental factor affecting autoimmune disease prevalence. *Experimental Biology and Medicine, 229*, 1136-1142.

[901] Holick, M.F. (2004). Vitamin D: importance in the prevention of cancers, type 1 diabetes, heart disease, and osteoporosis. *American Journal of Clinical Nutrition, 79*, 362-371.

[902] Atkinson, M.A. & Leiter, E.H. (1999). The NOD mouse model of type 1 diabetes: as good as it gets? *Nature Medicine, 5*, 601-604.

[903] Zella, J.B. & DeLuca, H.F. (2003). Vitamin B and autoimmune diabetes. *Journal of Cellular Biochemistry, 88*, 216-222.

[904] Boonstra, A., Barrat, F.J., Crain, C., Heath, V.L., Savekoul, H.F. & O'Garra, A. (2001). 1alpha,25-Dihydroxyvitamin D3 has a direct effect on naive CD4(+) T cells to enhance the development of Th2 cells. *Journal of Immunology, 167*, 4974-4980.

[905] Cantorna, M.T., Woodward, W.D., Hayes, C.E. & DeLuca, H.F. (1998). 1,25-dihydroxyvitamin D3 is a positive regulator for the two anticephalitogenic cytokines TGF-beta 1 and IL-4. *Journal of Immunology, 160*, 5314-5319.

[906] Berer, A., Stokl, J., Majdic, O., Wagner, T., Kollars, M., Lechner, K., Geissler, K. & Oehler, L. (2000). 1,25-dihydroxyvitamin D_3 inhibits dendritic cell differentiation and maturation in vitro. *Experimental Hematology, 28*, 575-583.

[907] Gregori, S., Giarratana, N., Smiroldo, S., Uskokovic, M. & Adorini, L.A. (2002). 1alpha,25-dihydroxyvitamin D(3) analog enhances regulatory T-cells and arrests autoimmune diabetes in NOD mice. *Diabetes, 51*, 1367-1374.

[908] Veldman, C.M., Cantorna, M.T & DeLuca, H.F. (2000). Expression of 1,25-dihydroxyvitamin D(3) receptor in the immune system. *Archives of Biochemistry and Biophysics, 374*, 334-338.

[909] Mathieu, C., Van Etten, E., Gysemans, C., Decalonne, B., Kato, S., Laureys, J., Depovere, J., Valckx, D., Verstuyf, A. & Bouillon, R. (2001). In vitro and in vivo analysis of the immune system of vitamin D receptor knockout mice. *Journal of Bone and Mineral Research, 16*, 2057-2065.

[910] Griffin, M.D., Lutz, W., Phan, V.A., Bachman, L.A., McKean, D.J. & Kumar, D. (2001). Dendritic cell modulation by 1alpha,25 dihydroxyvitamin D3 and its analogs: a vitamin D receptor-dependent pathway that promotes a persistent state of immaturity in vitro and in vivo. *Proceedings of the National Academy of Sciences of USA, 98*, 6800-6815.

[911] Panda, D.K., Miao, D., Tremblay, M.L., Sirous, J., Farookhi, R., Hendy, G.N. & Goltzman, D. (2001). Targeted ablation of the 25-hydroxyvitamin D 1alpha - hydroxylase enzyme: evidence for skeletal, reproductive, and immune dysfunction. *Proceedings of the National Academy of Sciences of USA, 98*, 7498-7503.

[912] Bhall, A.K., Amento, E.P., Serog, B. & Glimcher, L.H. (1984). 1,25-dihydroxyvitamin D3 inhibits antigen-induced T cell activation. *Journal of Immunology, 133*, 1748-1754.

[913] May, E., Asadullah, K. & Zugel, U. (2004). Immunoregulation through 1,25-dihydroxyvitamin D3 and its analogs. Current Drug Targets. *Inflammation and Allergy, 3*, 377-393.

[914] Miyamoto, K., Kesterson, R.A., Yamamoto, H., Taketani, Y., Nishiwaki, E., Tatsumi, E., Inoue, Y., Morita, K., Takeda, E. & Pike, J.W. (1997). Structural organization of the human vitamin receptor chromosomal gene and its promoter. *Molecular Endocrinology, 11*, 1165-1179.

[915] Uitterlinden, A.G., Fang, Y., van Meurs J.B.J., Pols, H.A.P., van Leeuwen, J.P.T.M. (2004). Genetics and biology of vitamin D receptor polymorphisms. *Gene, 338*, 143-156.

[916] Hauache, O.M., Lazaretti-Castro, M., Andreoni, S., Gimeno, S.G., Brandao, C., Ramalho, A.C., Kasamatsu, T.S., Kunii, I., Hayashi, L.F., Dib, S.A. & Vieira, J.G. (1998). Vitamin D receptor gene polymorphism: correlation with bone mineral density in a Brazilian population with insulin-dependent diabetes mellitus. *Osteoporosis International, 8*, 204-210.

[917] Ban, Y., Taniyama, M., Yanagawa, T., Yamada, S., Maruyama, T., Kasuga, A. & Ban, Y. (2001). Vitamin D receptor initiation codon polymorphism influences genetic susceptibility to type 1 diabetes mellitus in the Japanese population. *BMC Medical Genetics*, 2:7.

[918] Fassbender, W.J., Goertz ,B., Weismuller, K., Steinhauer, B., Stracke, H., Auch, D., Linn, T. & Bretzel, R.G. (2002) VDR gene polymorphisms are overrepresented in German patients with type 1 diabetes compared to healthy controls without effect on

biochemical parameters of bone metabolism. *Hormone and Metabolic Research, 34*, 330-337.

[919] Gyorffy, B., Vasarhelyi, B., Krikovszky, D., Madacsy, L., Tordai, A., Tulassay, T. & Szabo, A. (2002). Gender-specific association of vitamin D receptor polymorphism combinations with type 1 diabetes mellitus. *European Journal of Endocrinology, 147*, 803-808.

[920] Skrabic, V., Zemunik, T., Situm, M. & Terzic, J. (2003). Vitamin D receptor polymorphism and susceptibility to type 1 diabetes in the Dalmatian population. *Diabetes Research and Clinical Practice, 59*, 31-35.

[921] Motohashi, Y., Yamada, S., Yanagawa, T., Maruyama, T., Suzuki, R., Niino, M., Fukazawa, T., Kasuga, A., Hirose, H., Matsubara, K., Shimada, A. & Saruta, T. (2003). Vitamin D receptor gene polymorphism affects onset pattern of type 1 diabetes. *Journal of Clinical Endocrinology and Metabolism, 88*, 3137-3140.

[922] Turpeinen, H., Hermann, R., Vaara, S., Laine, A.P., Simell, O., Knip, M., Veijola, R. & Ilonen, J. (2003). Vitamin D receptor polymorphisms: no association with type 1 diabetes in the Finnish population. *European Journal of Endocrinology, 149*, 591-596.

[923] Bianco, M.G., Minicucci, L., Calevo, M.G. & Lorini, R. (2004). Vitamin D receptor polymorphisms: are they really associated with type 1 diabetes? *European Journal of Endocrinology, 151*, 641-642.

[924] Zemunik, T., Skrabic, V., Boraska, V., Diklic, D., Terzic, I.M., Capkun, V., Peruzovic, M. & Terzic, J. (2005). FokI polymorphism, vitamin D receptor, and interleukin-1 receptor haplotypes are associated with type 1 diabetes in the Dalmatian population. *Journal of Molecular Diagnostics, 7*, 600-604.

[925] McDermott, M.F., Ramachandran, A., Ogunkolade, B.W., Aganna, E., Curtis, D., Boucher, B.J., Snehalatha, C. & Hitman, G.A. (1997). Allelic variation in the vitamin D receptor influences susceptibility to IDDM in Indian Asians. *Diabetologia, 40*, 971-975.

[926] Guja, C., Marshall, S., Welsh, K., Merriman, M., Smith, A. & Todd, J.A. & Ionescu-Tirgoviste, C. (2002). The study of CTLA-4 and vitamin D receptor polymorphisms in the Romanian type 1 diabetes population. *Journal of Cellular and Molecular Biology, 6*, 75-81.

[927] Eerligh, P., Koeleman, B.P., Dudbridge, F., Jan Bruining, G., Roep, B.O. & Giphart, M.J. (2004). Functional genetic polymorphisms in cytokines and metabolic genes as additional genetic markers for susceptibility to develop type 1 diabetes. *Genes and Immunity, 5*, 36-40.

[928] Angel, B., Santos, J.L., Carrasco, E., Albala, C. & Perez-Bravo, F. (2004). Vitamin D receptor polymorphism and susceptibility to type 1 diabetes in Chilean subjects: a case-parent study. *European Journal of Epidemiology, 19*, 1085-1087.

[929] San-Pedro, J.I., Bilbao, J.R., Perez de Nanclares, G., Vitoria, J.C., Martul, P. & Castano, L. (2005). Heterogeneity of vitamin D receptor gene association with celiac disease and type 1 diabetes mellitus. *Autoimmunity, 38*, 439-444.

[930] Pani, M.A., Knapp, M., Donner, H., Braun, J., Baur, M.P., Usadel, K.H. & Badenhoop, K. (2000). Vitamin D receptor allele combinations influence genetic susceptibility to type 1 diabetes in Germans. *Diabetes, 49*, 504-507.

[931] Morrison, N.A., Qi, J.C., Tokita, A., Kelly, P.J., Crofts, L., Nguyen, T.V., Sambrook, P.N. & Eisman, J.A. (1994). Prediction of bone density from vitamin D receptor alleles. *Nature, 367*, 284-287.

[932] Nejentsev, S., Cooper, J.D., Godfrey, L., Howson, J.M., Rance, H., Nutland, S., Walker, N.M., Guja, C., Ionescu-Tirgoviste, C., Savage, D.A., Undlien, D.E., Ronningen, K.S., Tuomilehto-Wolf, E., Tuomilehto, J., Gillespiem K.M., Ring, S.M., Strachan, D.P., Widmer, B., Dunger, D. & Todd, J.A. (2004). Analysis of the vitamin D receptor gene sequence variants in type 1 diabetes. *Diabetes, 53*, 2709-2712.

[933] Poon, A.H., Laprise, C., Lemire, M., Montpetit, A, Sinnett, D., Schurr, E. & Hudson, T.J. (2004). Association of vitamin D receptor genetic variants with susceptibility to asthma and atopy. *American Journal of Respiratory and Critical Care Medicine. 170*, 967-973.

[934] Jurutka, P.W., Remus, L.S., Whitfield, G.K., Thompson, P.D., Hsieh, J.C., Zitzer, H., Tavakkoli, P., Galligan, M.A., Dang, H.T., Haussler, C.A. & Haussler, M.R. (2000). The polymorphic N terminus in human vitamin D receptor isoforms influences transcriptional activity by modulating interaction with transcription factor IIB. *Molecular Endocrinology, 14*, 401-420.

[935] Arai, H., Miyamoto, K., Taketani, Y., Yamamoto, H., Iemori, Y., Morita, K., Tonai, T., Nishsho, T., Mori, S. & Takeda, E. (1997). A vitamin D receptor gene polymorphism in the translation initiation codon: effect on protein activity and relation to bome mineral density in Japanese women. *Journal of Bone and Mineral Research, 12*, 915-921.

[936] Whitefield, G.K., Remus, L.S., Jurutka, P.W., Zitzer, H., Oza, A.K., Dang, H.T., Haussler, C.A., Galligan, M.A., Thatcher, M.L., Encinas, D.C. & Haussler, M.R. (2001). Functionally relevant polymorphisms in the human nuclear vitamin D receptor gene. *Molecular and Cellular Endocrinology, 177*, 145-159.

[937] Colin, E.M., Weel, A.E., Uitterlinden, A.G., Buurman, C.J., Birkenhager, J.C., Pols, H.A. & van Leeuwen, J.P. (2000). Consequences of vitamin D receptor gene polymorphisms for growth inhibition of cultured human peripheral blood mononuclear cells by 1, 25-dihydroxyvitamin D3. *Clinical Endocrinology (Oxford), 52*, 211-216.

[938] Wong, H.L., Seow, A., Arakawa, K., Lee, H.P., Yu, M.C. & Ingles, S.A. (2003). Vitamin D receptor start codon polymorphism and colorectal cancer risk: effect modification by dietary calcium and fat in Singapore Chinese. *Carcinogenesis, 24*, 1091-1095.

[939] Ogunkolade, B.W., Boucher, B.J., Prahl, J.M., Bustin, S.A., Burrin, J.M, Noonan, K., North, B.V., Mannan, N., McDermott, M.F., DeLuca, H.F. & Hitman, G.A. (2002). Vitamin D receptor (VDR) mRNA and VDR protein levels in relation to vitamin D status, insulin secretory capacity, and VDR genotype in Bangladeshi Asians. *Diabetes, 51*, 2294-2300.

[940] Valdivielso, J.M. & Fernandez, E (2006). Vitamin D receptor polymorphisms and diseases. *Clinica Chimica Acta, 371*, 1-12.

[941] Durrin, L.K., Haile, R.W., Ingles, S.A. & Coetzee, G.A. (1999). Vitamin D receptor 3'-untranslated region polymorphisms: lack of effect on mRNA stability. *Biochimica et Biophysica Acta, 1453*, 311-320.

[942] Verbeek, W., Gombart, A.F,, Shiohara, M., Campbell, M. & Koeffler, H.P. (1997). Vitamin D receptor: no evidence for allele-specific mRNA stability in cells which are heterozygous for the Taq I restriction enzyme polymorphism. *Biochemical and Biophysical Research Communications, 238*, 77-80.

[943] Morrison, N.A., Yeoman, R., Kelly, P.J. & Eisman, J.A. (1992). Contribution of trans-acting factor alleles to normal physiological variability: vitamin D receptor gene polymorphism and circulating osteocalcin. *Proceedings of the National Academy of Sciences of USA, 89*, 6665-6669.

[944] Carling, T., Ridefelt, P., Hellman, P., Rastad, J. & Akerstrom, G. (1997). Vitamin D receptor polymorphisms correlate to parathyroid cell function in primary hyperparathyroidism. *Journal of Clinical Endocrinology and Metabolism, 82*, 1772-1775.

[945] Arai, H., Miyamoto, K.I., Yoshida, M., Yamamoto, H., Taketani, Y., Morita, K., Kubota, M., Yoshida, S., Ikeda, M., Watabe, E., Kanemasa, Y. & Takeda, E. (2001). The polymorphism in the caudal-related homeodomain protein Cdx-2 binding element in the human vitamin D receptor gene. *Journal of Bone and Mineral Research, 16*, 1256-1264.

[946] Fang, Y., van Meurs, J.B., d'Alesio, A., Jhamai, M., Zhao, H., Rivadeneira, F., Hofman, A., van Leeuwen, J.P., Jehan, F., Pols, H.A. & Uitterlinden, A.G. (2005). Promoter and 3'-untranslated-region haplotypes in the vitamin d receptor gene predispose to osteoporotic fracture: the Rotterdam study. *American Journal of Human Genetics, 77*, 807-823.

[947] Nejentsev, S., Godfrey, L., Snook, H., Rance, H., Nutland, S., Walker, N.M., Lam, A.C., Guja, C., Ionescu-Tirgoviste, C., Undlien, D.E., Ronningen, K.S., Tuomilehto-Wolf, E., Tuomilehto, J., Newport, M.J., Clayton, D.G. & Todd, J.A. (2004). Comparative high-resolution analysis of linkage disequilibrium and tag single nucleotide polymorphisms between populations in the vitamin D receptor gene. *Human Molecular Genetics, 13*, 1633-1339.

[948] Copeman, J.B., Cucca, F., Hearne, C.M., Cornall, R.J., Reed, P.W., Ronningen, K.S., Undlien, D.E., Nistico, L., Buzzetti, R. &Tosi, R. (1995). Linkage disequilibrium mapping of a type 1 diabetes susceptibility gene (IDDM7) to chromosome 2q31-q33. *Nature Genetics, 9*, 80-85.

[949] Owerbach, D., & Gabbay, K.H. (1995). The HOXD8 locus (2q31) is linked to type I diabetes: interaction with chromosome 6 and 11 disease susceptibility genes. *Diabetes, 44*, 132-136.

[950] Luo, D.F., Maclaren, N.K., Huang, H.S., Muir, A. & She, J.X. (1995). Intrafamilial and case-control association analysis of D2S152 in insulin-dependent diabetes. *Autoimmunity, 21*, 143-147.

[951] Luo, D.F., Buzzetti, R., Rotter, J.I., Maclaren, N.K., Raffel, L.J., Nistico, L., Giovannini, C., Pozzilli, P., Thomson, G. & She, J.X. (1996). Confirmation of three susceptibility genes to insulin-dependent diabetes mellitus: IDDM4, IDDM5 and IDDM8. *Human Molecular Genetics, 5*, 693-698.

[952] Esposito, L., Hill, N.J., Pritchard, L.E., Cucca, F., Muxworthy, C., Merriman, M.E., Wilson, A., Julier, C., Delepine, M., Tuomilehto, J., Tuomilehto-Wolf, E., Ionesco-

Tirgoviste, C., Nistico, L., Buzzetti, R., Pozzilli, P. Ferrari, M., Bosi, E., Pociot, F., Nerup, J., Bain, S.C. &Todd, J.A. (1998). Genetic analysis of chromosome 2 in type 1 diabetes: analysis of putative loci IDDM7, IDDM12, and IDDM13 and candidate genes NRAMP1 and IA-2 and the interleukin-1 gene cluster. IMDIAB Group. *Diabetes, 47*, 1797-1799.

[953] Kristiansen, O.P., Pociot, F., Bennett, E.P., Clausen, H., Johannesen, J., Nerup, J. & Mandrup-Poulsen, T. (2000). IDDM7 links to insulin-dependent diabetes mellitus in Danish multiplex families but linkage is not explained by novel polymorphisms in the candidate gene GALNT3. The Danish Study Group of Diabetes in Childhood and The Danish IDDM Epidemiology and Genetics Group. *Human Mutation, 15*, 295-296.

[954] Naya, F.J., Stellrecht, C.M. & Tsai, M.J. (1995). Tissue-specific regulation of the insulin gene by a novel basic helix-loop-helix transcription factor. *Genes and Development, 9*, 1009–1019.

[955] Iwata, I., Nagafuchi, S., Nakashima, H., Kondo, S., Koga, T., Yokogawa, Y., Akashi, T., Shibuya, T., Umeno, Y., Okeda, T., Shibata, S., Kono, S., Yasunami, M., Ohkubo, H. & Niho, Y. (1999). Association of polymorphism in the NeuroD/BETA2 gene with type 1 diabetes in the Japanese. *Diabetes, 48*, 416-419.

[956] Dupont, S., Dina, C., Hani, E.H. & Froguel, P. (1999). Absence of replication in the French population of the association between beta 2/NEUROD-A45T polymorphism and type 1 diabetes. *Diabetes and Metabolism, 25*, 516-517.

[957] Hansen, L., Jensen, J.N., Urioste, S., Petersen H.V., Pociot, F., Eiberg, H., Kristiansen, O.P., Hansen, T., Serup, P., Nerup, J. & Pedersen, O. (2000). NeuroD/BETA2 gene variability and diabetes: no associations to late-onset type 2 diabetes but an A45 allele may represent a susceptibility marker for type 1 diabetes among Danes. Danish Study Group of Diabetes in Childhood, and the Danish IDDM Epidemiology and Genetics Group. *Diabetes, 49*, 876-878.

[958] Malecki, M.T., Klupa, T., Moczulski, D.K. & Rogus, J.J. (2003). The Ala45Thr polymorphism of BETA2/NeuroD1 gene and susceptibility to type 1 diabetes mellitus in caucasians. *Experimental and Clinical Endocrinology and Diabetes, 111*, 251-254.

[959] Reed, P., Cucca, F., Jenkins, S., Merriman, M., Wilson, A., McKinney, P., Bosi, E., Joner, G., Ronningen, K., Thorsby, E., Undlien, D., Merriman, T., Barnett, A., Bain, S. & Todd, J. (1997). Evidence for a type 1 diabetes susceptibility locus (IDDM10) on human chromosome 10p11-q11. *Human Molecular Genetics, 6*, 1011-1016.

[960] Mein, C.A., Esposito, L., Dunn, M.G., Johnson, G.C., Timms, A.E., Goy, J.V., Smith, A.N., Sebag-Montefiore, L., Merriman, M.E., Wilson, A.J., Pritchard, L.E., Cucca, F., Barnett, A.H., Bain, S.C. & Todd, J.A. (1998). A search for type 1 diabetes susceptibility genes in families from the United Kingdom. *Nature Genetics, 19*, 231-214.

[961] Johnson, G.C., Koeleman, B.P. & Todd, J.A. (2002). Limitations of stratifying sib-pair data in common disease linkage studies: an example using chromosome 10p14-10q11 in type 1 diabetes. *American Journal of Medical Genetics, 113*, 158-166.

[962] Chistiakov, D.A., Seryogin, Y., Savostanov, K.V., Zilberman, L.I., Titovich, E.V., Kuraeva, T.L., Dedov, I.I. & Nosikov, V.V. (2004) Evidence for a type 1 diabetes

susceptibility locus (IDDM10) on chromosome 10p11-q11 in a Russian population. *Scandinavian Journal of Immunology, 60*, 316-323.

[963] Nerup, J., Pociot, F. & European Consortium for IDDM Studies. (2001). A genomewide scan for type 1-diabetes susceptibility in Scandinavian families: identification of new loci with evidence of interactions. *American Journal of Human Genetics, 69*, 1301-1313.

[964] Vaessen, N., Heutink, P., Houwing-Duistermaat, J.J., Snijders, P.J., Rademaker, T., Testers, L., Batstra, M.R., Sandkuijl, L.A., van Duijn, C.M. & Oostra, B.A. (2002). Genome-wide search for linkage-disequilibrium with type 1 diabetes in a recent genetically isolated population from the Netherlands. *Diabetes, 51*, 856-859.

[965] Wapelhorst, B., Bell, G.I., Risch, N., Spielman, R.S. & Concannon, P. (1995). Linkage and association studies in insulin-dependent diabetes with a new dinucleotide repeat polymorphism at the GAD65 locus. *Autoimmunity, 21*, 127-130.

[966] Rambrand, T., Pociot, F., Ronningen, K., Nerup, J. & Michelsen, B.K. (1997). Genetic markers for glutamic acid decarboxylase do not predict insulin-dependent diabetes mellitus in pairs of affected siblings. The Danish Study Group of Diabetes in Childhood. *Human Genetics, 99*, 177-185.

[967] Johnson, G.C., Payne, F., Nutland, S., Stevens, H., Tuomilehto-Wolf, E., Tuomilehto, J. & Todd, J.A. (2002). Comprehensive, statistically powered analysis of GAD2 in type 1 diabetes. *Diabetes, 51*, 2866-2870.

[968] Dubois-Laforgue, D., Hendel, H., Caillat-Zucman, S., Zagury, J.F., Winkler, C., Boitard, C. & Timsit, J. (2001). A common stromal cell-derived factor-1 chemokine gene variant is associated with the early onset of type 1 diabetes. *Diabetes, 50*, 1211.

[969] Ide, A., Kawasaki, E., Abiru, N., Sun, F., Fukushima, T., Takahashi, R., Kuwahara, H., Fujita, N., Kita, A., Oshima, K., Uotani, S., Yamasaki, H., Yamaguchi, Y., Kawabata, Y., Fujisawa, T., Ikegami, H. & Eguchi K. (2003). Stromal-cell derived factor-1 chemokine gene variant is associated with type 1 diabetes age at onset in Japanese population. *Human Immunology, 64*, 973-978.

[970] Kawasaki, E., Ide, A., Abiru, N., Kobayashi, M., Fukushima, T., Kuwahara, H., Kita, A., Uotani, S., Yamasaki, H. & Eguchi, K. (2004). Stromal cell-derived factor-1 chemokine gene variant in patients with type 1 diabetes and autoimmune thyroid disease. *Annals of the New York Academy of Sciences, 1037*, 79-83.

[971] Leonard, W.J., Depper, J.M., Kanehisa, M., Kronke, M., Peffer, N.J., Svetlik, P.B., Sullivan, M & Greene, W.C. (1985). Structure of the human interleukin-2 receptor gene. *Science,* 230, 633-639.

[972] Vella, A., Cooper, J.D., Lowe, C.E., Walker, N., Nutland, S., Widmer, B., Jones, R., Ring, S.M., McArdle, W., Pembrey, M.E., Strachan, D.P., Dunger, D.B., Twells, R.C., Clayton, D.G. & Todd JA. (2005). Localization of a type 1 diabetes locus in the IL2RA/CD25 region by use of tag single-nucleotide polymorphisms. *American Journal of Human Genetics, 76*, 773-779.

[973] Podolin, P.L., Wilusz, M.B., Cubbon, R.M., Pajvani, U., Lord, C.J., Todd, J.A., Peterson, L.B., Wicker, L.S. & Lyons, P.A. (2000). Differential glycosylation of interleukin 2, the molecular basis for the NOD Idd3 type 1 diabetes gene? *Cytokine, 12*, 477-482.

[974] Pearson, T., Weiser, P., Markees, T.G., Serreze, D.V., Wicker, L.S., Peterson, L.B., Cumisky, A.M., Shultz, L.D., Mordes, J.P., Rossini, A.A. & Greiner, D.L. (2004). Islet allograft survival induced by costimulation blockade in NOD mice is controlled by allelic variants of Idd3. *Diabetes, 53*, 1972-1978.

[975] Gordon, E.J., Wicker, L.S., Peterson, L.B., Serreze, D.V., Markees, T.G., Shultz, L.D., Rossini, A.A., Greiner, D.L. & Mordes, J.P. (2005). Autoimmune diabetes and resistance to xenograft transplantation tolerance in NOD mice. *Diabetes, 54*, 107-115.

[976] Delepine, M., Pociot, F., Habita, C., Hashimoto, L., Froguel, P., Rotter, J., Cambon-Thomsen, A., Deschamps, I., Djoulah, S., Weissenbach, J., Nerup, J., Lathrop, M. & Julier, C. (1997). Evidence of a non-MHC susceptibility locus in type I diabetes linked to HLA on chromosome 6. *Nature Genetics, 19*, 292-296.

[977] Concannon, P., Gogolin-Ewens, K.J., Hinds, D.A., Wapelhorst, B., Morrison, V.A., Stirling, B., Mitra, M., Farmer, J., Williams, S.R., Cox, N.J., Bell, G.I., Risch, N. & Spielman, R.S. (1998). A second-generation screen of the human genome for susceptibility to insulin-dependent diabetes mellitus. *Nature Genetics, 19*, 292-296.

[978] Barber MJ, Todd JA, Cordell HJ. (2006). A multimarker regression-based test of linkage for affected sib-pairs at two linked loci. Genetic Epidemiology, 30, 191-208.

[979] Chistiakov, D.A., Chernisheva, A., Savost'anov, K.V., Turakulov, R.I., Kuraeva, T.L., Dedov, I.I., Nosikov, V.V. (2005). Lack of association between genetic markers on chromosome 16q22-Q24 and type 1 diabetes in Russian affected families. *Croatian Medical Journal, 46*, 670-677.

[980] Hirai, K., Suzuki, S., Kasuga, S. & Chiba, M. (1998). Association of DT-diaphorase Pro187Ser mutation with insulin-dependent diabetes mellitus in Japanese. *Diabetes, 47*, 696.

[981] Kadlubar, F.F., Anderson, K.E.,Haussermann, S., Lang, N.P., Barone, G.W.,Thompson, P.A., MacLeod, S.L., Chou, M.W., Mikhailova, M., Plastaras, J., Marnett, L.J., Nair, J., Velic, I. & Bartsch, H. (1998). Comparison of DNA adduct levels associated with oxidative stress in human pancreas. *Mutation Research, 405*, 125-133.

[982] Kristiansen, O.P., Larsen, Z.M., Johannesen, J., Nerup, J., Mandrup-Poulsen, T. & Pociot, F. (1999). No linkage of P187S polymorphism in NAD(P)H:quinone oxidoreductase (NQO1/DIA4)and type 1 diabetes in the Danish population. DIEGG and DSGD. Danish IDDM Epidemiology and Genetics Group and The Danish Study Group of Diabetes in Childhood. *Human Mutation, 14*, 67-70.

[983] King, A.L., Yiannakou, J.Y.,Brett, P.M.,Curtis, D., Morris, M.A., Dearlove, A.M., Rhodes, M., Rosen-Bronson, S., Mathew, C., Ellis, H.J. & Ciclitira, P.J. (2000). A genome-wide family-based link- age study of coeliac disease. *Annals of Human Genetics, 64*, 479-490.

[984] Ober, C., Tsalenko, A. Parry, R. & Cox, N.J. (2000). A second-generation genomewide screen for asthma-susceptibility alleles in a founder population. *American Journal of Human Genetics, 67*, 1154-1162.

[985] Fisher, S.A., Lanchbury, J.S. & Lewis, C.M (2003). Meta-analysis of four rheumatoid arthritis genome-wide linkage: confirmation of a susceptibility locus on chromosome 16. *Arthritis and Rheumatism, 48*, 1200-206.

[986] van Tilburg, J.H., Sandkuijl, L.A., Strengman, E., van Someren, H., Rigters-Aris, C.A., Pearson, P.L., van Haeften, T.W. & Wijmenga, C. (2003). A genome-wide scan in type 2 diabetes mellitus provides independent replication of a susceptibility locus on 18p11 and suggests the existence of novel Loci on 2q12 and 19q13. *Journal of Clinical Endocrinology and Metabolism, 88*, 2223-2230.

[987] Chen, C.H., Chang, C.J., Yang, W.S., Chen, C.L. & Fann, C.S. (2003). A genome-wide scan using tree-based association analysis for candidate loci related to fasting plasma glucose levels. *BMC Genetics*, 4:S65.

[988] An, P., Freedman, B.I., Hanis, C.L., Chen, Y.D., Weder, A.B., Schork, N.J., Boerwinkle, E., Province, M.A., Hsiung, C.A., Wu, X., Quertermous, T. & Rao, D.C. (2005). Genome-wide linkage scans for fasting glucose, insulin, and insulin resistance in the National Heart, Lung, and Blood Institute Family Blood Pressure Program: evidence of linkages to chromosome 7q36 and 19q13 from meta-analysis. *Diabetes, 54*, 909-914.

[989] Groop, L.C., Kankuri, M., Schalin-Jantti, C., Ekstrand, A., Nikula-Ijas, P., Widen, E., Kuismanen, E., Eriksson, J., Franssila-Kallunki, A. & Saloranta, C. (1993). Association between polymorphism of the glycogen synthase gene and non-insulin-dependent diabetes mellitus. *New England Journal of Medicine, 328*, 10-14.

[990] Majer, M., Mott, D.M., Mochizuki, H., Rowles, J.C., Pedersen, O., Knowler, W.C., Bogardus, C. & Prochazka, M. (1996). Association of the glycogen synthase locus on 19q13 with NIDDM in Pima Indians. *Diabetologia, 39*, 314-321.

[991] Orho-Melander, M., Almgren, P., Kanninen, T., Forsblom, C. & Groop, L.C. (1999). A paired-sibling analysis of the XbaI polymorphism in the muscle glycogen synthase gene. *Diabetologia, 42*, 1138-1145.

[992] Study Group for the Identification of Type 2 Diabetes Genes in Japanese (2000). The Met416-->Val variant in the glycogen synthase gene: the prevalence and the association with diabetes in a large number of Japanese individuals. *Diabetes Care, 23*, 1709-1710.

[993] Naumova, A.K., Leppert, M., Barker, D.F., Morgan, K. & Sapienza, C. (1998) Parental origin-dependent, male offspring-specific transmission-ratio distortion at loci on the human X chromosome. *American Journal of Human Genetics, 62*, 1493–1499.

[994] Zavattari, P., Esposito, L., Nutland, S., Todd, J.A. & Cucca, F. (2000). Transmission-ratio distortion at Xp11.4-p21.1 in type 1 diabetes. *American Journal of Human Genetics, 66*, 330-332.

[995] Todd, J.A. (2006). Statistical false positive or true disease pathway? *Nature Genetics, 38*, 731-733.

[996] Smyth, D.J., Cooper, J.D., Bailey, R., Field, S., Burren, O., Smink, L.J., Guja, C., Ionescu-Tirgoviste, C., Widmer, B., Dunger, D.B., Savage, D.A., Walker, N.M., Clayton, D.G. & Todd, J.A. (2006). A genome-wide association study of nonsynonymous SNPs identifies a type 1 diabetes locus in the interferon-induced helicase (IFIH1) region. *Nature Genetics, 38*, 617-619.

[997] Kang, D.C., Gopalkrishnan, R.V., Wu, Q., Jankowsky, E., Pyle, A.M. & Fisher, P.B. (2002). Mda-5: an interferon-inducible putative RNA helicase with double-stranded

RNA-dependent ATPase activity and melanoma growth-suppressive properties. *Proceedings of the National Academy of Sciences of USA 99*, 637-642.

[998] Yui, M.A. & Rothenberg, E.V. (2004). Deranged early T cell development in immunodeficient strains of nonobese diabetic mice. *Journal of Immunology, 173*, 5381-5391.

[999] Teutsch, S.M., Booth, D.R., Bennetts, B.H., Heard, R.N. & Stewart, G.J. (2003). Identification of 11 novel and common single nucleotide polymorphisms in the interleukin-7 receptor-alpha gene and their associations with multiple sclerosis. *European Journal of Human Genetics, 11*, 509-515.

[1000] Booth, D.R., Arthur, A.T., Teutsch, S.M., Bye, C., Rubio, J., Armati, P.J., Pollard, J.D., Heard, R.N. & Stewart, G.J.; The Southern MS Genetics Consortium (2005). Gene expression and genotyping studies implicate the interleukin 7 receptor in the pathogenesis of primary progressive multiple sclerosis. *Journal of Molecular Medicine, 83*, 822-830.

[1001] Dittmar, M. & Kanaly, G.J. (2005). Polyglandular autoimmune syndromes: immunogenetics and long-term follow-up. *Journal of Clinical Endocrinology and Metabolism, 88*, 1983-2992.

[1002] Betterle, C., Greggio, N.A. & Volpato, M. (1998) Clinical review 93: autoimmune polyglandular syndrome type 1. *Journal of Clinical Endocrinology and Metabolism, 83*, 1049-1055.

[1003] Betterle, C., Volpato, M., Greggio, A.N. & Presotto, F. (1996). Type 2 polyglandular autoimmune disease (Schmidt's syndrome). *Journal of Pediatric Endocrinology Metabolism, 9*, 113-123.

[1004] Bjorses, P., Aaltonen, J., Horelli-Kuitunen, N., Yaspo, M.L. & Peltonen, L. (1998). Gene defect behind APECED: a new clue to autoimmunity. *Human Molecular Genetics, 7*, 1547-1553.

[1005] The Finnish-German APECED Consortium (1997). An autoimmune disease, APECED, caused by mutations in a novel gene featuring two PHD-type zinc-finger domains. Autoimmune Polyendocrinopathy-Candidiasis-Ectodermal Dystrophy. *Nature Genetics, 17*, 399-403.

[1006] Pearce, S.H., Cheetham, T., Imrie, H., Vaidya, B., Barnes, N.D., Bilous, R.W., Carr, D., Meeran, K., Shaw, N.J., Smith, C.S., Toft, A.D. Williams, G. & Kendall-Taylor, P. (1998). A common and recurrent 13-bp deletion in the autoimmune regulator gene in British kindreds with autoimmune polyendocrinopathy type 1. *American Journal of Human Genetics, 63*, 1675-1684.

[1007] Meyer, G., Donner, H., Herwig, J., Bohles, H., Usadel, K.H. & Badenhoop, K. (2001). Screening for an AIRE-1 mutation in patients with Addison's disease, type 1 diabetes, Graves' disease and Hashimoto's thyroiditis as well as in APECED syndrome. *Clinical Endocrinology (Oxford), 54*, 335-338.

[1008] Partanen, J., Peterson, P., Westman, P., Aranko, S. & Krohn, K. (1994). Major histocompatibility complex class II and III in Addison's disease. MHC alleles do not predict autoantibody specificity and 21-hydroxylase gene polymorphism has no independent role in disease susceptibility. *Human Immunology, 41*, 135-140.

[1009]Cofie, D.Q., Rogers, R., Draelos, M.T., Olansky, L. & Scofield, R.H. (1995). Syndrome of type II polyglandular autoimmunity associated with HLA-DR4 in a large kindred, including HLA-DR3/DR4 heterozygosity in the probands, identical twins with identical manifestations. *Endocrine Practice, 1*, 395-398.

[1010]Huang, W., Connor, E., Rosa, T.D., Muir, A., Schatz, D., Silverstein, J., Crockett, S., She, J.X. & Maclaren, N.K. (1996). Although DR3-DQB1*0201 may be associated with multiple component diseases of the autoimmune polyglandular syndromes, the human leukocyte antigen DR4-DQB1*0302 haplotype is implicated only in beta-cell autoimmunity. *Journal of Clinical Endocrinology and Metabolism, 81*, 2559-2563.

[1011]Wallaschowski, H., Meyer, A., Tuschy, U. & Lohmann, T. (2003). HLA-DQA1*0301-associated susceptibility for autoimmune polyglandular syndrome type II and III. *Hormone and Metabolic Research, 35*, 120-124.

[1012]Takamatsu, K., Nishiyama, T., Nakauchi, Y., Yamano, T. & Ohno, F. (1989). A case of insulin dependent diabetes mellitus associated with relapsing polychondritis, Hashimoto's thyroiditis and pituitary adrenocortical insufficiency in succession. *Japan Journal of Medicine, 28*, 232-236.

[1013]Myhre, A.G., Undlien, D.E., Lovas, K., Uhlving, S., Nedrebo, B.G., Fougner, K.J., Trovik, T., Sorheim, J.L. & Husebye, E.S. (2002). Autoimmune adrenocortical failure in Norway autoantibodies and human leukocyte antigen class II associations related to clinical features. *Journal of Clinical Endocrinology and Metabolism, 87*, 618-823.

[1014]Kemp, E.H., Ajjan, R.A., Husebye, E.S., Peterson, P., Uibo, R., Imrie, H., Pearce, S.H., Watson, P.F. & Weetman, A.P. (1998) A cytotoxic T lymphocyte antigen-4 (CTLA-4) gene polymorphism is associated with autoimmune Addison's disease in English patients. *Clinical Endocrinology (Oxford), 49*, 609-613.

[1015]Vaidya, B., Imrie, H., Geatch, D.R., Perros, P., Ball, S.G., Baylis, P.H., Carr, D., Hurel, S.J., James, R.A., Kelly, W.F., Kemp, E.H., Young, E.T., Weetman, A.P., Kendall-Taylor, P. & Pearce, S.H. (2000) Association analysis of the cytotoxic T lymphocyte antigen-4 (CTLA-4) and autoimmune regulator-1 (AIRE-1) genes in sporadic autoimmune Addison's disease. *Journal of Clinical Endocrinology and Metabolism, 85*, 688-689.

[1016]Kemp, E.H., Ajjan, R.A., Waterman, E.A., Gawkrodger, D.J., Cork, M.J., Watson, P.F. & Weetman, A.P. (1999). Analysis of a microsatellite polymorphism of the cytotoxic T-lymphocyte antigen-4 gene in patients with vitiligo, *British Journal of Dermatology, 140*, 73–78.

[1017]Einarsdottir, E., Soderstrom, I., Logfren-Burstrom, A., Haraldsson, S., Nillson-Qrdnor, S., Penha-Goncalves, C., Lind, L., Holmgren, G., Holmsberg, M., Asplund, K. & Holmsberg, D. (2003). The CTLA4 region as a general autoimmunity factor: an extended pedigree provides evidence for synergy with the HLA locus in the etiology of type 1 diabetes mellitus, Hashimoto's thyroiditis and Graves' disease. *European Journal of Human Genetics, 11*, 81-84.

[1018]Jenkins, R.C. & Weetman, A.P. (2002). Disease associations with autoimmune thyroid disease. *Thyroid, 12*, 977-988.

[1019]Hollowell, J.G., Staehling, N.W., Flanders, W.D., Hannon, W.H., Gunter, E.W., Spencer, C.A. & Braverman, L.E. (2002). Serum TSH, T_4, and thyroid antibodies in the United States population (1988 to 1994): National Health and Nutrition Examination Survey (NHANES III). *Journal of Clinical Endocrinology and Metabolism, 87*, 489-499.

[1020]Ai, J., Leonhardt, J.M. & Heymann, W.R. (2003). Autoimmune thyroid diseases: etiology, pathogenesis, and dermatologic manifestations. *Journal of American Academy of Dermatology, 48*, 641-662.

[1021]Holl, R.W., Bohm, B., Loos, U., Grabert, M., Heinze, E. & Homoki, J. (1999). Thyroid autoimmunity in children and adolescents with type 1 diabetes mellitus. Effect of age, gender and HLA type. *Hormone Research, 52*, 113-118.

[1022]De Block, C.E., De Leeuw, I.H., Vertommen, J.J., Rooman, R.P., Du Caju, M.V., Van Campenhout, C.M., Weyler, J.J., Winnock, F., Van Autreve, J. & Gorus F.K.; Belgian Diabetes Registry (2001). Beta-cell, thyroid, gastric, adrenal and coeliac autoimmunity and HLA-DQ types in type 1 diabetes. *Clinical and Experimental Immunology, 126*, 236-241.

[1023]Kordonouri, O., Klinghammer, A., Lang, E.B., Gruters-Kieslich, A., Grabert, M. & Holl, R.W. (2002). Thyroid autoimmunity in children and adolescents with type 1 diabetes: a multicenter survey. *Diabetes Care 25*, 1346-1350.

[1024]Kucera, P., Novakova, D., Beharova, M., Novak, J., Tlaskalova-Hogenova, H. & Andel, M. (2003). Gliadin, endomysial and thyroid antibodies in patients with latent autoimmune diabetes in adults. *Clinical and Experimental Immunology, 133*, 139-143.

[1025]Vondra, K., Vrbikova, J. & Dvorakova, K. (2005). Thyroid gland diseases in adult patients with diabetes mellitus. *Minerva Endocrinology, 30*, 217-236.

[1026]Maclaren, N.K. & Riley, W.J. (1985). Thyroid, gastric, and adrenal autoimmunities associated with insulin-dependent diabetes mellitus. *Diabetes Care, 8*, 34-38.

[1027]Hansen, D., Bennebaek, F.N., Hoier-Madsen, M., Hegedus, L. Jacobsen, B.B. (2003). A prospective study of thyroid function, morphology and autoimmunity in young patients with type 1 diabetes. *European Journal of Endocrinology, 148*, 245-251.

[1028]Robert, P., Gallas, J., Stolk, R.P., Bakker, K., Endert, E. & Wiesinga, W.M. (2002). Thyroid dysfuncation during pregnancy and in the first pospartum year in women with diabetes mellitus type 1. *European Journal of Endocrinology, 147*, 443-451.

[1029]Burek, C.L., Rose, N.R., Guire, K.E. & Hoffman, W.H. (1990). Thyroid autoantibodies in black and in white children and adolescents with type 1 diabetes mellitus and their first-degree relatives. *Autoimmunity, 7*, 157-167.

[1030]Maugendre, D., Verite, F., Guilhem, I., Genetet, B., Allanic, H. & Delamaire, H. (1997). Anti-pancreatic autoimmunity and Graves' disease: study of a cohort of 600 Caucasian patients. *European Journal of Endocrinology, 137*, 503-510.

[1031]Silva, R.S., Sallorenzo, C., Kater, C.E., Dib, S.A. & Falorni, A. (2003). Autoantibodies against glutamic acid decarboxylase and 21-hydroxylase in Brazilian patients with type 1 diabetes or autoimmune thyroid diseases. *Diabetes Nutrition and Metabolism, 16*, 160-168.

[1032]Sumnik, Z., Drevinek, P., Snajderova, M., Krolouskova, S., Sedlakova, P., Pechova, M., Vavrinec, J. & Cinek, O. (2003). HLA-DQ polymorphisms modify the risk of thyroid autoimmunity in children with type 1 diabetes mellitus. *Journal of Pediatric Endocrinology and Metabolism, 16*, 851-858.

[1033]Tait, K.F., Marshall, T., Berman, J., Carr-Smith, J., Rowe, B., Todd, J.A., Bain, S.C., Barnett, A.H. & Gough, S.C. (2004). Clustering of autoimmune disease in parents of siblings from the Type 1 diabetes Warren repository. *Diabetic Medicine, 21*, 358-362.

[1034]Hanukoglu, A., Mizrachi, A., Dalai, I., Admoni, O., Rakover, Y., Bistritzer, Z., Levine, A., Somekh, E., Lehmann, D., Tuval, M., Boaz, M. & Golander, A. (2003). Extrapancreatic autoimmune manifestations in type 1 diabetes patients and their first-degree relatives: a multicenter study. *Diabetes Care, 26*, 1235-1240.

[1035]Devendra, D., & Eisenbarth, G.S. (2003). 17. Immunologic endocrine disorders. *Journal of Allergy and Clinical Immunology, 111 (Suppl.2)*, S624-S636.

[1036]Larsen, C.E. & Alper, C.A. (2004). The genetics of HLA-associated disease. *Current Opinion in Immunology, 16*, 660-667.

[1037]Levin, L. & Tomer, Y. (2003). The etiology of autoimmune diabetes and thyroiditis: evidence for common genetic susceptibility. *Autoimmunity Reviews, 2*, 377-386.

[1038]Moens, H., Farid, N.R., Sampson, L., Noel, E.L. & Barnard, J.M. (1978). Hashimoto's thyroiditis is associated with HLA-DRw3. *New England Journal of Medicine, 299*, 133–134.

[1039]Tandon, N., Zhang, L. & Weetman, A.P. (1991). HLA associations with Hashimoto's thyroiditis. *Clinical Endocrinology (Oxford), 34*, 383–386.

[1040]Ban, Y., Davies, T.F., Greenberg, D.A., Concepcion, E.S. & Tomer, Y. (2002). The influence of human leukocyte antigen (HLA) genes on autoimmune thyroid disease (AITD): results of studies in HLA-DR3 positive AITD families. *Clinical Endocrinology (Oxford), 57*, 81–88.

[1041]Gonzales-Trevino, O., Yamamoto-Furusho, J.K. & Cutino-Moguel, T. (2005). Genetic analysis of families with autoimmune disabetes and thyroiditis; evidence for common and unique genes. *Journal of Clinical Endocrinology and Metabolism, 90*, 4904-4911.

[1042]Kong, Y.C., Lomo, L.C. & Motte, R.W. (1996). HLA-DRB1 polymorphism determines susceptibility to autoimmune thyroiditis in transgenic mice: definitive association with HLA-DRB1*0301 (DR3) gene. *Journal of Experimental Medicine, 184*, 1167-1172.

[1043]Flynn, J.C., Wan, Q., Panos, J.C., McCormick, D.J., Giraldo, A.A., David, C.S. & Kong, Y.C. (2002). Coexpression of susceptible and resistant HLA class II transgenes in murine experimental autoimmune thyroiditis: DQ8 molecules downregulate DR3-mediated thyroiditis. *Journal of Autoimmunity, 18*, 213-220.

[1044]Deschamps, I., Beressi, J.P., Khalil, I., Robert, J.J. & Hors, J. (1991). The role of genetic predisposition to type I (insulin-dependent) diabetes mellitus. *Annals of Medicine, 23*, 427-435.

[1045]Marsh, S.G., Albert, E.D., Bodmer, W.F., Bontrop, R.E., Dupont, B., Erlich, H.A., Geraghty, D.E., Hansen, J.A., Hurley, C.K., Mach, B., Mayr, W.R., Parham, P., Petersdorf, E.W., Sasazuki, T., Schreuder, G.M., Strominger, J.L., Svejgaard, A., Terasaki, P.I. & Trowsdale, J. (2005). Nomenclature for factors of the HLA system, 2004. *Tissue Antigens, 65*, 301-369.

[1046]Ban, Y., Davies, T.F., Greenberg, D.A., Concepcion, E.S., Osman, R., Oashi, T. & Tomer, Y. (2004). Arginine at position 74 of the HLA-DR β1 chain is associated with Graves' disease. *Genes and Immunity, 5*, 203-208.

[1047] Simmonds, M.J., Howson, J.M., Heward, J.M., Cordell, H.J., Foxall, J. Carr-Smith, J., Gibson, S.M., Walker, N., Tomer, Y., Franklyn, J.A., Todd, J.A. & Gough, S.C. (2005). Regression mapping of association between the human leukocyte antigen region and Graves disease. *American Journal of Human Genetics, 76*, 157-163.

[1048] Orhan, Y., Azezli, A., Carin, M., Aral, F., Sencer, E. & Molvalivar, S. (1993). Human lymphocyte antigens (HLA) and Graves' disease in Turkey. *Journal of Clinical Immunology, 13*, 339-343.

[1049] Chen, Q.Y., Huang, W., She, J.X , Baxter, F., Volpe, R. & Maclaren, N.K. (1999). HLA-DRB1*08, DRB1*03/DRB3*0101, and DRB3*0202 are susceptibility genes for Graves' disease in North American Caucasians, whereas DRB1*07 is protective. *Journal of Clinical Endocrinology and Metabolism, 84*, 3182-3186.

[1050] Sumnik, Z., Drevinek, P., Snajderova, M., Kolouskova, S., Sedlakova, P., Pechova, M., Vavrinec, J. & Cinek, O. (2003). HLA-DQ polymorphisms modify the risk of thyroid autoimmunity in children with type 1 diabetes mellitus. *Journal of Pediatric Endocrinology and Metabolism, 16*, 851-858.

[1051] Awata, T., Katsuren, E., Matsumoto, C., Nagayama, I., Uchigata, Y., Kuzuya, N. & Kanazawa, K. (1995). Absence of shared HLA class II (DR, DQ)-linked genetic basis between IDDM and autoimmune thyroid disease in Japanese, *Diabetes Care, 18*, 582-583.

[1052] Djilali-Saiah, I., Bertin, E., Larger, E., Timsit, J., Assan, R., Boitard, C., Bach, J.F. & Caillat-Zucman S. (1998). Major histocompatibility class II genes polymorphism in insulin dependent diabetes mellitus with or without associated thyroid autoimmunity. *Human Immunology, 59*, 176-182.

[1053] Chikuba, N., Akazawa, S., Yamaguchi, Y., Kawasaki, E., Takino, H., Yoshimoto, M., Ohe, N., Yamashita, K., Yano, A. & Nagataki, S. (1995). Immunogenetic heterogeneity in type 1 (insulin-dependent) diabetes among Japanese - class II antigen and autoimmune thyroid disease. *Diabetes Research and Clinical Practice, 27*, 31-37.

[1054] Chuang, L.M., Wu, H.P., Chang, C.C., Tsai, M.W , Chang, H.M., Tai, T.Y. & Lin, B.J. (1996). HLA DRB1/DQA1/DQB1 haplotype determines thyroid autoimmunity in patients with insulin-dependent diabetes mellitus. *Clinical Endocrinology (Oxford), 45*, 631-636.

[1055] Kim, E.Y., Shin, C.H. & Yang, S.W. (2003). Polymorphisms of HLA class II predispose children and adolescents with type 1 diabetes mellitus to autoimmune thyroid disease. *Autoimmunity, 36*, 177-181.

[1056] Santamaria, P., Barbosa, J.J., Lindstrom, A.L., Lemke, T.A., Goetz, F.C. & Rich, S.S. (1994). HLA-DQB1-asociated susceptibility that distinguishes Hashimoto's thyroiditis from Graves' disease in type 1 diabetic patients. *Journal of Clinical Endocrinology and Metabolism, 78*, 878-883.

[1057] Payami, H., Joe, S. & Thomson, G. (1989). Autoimmune thyroid disease in Type 1 diabetes. *Genetic Epidemiology, 6*, 137-141.

[1058] Torfs, C.P., King, M.C., Bing, H , Malmgren, J. & Grumet, F.C. (1986). Genetic interrelationship between insulin-dependent diabetes mellitus, the autoimmune thyroid diseases and rheumatoid arthritis. *American Journal of Human Genetics, 38*, 170-187.

[1059]Levin, L., Ban, Y., Concepcion, E., Davies, T.F., Greenberg, D.A. & Tomer, Y. (2004). Analysis of HLA genes in families with autoimmune diabetes and thyroiditis. *Human Immunology, 65*, 640-647.

[1060]Golden, B., Levin, L., Ban, Y., Concepcion, E., Greenberg, D.A. & Tomer, Y. (2005). Genetic analysis of families with autoimmune disabetes and thyroiditis; evidence for common and unique genes. *Journal of Clinical Endocrinology and Metabolism, 90*, 4904-4911.

[1061]Vaidya, B. & Pearce, S. (2004). The emerging role of the CTLA-4 gene in autoimmune endocrinopathies. *European Journal of Endocrinology, 150*, 619-626.

[1062]Donner, H., Rau, H., Walfish, P.G., Braun, J., Siegmund, T., Finke, R., Herwig, J., Usadel, K.H. & Badenhoop, K. (1997). CTLA4 alanine-17 confers genetic susceptibility to Graves' disease and to type 1 diabetes mellitus. *Journal of Clinical Endocrinology and Metabolism, 82*, 143-146.

[1063]Takara, M., Komiya, I., Kinio, Y., Tomoyose, T., Yamashiro, S., Akamine, H., Masuda, M. & Takasu, N. (2000). Association of CTLA-4 gene A/G polymorphism in Japanese type 1 diabetic patients with younger age of onset and autoimmune thyroid disease. *Diabetes Care, 23*, 975-978.

[1064]Mochizuki, M., Amemiya, S., Kobayashi, K., Kobayashi, K., Shimura, Y., Ishihara T., Nakagomi, Y., Onigata, K., Tamai, S., Kasuga, A. & Nanazawa, S. (2003). Association of the CTLA-4 gene 49 A/G polymorphism with type 1 diabetes and autoimmune thyroid disease in Japanese children. *Diabetes Care, 26*, 843-847.

[1065]Oaks, M.K. & Hallett, K.M. (2000). Cutting edge: a soluble form of CTLA-4 in patients with autoimmune thyroid disease. *Journal of Immunology, 164*, 568-572.

[1066]Velaga, M.R., Wilson, V., Jennings, C.E., Owen, C.J., Herington, S., Donaldson, P.T., Ball, S.G., James, R.A., Quinton, R., Perros, P. & Pearce, S.H. (2004). The codon 620 tryptophan allele of the lymphoid tyrosine phosphatase (LYP) gene is a major determinant of Graves' disease. *Journal of Clinical Endocrinology and Metabolism, 89*, 5862-5865.

[1067]Skorka, A., Bednarczuk, T., Bar-Andziak, E., Nauman, J. & Ploski, R. (2005). Lymphoid tyrosine phosphatase (PTPN22/LYP) variant and Graves' disease in a Polish population: association and gene dose-dependent correlation with age of onset. *Clinical Endocrinology (Oxford), 62*, 679-682.

[1068]Ban, Y., Tozaki, T., Taniyama, M., Tomita, M. & Ban, Y. (2005). The codon 620 single nucleotide polymorphism of the protein tyrosine phosphatase-22 gene does not contribute to autoimmune thyroid disease susceptibility in the Japanese. *Thyroid, 15*, 1115-1118.

[1069]Imrie, H., Vaidya, B., Perros, P., Kelly, W.F., Toft, A.D., Young, E.T., Kendall-Taylor, P. & Pearce, S.H. (2001). Evidence for a Graves' disease susceptibility locus at chromosome Xp11 in a United Kingdom population. *Journal of Clinical Endocrinology and Metabolism, 86*, 626-630.

[1070]Lind, P., Landsteger, W., Molnar, M., Gallowitsch, H.J., Mikosch, P. & Gomez, I. (1998). Epidemiology of thyroid diseases in iodine sufficiency. *Thyroid, 8*, 1179-1183.

[1071]Taylor, J.C., Gough, S.C., Hunt, P.J., Brix, T.H., Chatterjee, K., Connell, J.M., Franklyn, A., Hedegus, L., Robinson, B.G., Wiersinga, W.M., Wass, J.A., Zabaneh,

D., Mackay, I. & Weetman, A.P. (2006). A genome-wide screen in 1,119 relative pairs with autoimmune thyroid disease. *Journal of Clinical Endocrinology and Metabolism, 91*, 646-653.

[1072]Gangloff, S.C. & Guenounou, M. (2004). Toll-like receptors and immune response in allergic disease. *Clinical Reviews in Allergy and Immunology 26*, 115-125.

[1073]Sakai, K., Shirasawa, S., Ishikawa, N., Ito, K., Tamai, H., Kuma, K., Akamizu, T., Tanimura, M., Furugaki, K., Yamamoto, K. & Sasazuki, T. (2001). Identification of susceptibility loci for autoimmune thyroid disease to 5q31-q33 and Hashimoto's thyroiditis to 8q23-q24 by multipoint affected sib-pair linkage analysis in Japanese. *Human Molecular Genetics, 10*, 1379-1386.

[1074]Akamizu, T., Hiratani, H., Ikegami, S., Rich, S. & Bowden, D.W. (2003). Association study of autoimmune thyroid disease at 5q23-q33 in Japanese patients, *Journal of Human Genetics, 48*, 236-242.

[1075]Jin, Y., Teng, W., Ben, S., Xiong, X., Zhang, J., Xu, S., Shugart, Y.Y., Jin, L., Chen, J. & Huang, W. (2003). Genome-wide scan of Graves' disease: evidence for linkage on chromosome 5q31 in Chinese Han pedigrees. *Journal of Clinical Endocrinology and Metabolism, 88*, 1798-1803.

[1076]Morahan, G., Huang, D., Ymer, S.I., Cancilla, M.R., Stephen, K., Dabadghao, P., Werther, G., Tait, B.D., Harrison, L.C. & Colman, P.G. (2001). Linkage disequilibrium of a type 1 diabetes susceptibility locus with a regulatory IL12B allele. *Nature Genetics, 27*, 218-221.

[1077]Vitoria, J.C., Castano, L., Rica, I., Bilbao, J.R., Arrieta, A. & Garcia-Masdevall, M.D. (1998). Association of insulin-dependent diabetes mellitus and celiac disease: a study based on serologic markers. *Journal of Pediatric Gastroenterology and Nutrition, 27*, 47-52.

[1078]Carlsson, A.K., Axelsson, I.E., Borulf, S.K., Bredberg, A.C., Lindberg, B.A., Sjoberg, K.G. & Ivarsson, S.A. (1999). Prevalence of IgA-antiendomysium and IgA-antigliadin autoantibodies at diagnosis of insulin-dependent diabetes mellitus in Swedish children and adolescents. *Pediatrics, 103*, 1248-1252.

[1079]Aktay, A.N., Lee, P.C., Kumar, V., Parton, E., Wyatt, D.T. & Werlin, S.L. (2001). The prevalence and clinical characteristics of celiac disease in juvenile diabetes in Wisconsin. *Journal of Pediatric Gastroenterology and Nutrition, 33*, 462-465.

[1080]Barera, G., Bonfanti, R., Viscardi, M., Bazzigaluppi, E., Calori, G., Meschi, F., Bianchi, C. & Chiumello, G. (2002). Occurrence of celiac disease after onset of type 1 diabetes: a 6-year prospective longitudinal study. *Pediatrics, 109*, 833-838.

[1081]Williams, A.J., Norcross, A.J., Lock, R.J., Unsworth, D.J., Gale, E.A. & Bingley, P.J. (2001). The high prevalence of autoantibodies to tissue transglutaminase in first-degree relatives of patients with type 1 diabetes is not associated with islet autoimmunity. *Diabetes Care, 24*, 504-509.

[1082]Dewar, D.H. & Ciclitira, P.J. (2005). Clinical features and diagnosis of celiac disease. *Gastroenterology, 128 (Suppl.1)*, S19-S24.

[1083]Dieterich, W., Laag, E., Schopper, H., Volta, U., Ferguson, A., Gilett, H., Riecken, E.O. & Schuppan, D (1998). Autoantibodies to tissue transglutaminase as predictors of celiac disease. *Gastroenterology, 115*, 1317-1321.

[1084]Bao, F., Yu, L., Babu, S., Hoffenberg, E.J., Rewers, M. & Eisenbarth, G.S. (1999). One third of HLA DQ2 homozygous patients with type 1 diabetes express celiac disease-associated transglutaminase autoantibodies. *Journal of Autoimmunity, 13*, 143-148.

[1085]Schuppan, D. & Hahn, E.G. (2001). Celiac disease and its link to type 1 diabetes mellitus. *Journal of Pediatric Endocrinology and Metabolism, 14*, 597-605.

[1086]Fasano, A. & Shea-Donohue, T. (2005). Mechanisms of disease: the role of intestinal barrier function in the pathogenesis of gastrointestinal autoimmune diseases. *Gastroenterology and Hepathology, 2*, 416-422.

[1087]Petronzelli, F., Bonamico, M., Ferrante, P., Grillo, R., Mora, B., Mariani, P., Apollonio, I., Gemme, G. & Mazzilli, M.C. (1997). Genetic contribution of the HLA region to the familial clustering of coeliac disease. *Annals of Human Genetics, 61*, 307-317.

[1088]Hue, S., Monteiro, R.C., Berrih-Aknin, S. & Caillat-Zucman, S. (2003). Potential role of NKG2D/MHC class I-related chain Aonteraction in intrathymic maturation of single-positive CD8 T cells. *Journal of Immunology, 171*, 1909-1917.

[1089]Gupta, M., Nikitina-Zake, L., Zarghami, M., Landin-Olsson, M., Kockum, I., Lernmark, A. & Sanjeevi, C.B. (2003). Association between the transmembrane polymorphism of MHC class I chain-related gene A (MICA-A) and type 1 diabetes mellitus in Sweden. *Human Immunology, 64*, 553-561.

[1090]Zake. L.N., Ghaderi, M., Park, Y.S., Babu, S., Eisenbarth, G., Sanjjevi, C.B. (2002). MHC class I chain-related gene alleles 5 and 5.1 are transmitted more frequently to type 1 diabetes offspring in HBDI families. *Annals of New York Academy of Sciences. 958*, 309-311.

[1091]Bilbao, J.R., Martin-Pagola, A., Vitoria, J.C., Zubillaga, P., Ortiz, L. & Castano, L. (2002). HLA-DRB1 and MHC class I chain-related A haplotypes in Basque families with celiac disease. *Tissue Antigens, 60*, 71-76.

[1092]Rueda, B., Pascual, M., Lopez-Nevot, M.A., Koeleman, B.P., Ortega, E. , Maldonado, J., Lopez, M & Martin, J. (2003). Association of MICA-A5.1 allele with susceptibility to celiac disease in a family study. *American Journal of Gastroenterology, 98*, 359-362.

[1093]Naluai, A.T., Nilsson ,S., Samuelsson, L., Gudjonsdottir, A.H., Ascher, H., Ek, J., Hallberg, B., Kristiansson, B., Martinsson, T., Nerman, O., Sollid, L.M. & Wahlstrom, J. (2000). The CTLA4/CD28 gene region on chromosome 2q33 confers susceptibility to celiac disease in a way possibly distinct from that of type 1 diabetes and other chronic inflammatory disorders. *Tissue Antigens, 56*, 350-355.

[1094]Zhernakova, A., Eerligh, P., Barrera, P., Weseloy, J.Z., Huizinga, T.W., Roep, B.O., Wijmenga, C. & Koeleman, B.P. (2005). CTLA4 is differentially associated with autoimmune diseases in the Dutch population. *Human Genetics, 118*, 58-66.

[1095]Yu, L., Brewer, K.W., Gates, S., Wu, A., Wang, T., Babu, S.R., Gottlieb, P.A., Freed, B.M., Noble, J., Erlich, H.A., Rewers, M.J. & Eisenbarth, G.S. (1999). DRB1*04 and DQ alleles: expression of 21-hydroxylase autoantibodies and risk of progression to Addison's disease. *Journal of Clinical Endocrinology and Metabolism, 84*, 328-335.

[1096]Barker, J.M., Ide, A., Hostetler, C., Yu, L., Miao, D., Fain, P.R., Eisenbarth, G.S. & Gottlieb, P.A. (2005). Endocrine and immunogenetic testing in individuals with type 1 diabetes and 21-hydroxylase autoantibodies: Addison's disease in a high-risk population. *Journal of Clinical Endocrinology and Metabolism, 90*, 128-134.

[1097]Falorni, A., Laureti, S., Nikoshkov, A., Picchio, M.L., Hallengren, B., Vandewalle, C.L., Gorus, F.K., Tortoioli, C., Luthman, H., Brunetti, P. & Santeusanio, F. (1997). 21-hydroxylase autoantibodies in adult patients with endocrine autoimmune diseases are highly specific for Addison's disease. Belgian Diabetes Registry. *Clinical and Experimental Immunology, 107*, 341-346.

[1098]Peterson, P., Salmi, H., Hyoty, H., Miettinen, A., Ilonen, J., Reijonen, H., Knip, M., Akerblom, H.K. & Krohn, K. (1997). Steroid 21-hydroxylase autoantibodies in insulin-dependent diabetes mellitus. Childhood Diabetes in Finland (DiMe) Study Group. *Clinical Immunology and Immunopathology 82*, 37-42.

[1099]Zelissen, P.M., Bast, E.J. & Croughs, R.J. (1995). Associated autoimmunity in Addison's disease. *Journal of Autoimmunity, 8*, 121-130.

[1100]Myhre, A.G., Undlien, D.E., Lovas, K., Uhlving, S., Nedrebo, B.G., Fougner, K.J., Trovik, T., Sorheim, J.I. & Husebye, E.S. (2002). Autoimmune adrenocortical failure in Norway autoantibodies and human leukocyte antigen class II associations related to clinical features. *Journal of Clinical Endocrinology and Metabolism, 87*, 618-623.

[1101]Blomhoff, A., Lie, B.A., Myhre, A.G., Kemp, E.H., Weetman, A.P., Akselsen, H.E., Huseby, E.S. & Undlien, D.E. (2004). Polymorphisms in the cytotoxic T lymphocyte antigen-4 gene region confer susceptibility to Addison's disease. *Journal of Clinical Endocrinology and Metabolism, 89*, 3474-3476.

[1102]Devendra, D., Liu, E. & Eisenbarth, G.S. (2004) Type 1 diabetes: recent developments, *British Medical Journal, 328*, 750–754.

[1103]Butler, A.E., Janson, J., Bonner-Weir, S., Ritzel, R., Rizza, R.A. & Butler, P.C. (2003). β-Cell deficit and increased β cell apoptosis in humans with type 2 diabetes. *Diabetes, 52*, 102–110.

[1104]Beattie, G.M., Montgomery, A.M.P., Lopez, A.D., Hao, E., Perez, B., Just, M.L., Lakey, J.R.T., Hart M.E., & Hayek, A. (2002). A novel approach to increase human islet cell mass while preserving β cell function, *Diabetes, 51*, 3435–3439.

[1105]Korbutt, G.S., Elliott, J.F., Ao, Z., Smith, D.K., Warnock, G.L. & Rajotte, R.V. (1996). Large scale isolation, growth, and function of porcine neonatal islet cells. *Journal of Clinical Investigations, 97*, 2119-2129.

[1106]Cantarovich, D., Blancho, G., Potiron, N., Jugeau, N., Fiche, M., Chagneau, C., Letessier, E., Boeffard, F., Loth, P., Karam, G., Soulillou, J.P. & Le Mauff, B. (2002). Rapid failure of pig islet transplantation in non human primates. *Xenotransplantation, 9*, 25-35.

[1107]Cicalese, L., Giacomoni, A., Rastellini, C. & Benedetti, E. (1999). Pancreatic transplantation: a review. *International Surgery, 84*, 305-312.

[1108]Efrat, S. (2002). Cell replacement therapy for type 1 diabetes. *Trends in Molecular Medicine, 8*, 334-339.

[1109]de la Tour, D., Halvorsen, T., Demeterco, C., Tyrberg, E., Itkin-Ansari, P., Loy, M., Yoo, S.J., Hao, E., Bossie, S. & Levine, F. (2001). Beta-cell differentiation from a human pancreatic cell line in vitro and in vivo. *Molecular Endocrinology, 15*, 476-483.

[1110]Weir, G.C. (2004). Can we make surrogated β-cells better than the original? *Seminars in Cell and Developmental Biology, 15*, 347–357.

[1111]Soria, B., Roche, E., Berna, G., Leon-Quinto, T., Reig, J.A., & Martin, F. (2000). Insulin-secreting cells derived from embryonic stem cells normalize glycemia in streptozotocin-induced diabetic mice. *Diabetes, 49*, 157–162.

[1112]Lumelsky, N., Blondel, O., Laeng, P., Velasco, I., Ravin, R. & McKay, R. (2001). Differentiation of embryonic stem cells to insulin-secreting structures similar to pancreatic islets. *Science, 292*, 1389–1394.

[1113]Leon-Quinto, T., Jones, J., Skoudy, A., Burcin, M. & Soria, B. (2004). In-vitro directed differentiation of mouse embryonic stem cells into insulin-producing cells. *Diabetologia, 47,* 1442–1451.

[1114]Assady, S., Maor, G., Amit, M., Itskovitz-Eldor, J., Skorecki, K. & Tzukerman, M. (2001). Insulin production by human embryonic stem cells. *Diabetes, 50*, 1691–1697.

[1115]Segev, H., Fishman, B., Ziskind, A., Shulman, M. & Itskovitz-Eldor, J. (2004). Differentiation of human embryonic stem cells into insulin-producing clusters. *Stem Cells, 22*, 265–274.

[1116]Blyszczuk, P., Cryz, J., Kania, G., Wagner, M., Roll, U., St-Ogne, L. & Wobbus, A.M. (2003). Expresion of Pax4 in embryonic stem cells promotes differentiation of nestin-positive progenitor and insulin-producing cells. *Proceedings of the National Academy of sciences of USA, 100*, 998-1003.

[1117]Miyazaki, S., Yamato, E. & Miyazaki, J. (2004). Regulated expression of pdx-1 promotes in vitro differentiation of insulin-producing cells from embryonic stem cells. *Diabetes, 53*, 1030-1037.

[1118]Tourrel, C., Bailbe, D., Meile, M.J., Kergoat, M., Portha, B. (2001). Glucagon-like peptide-1 and exendin-4 stimulate beta-cell neogenesis in streptozotocin-treated newborn rats resulting in persistently improved glucose homeostasis at adult age. *Diabetes, 50*, 1562-1570.

[1119]Finegood, D.T., Scaglia, L. & Bonner-Weir, S. (2001). Dynamics of beta-cell in the growing rat pancreas. Estimation with a simple mathematical model. *Diabetes, 44*, 249-256.

[1120]Sharma, A., zangen, D.H., Reitz, P., Taneja, M., Lissaeur, M.E., Miller, C.P., Weir, G.C., Habener, J.F. & Bonner-Wejr, S. (1999). The homeodomain protein IDX-1 increases after an early burst of proliferation during pancreatic regeneration. *Diabetes, 48*, 507-513.

[1121]Ramiya, V.K., Maraist, M., Arfors, K.E., Schatz, D.A., Peck, A.B. & Cornelius, J.G. (2000). Reversal of insulin-dpendent diabetes using islets generated in vitro from pancreatic stem cells. *Nature Medicine, 6*, 278-282.

[1122]Bonner-Weir, S., Taneja, M., Weir, G.C., Tatarkiewicz, K., Song, K.H., Sharma, A & O'Neil, J.J. (2000). In vitro cultivation of human islets from expanded ductal tissue. *Proceedings of the National Academy of USA, 97*, 7999-8004.

[1123]Tang, D., Cao, L., Burkhardt, B.R., Xia, C., Litherland, S.A. & Atkinson, M.A. (2004). In vivo and in vivo characterization of insulin-producing cells obtained from murine bone marrow. *Diabetes, 53*, 1721-1732.

[1124]Hess, D., Li, L., Martin, M., Sakano, S., Hill, D., Strutt, B., Thyssen, S., Gray, D.A. & Bhatia, M. (2003). Bone marrow-derived stem cells initiate pancreatic regeneration. *Nature Biotechnology, 21*, 763-760.

[1125]Ianus, A., Holz, G.G., Theise, N.D. & Hussain, M.A. (2003). In vivo derivation of glucose-competent pancreatic endocrine cells from bone marrow without evidence of cell fusion. *Journal of Clinical Investigations, 111*, 843-850.

[1126]Halban, P.A., Khan, S.E., Lernmark, A., Rhodes, C.J. (2001). Gene and cell-replacement therapy in the treatment of type 1 diabetes. How high must the standards be set? *Diabetes, 50*, 2181-2191.

[1127]Easom, R.A. (2000). Beta-granule transport and exocytosis. *Seminars in Cell and Developmental Biology, 11*, 253-266.

[1128]Hughes, S.D., Johnson, J.H., Quaade, C. & Newgard, C.B. (1992). Engineering of glucose-stimulated insulin secretion and biosynthesis in onon-ilset cells. *Proceedings of the National Academy of Sciences of USA, 89*, 683-692.

[1129]Hughes, S.D., Quaade, C., Johnson, J.H., Ferber, S. & Newgard, C.B. (1993). Transfection of AtT-20ins cells with GLUT-2 but not GLUT-1 confers glucose-stimulated insulin secretion. Relationship ro glucose metabolism. *Journal of Biological Chemistry, 268*, 15202-15212.

[1130]Cheung, A.T., Dayanandan, B., Lewis, J.T., Korbutt, G.S., Rajotte, R.V., Bryer-Ash, M., Boylan, M.O., Wolfe, M.M. & Kieffer, T.J. (2000). Glucose-dependent insulin release from genetically engineered K cells. *Science, 290*, 1959-1962.

[1131]Corbett, J.A. (2001). K cells: a novel target for insulin gene therapy for the prevention of diabetes. *Trends in Endocrinology and Metabolism. 12*, 140-142.

[1132]Gould, G.W. & Holman, G.D. (1993). The glucose transporter family: structure, function and tissue-specific expression. *Biochemical Journal, 295*, 329-341.

[1133]Dong, H. & Woo, S. L. (2001). Hepatic insulin production for type 1 diabetes. *Trends in Endocrinology and Metabolism, 12*, 441-446.

[1134]Chen, R., Meseck, M.L. & Woo, S.L. (2001). Auto-regulated hepatic insulin gene expression in type 1 diabetic rats. *Molecular Therapy, 3*, 584-590.

[1135]Lee, H.C., Kim, S.J., Kim, K.S., Shin, H.C. & Yoon, J.W. (2000). Remission in models of type 1 diabetes by gene therapy using a single-chain insulin analogue. *Nature, 408*, 483-488.

[1136]Olson, D.E., Paveglio, S.A., Huey, P.U., Porter, M.H. & Thule, P.M. (2003). Glucose-responsive hepatic insulin gene therapy of spontaneous diabetic BB/Wor rats. *Human Gene Therapy, 14*, 1401-1413.

[1137]Wanke, I.E. & Wong, N.C. (1997). Specific problems facing gene therapy for insulin-dependent diabetes mellitus: glucose-regulated insulin secretion from hepatocytes. *Proceedings of the Western Pharmacology Society, 40*, 131-133.

[1138]Rivera, V.M., Wang, X., Wardwell, S., Courage, N.L., Volchuk, A., Keenan, T., Holt, D.A., Gilman, M., Orci, L., Cerasoli, F., Jr., Rotman, A.E. & Clackson, T. (2000).

Regulation of protein secretion through controlled aggregation in the endoplasmic reticulum. *Science, 287*, 826-830.

[1139]Yanagita, M., Hoshino, H., Nakayama, K. & Takeuchi, T. (1993). Processing of mutated proinsulin with tetrabasic cleavage sites to mature insulin reflects the expression of furin in nonendocrine cell lines. *Endocrinology, 133*, 639-644.

[1140]Thule, P.M. & Liu, J.M. (2000). Regulated hepatic insulin gene therapy of STZ-diabetic rats. *Gene Therapy, 7*, 1744-1752.

[1141]Auricchio, A., Gao, G.P., Yu, Q.C., Paper, S., Rivera, V.M., Clackon, T. & Wilson, J.M. (2002). Constitutive and regulated expression of processed insulin following in vivo hepatic gene transfer. *Gene Therapy, 9*, 963-971.

[1142]Alam, T. & Sollinger, H.W. (2002). Glucose-regulated insulin production in hepatocytes. *Transplantation, 74*, 1781-1787.

[1143]Shaw, J.A., Delday, M.I., Hart, A.W., Docherty, H.M., Martin, C.A. & Docherti, K. (2002). Secretion of bioactive human insulin following plasmid-mediated gene transfer to non-neuroendocrine cell lines, primary cultures and rat skeletal muscle in vivo. *Journal of Endocrinology, 172*, 653-672.

[1144]Contreras, J.L., Eckhoff, D.E., Cartner, S., Bilbao, G., Ricordi, C., Neville, D.M., Jr., Thomas, F.T. & Thomas, J.M. (2000). Long-term functional islet mass and metabolic function after xenoislet transplantation in primates. *Transplantation, 69*, 195–201.

[1145]Thomas, F.T., Ricordi, C., Contreras, J.L., Hubbard, W.J., Jiang, J.L., Eckhoff, D.E., Cartner, S., Bilbao, G., Neville, D.M., Jr. & Thomas, J.M. (1999). Reversal of naturally occuring diabetes in primates by unmodified islet xenografts without chronic immunosuppression. *Transplantation, 67*, 846–854.

[1146]Thomas, J.M., Contreras, J.L., Smyth, C.A., Smyth, C.A., Lobashevsky, A., Jenkins, S., Hubbard, W.J., Eckhoff, D.E., Stavrou, S., Neville, D.M., Jr. & Thomas, J.M. (2001). Successful reversal of streptozotocin-induced diabetes with stable allogeneic islet function in a preclinical model of type 1 diabetes. *Diabetes, 50*, 1227–1236.

[1147]Adams, A.B., Shirasugi, N., Durham, M.M., Strobert, E., Anderson, D., Rees, P., Cowan, S.R., Xu, H., Blinder, Y., Cheung, M., Hollenbaugh, D., Kenyon, N.S., Pearson, T.C. & Larsen, C.P. (2002). Calcineurin inhibitor-free CD28 blockade-based protocol protects allogeneic islets in nonhuman primates. *Diabetes, 51*, 265–270.

[1148]Calne, R., Moffatt, S.D., Friend, P.J., Jamieson, N.V., Bradley, J.A., Hale, G., Fifth, J., Bradley, J., Smith, K.G. & Waldmann, H. (1999). Campath IH allows low-dose cyclosporine monotherapy in 31 cadaveric renal allograft recipients. *Transplantation, 68*, 1613–1616.

[1149]Shapiro, A., Ryan, E. & Paty, B.W. (2003). Three year follow-up in clinical islet-alone transplant with the Edmonton Protocol, and preliminary impact of infliximab and Campath-1H. *American Journal of Transplantation, 3*, 296.

[1150]Orive, G., Hernandez, R.M., Gascon, A.R., Calafiore, R., Chang, T.M., De Vos, P., Hortelano, G., Hunkeler, D., Lacik, I., Shapiro, A.M. & Pedraz, J.L. (2003). Cell encapsulation: promise and progress. *Nature Medicine, 9*, 104–107.

[1151]Lakey, J.R., Mirbolooki, M.R. & Shapiro, A.M. (2006). Current status of clinical islet cell transplantation. *Methods in Molecular Biology, 333*, 47-104.

[1152]Lambert, A.P., Gillespie, K.M., Thomson, G., Gordell, H.J., Todd, J.A., Gale, E A. & Bingley, P.J. (2004). Absolute risk of childhood-onset type 1 diabetes defined by human leukocyte antigen class II genotype: a population-based study in the United Kingdom. *Journal of Clinical Endocrinology and Metabolism, 89*, 4037-4043.

[1153]Hermann, R., Bartsosas, C.S., Soltecz, G., Vazeou, A., Paschou, P., Bozas, E., Malamitsi-Puchner, A., Simell, O., Knip, M. & Ilonen, J. (2004). Genetic screening for individuals at high risk for type 1 diabetes in the general population using HLA Class II alleles as disease markers. A comparison between three European populations with variable rates of disease incidence. *Diabetes Metabolism Research and Reviews, 20*, 322-329.

[1154]Buzzetti, R., Galgani, A., Petroni, A., Del Buono, M.L., Erlich, H.A., Bugawan, T.L., Lorini, R., Meschi, F., Multari, G., Pozzilli, P., Locatelli, M., Botazzo, G. & Di Mario, U. (2004). Genetic prediction of type 1 diabetes in a population with low frequency of HLA risk genotypes and low incidence of the disease (the DIABFIN study). *Diabetes Metabolism Research and Reviews, 20*, 137-143.

[1155]Rewers, M., Bugawan, T.L., Norris, J.M., Blair, A., Beauty, B., Hoffmann, M., McDiffie, R.S., Jr., Hamman, R.F., Klingensmith, G., Eisenbarth, G.S. & Erlich, H.A. (1996). Newborn screening for HLA markers associated with IDDM: diabetes autoimmunity study in the young (DAISY). *Diabetologia, 39*, 807-812.

[1156]Kupila, A., Muona, P., Simell, T., Arvilommi, P., Savolainen, H., Hamalailen, A.M., Korhonen, S., Kimpimaki, T., Sjoroos, M., Ilonen, J., Knip, M. & Simell, O. (2001). Feasibility of genetic and immunological prediction of type I diabetes in a population-based birth cohort. *Diabetologia, 44*, 290-297.

[1157]Yu, J., Yu, L., Bugawan, T.L., Erlich, H.A., Barriga, K., Hoffman, M., Rewers, M. & Eisenbarth, G.S. (2000). Transient antiislet autoantibodies: infrequent occurrence and lack of association with "genetic" risk factors. *Journal of Clinical Endocrinology and Metabolism, 85*, 2421-2428.

[1158]Laine, A.P., Hermann, R., Knip, M., Simell, O., Akerblom, H.K. & Ilonen, J. (2004). The human leukocyte antigen genotype has a modest effect on the insulin gene polymorphism-associated susceptibility to type 1 diabetes in the Finnish population. *Tissue Antigens, 63*, 72-74.

[1159]Walter, M., Albert, E., Conrad, M., Keller, E., Hummel, M., Ferber, K., Barratt, B.J., Todd, J.A., Ziegler, A.G. & Bonifacio, E. (2003). IDDM2/insulin VNTR modifies risk conferred by IDDM1/HLA for development of Type 1 diabetes and associated autoimmunity. *Diabetologia, 46*, 712-720.

[1160]Ziegler, A.G., Schmid, S., Huber, D., Hummel, M. & Bonifacio, E. (2003). Early infant feeding and risk of developing type 1 diabetes-associated autoantibodies. *JAMA, 290*, 1721-1738.

[1161]Yu, L., Cuthbertson, D.D., Eisenbarth, G.S. & Krischer, J.P. (2002). Diabetes Prevention Trial 1: prevalence of GAD and ICA512 (IA-2) autoantibodies by relationship to proband. *Annals of New York Academy of Sciences, 958*, 254-258.

[1162]Bonifacio, E., Hummel, M., Walter, M., Schmid, S & Ziegler, A.G. (2004). IDDM1 and multiple family history of type 1 diabetes combine to identify neonates at high risk for type 1 diabetes. *Diabetes Care, 27*, 2695-2700.

[1163]Bingley, P.J., Bonifacio, E., Ziegler, A.G., Schatz, D.A. & Eisenbarth, G.S. (2001). Proposed guidelines on screening for risk of type 1 diabetes. *Diabetes Care, 24*, 398.

[1164]Mire-Sluis, A.R., Gaines Das, R. & Lernmark, A. (2000). The World Health Organization International Collaborative Study for islet cell antibodies. *Diabetologia, 43*, 1282-1292.

[1165]Bingley, P.J., Williams, A.J. & Gale, E.A. (1999). Optimized autoantibody-based risk assessment impending type 1 diabetes in siblings of patients. *Diabetes Care, 22*, 1796-1801.

[1166]Krischer, J.P., Cuthbertson, D.D., Yu, L., Orban, T., Maclaren, N., Jackson, R., Winter, W.E., Schatz, D.A., Palmer, J.P. & Eisenbarth, G.S. (2003). Screening strategies for the identification of multiple antibody-positive relatives of individuals with type 1 diabetes. *Journal of Clinical Endocrinology and Metaboilsm, 88*, 103-108.

[1167]Achenbach, P., Warncke, K., Reiter, J., Naserke, H.E., Williams, A.J., Bingley, P.J., Bonifacio, E. & Ziegler, A.G. (2004). Stratification of type 1 diabetes risk on the basis of islet autoantibody characteristics. *Diabetes, 53*, 384-392.

[1168]Achenbach, P., Koszwara, K., Knoppf, A., Naserke, H.E., Ziegler, A.G. & Bonifacio, E. (2004). Mature high-affinity immune responses to (pro)insulin anticipate the autoimmune cascade that leads to type 1 diabetes. *Journal of Clinical Investigations, 114*, 589-597.

[1169]Fourlanos, S., Narendran, P., Byrnes, G.B., Colman, P.G. & Harrison, L.C. (2004). Insulin resistance is a risk factor for progression to type 1 diabetes. *Diabetologia, 47*, 1161-1167.

[1170]Barker, J.M., Barriga, K.J., Yu, L., Miao, D., Erlich, H.A., Norris, J.M., Eisenbarth, G.S. & Rewers, M. (2004). Prediction of autoantibody positivity and progression to type 1 diabetes: Diabetes Autoimmunity Study in the Young (DAISY). *Journal of Clinical Endocrinology and Metaboilsm, 89*, 3896-3902.

[1171]Hummel, M., Bonifacio, E., Schmid, S., Walter, M., Knoppf, A. & Ziegler, A.G. (2004). Early appearance of islet autoantibodies predicts childhood type 1 diabetes in offspring of diabetic parents. *Annals of Internal Medicine, 140*, 882-886.

[1172]Decochez, K, De Leeuw, I.H., Keymeulen, B. Mathieu, C., Rottiers, R., Weets, I., Vandemeulebroucke, E., Truyen, I., Kaufman, L. Schuit, F.C., Pipeleers, D.G. & Gorus, F.K. (2002). IA-2 autoantibodies predict impending type I diabetes in siblings of patients. *Diabetologia, 45*, 1658-1666.

[1173]Kimpimaki, T., Kummala, P., Savola, K., Kupila, A., Korhonen, S., Simell, T., Ilonen, J., Simell, O. & Knip, M. (2002). Natural history of beta-cell autoimmunity in young children with increased genetic susceptibility to type 1 diabetes recruited from the general population. *Journal of Clinical Endocrinology and Metabolism, 87*, 4572-4579.

[1174]Kulmala, P., Savola, K., Reijonen, H., Veijola, R., Vahasalo, P., Karjalainen, J., Tuomilehto-Wolf, E., Ilonen, J., Tuomilehto, J., Akerblom, H.K. & Knip, M. (2000). Genetic markers, humoral autoimmunity, and prediction of type 1 diabetes in siblings of affected children. Childhood Diabetes in Finland Study Group. *Diabetes, 49*, 48-58.

[1175]Colman, P.G., Steele, C., Couper, J.J., Beresford, S.J., Powell, T., Kewming, T., Pollard, A., Gellert. S., Tait, B., Honeyman, M. & Harrison, L.C. (2000). Islet autoimmunity in infants with a Type I diabetic relative is common but is frequently restricted to one autoantibody. *Diabetologia, 43*, 203-209.

[1176]Diabetes Prevention Trial – Type 1 Diabetes Study Group. (2002). Effects of insulin in relatives of patients with type 1 diabetes mellitus. *New England Journal of Medicine, 346*, 1685-1691.

[1177]Keskinen, P., Korhonen, S., Kupila, A., Veijola, R., Erkkila, S., Savolainen, H., Arvilommi, P., Simell, T., Ilonen, J., Knip, M. & Simell, O. (2002). First-phase insulin response in young healthy children at genetic and immunological risk for Type I diabetes. *Diabetologia, 45*, 1639-1648.

[1178]DPT-1 Study Group (1994). The Diabetes Prevention Trail-type 1 diabetes (DPT-1). *Diabetes, 43 (Suppl.)*, 159A.

[1179]Thai, A.C. & Eisenbarth, G.S. (1993). Natural history of IDDM. *Diabetes Reviews, 1*, 1-14.

[1180]Virtanen, S.M., Salonen, S. & Salivahti, E. (1999). Feasibility of a randomized double-blind trial aiming at avoidance of cow's milk in infancy: the TRIGR project. *Diabetes Research and Clinical Practice, 44 (Suppl.)*, S7.

[1181]Akerblom, H.K., Virtanen, S.M., Ilonen, J., Savilahti, E., Vaarala, O., Reunanen, A., Teramo, K., Hamalainen, A.M., Paronen, J., Riikjarv, M.A., Ormisson, A., Ludvigsson, J., Dosch, H.M., Hakulinen, T. & Knip, M.; National TRIGR Study Groups (2005). Dietary manipulation of beta cell autoimmunity in infants at increased risk of type 1 diabetes: a pilot study. *Diabetologia, 48*, 829-837.

[1182]Burkart, V., Koike, T., Brenner, H.H. & Kolb, H. (1992). Oxygen radicals generated by the enzyme xanthine oxydase lyse rat pancreatic islet cells in vitro. *Diabetologia, 35*, 1028-1034.

[1183]Lampete, E.F., Klinghammer, A. & Scherbaum, W.A. (1998). The Deutsche Nicotinamide Intervention Study: an attempt to prevent type 1 diabetes. DENIS group. *Diabetes, 47*, 980-984.

[1184]Schatz, D.A. & Bingley, P.J. (2001). Update on major trials for the prevention of type 1 diabetes mellitus: the American Diabetes Prevention Trial (DPT-1) and the European Nicotinamide Diabetes Intervention Trial (ENDIT). *Journal of Pediatric Endocrinology and Metabolism, 14*, 619-622.

[1185]Gale, E.A., Bingley, P.J., Emmett, C.L. & Collier, T.; European Nicotinamide Diabetes Intervention Trial (ENDIT) Group (2004). European Nicotinamide Diabetes Intervention Trial (ENDIT): a randomised controlled trial of intervention before the onset of type 1 diabetes. *Lancet, 363*, 925-931.

[1186]Yu, L., Robles, D.T., Abiru, N., Kaur, P., Rewers, M., Kelemen, K. & Eisenbarth, G.S. (2000). Early expression of antiinsulin autoantibodies of humans and the NOD mouse: evidence for early determination of subsequent diabetes. *Proceedings of the National Academy of Sciences of USA, 97*, 1701-1706.

[1187]Bonifacio, E., Bingley, P.J., Shattock, M., Dean, B.M., Dunger, D., Gale, E.A. & Botazzo, G.F. (1990). Quantification of islet-cell antibodies and prediction of insulin-dependent diabetes. *Lancet, 335*, 147-149.

[1188]Chase, H.P., Cooper, S., Osberg, I., Stene, L.C., Barriga, K., Norris, J., Eisenbarth, G.S. & Rewers, M. (2004). Elevated C-reactive protein levels in the development of type 1 diabetes. *Diabetes, 53*, 2569-2573.

INDEX

A

B

D

E

F

G

H

I

J

K

L

M

N

Q

R

S

T

U

V

W

X

Y

Z